EVALUATING ADHD IN CHILDREN AND ADOLESCENTS

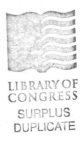

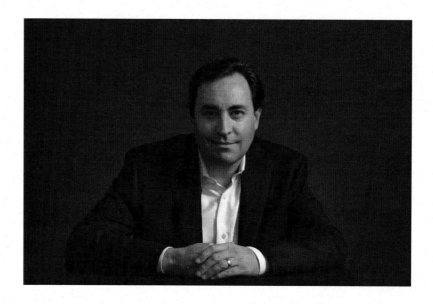

ABOUT THE AUTHOR

Gene Carroccia, Psy.D. earned his Bachelor of Arts in psychology from the University of Delaware in Newark, Delaware where he was inducted into Phi Beta Kappa. He obtained his doctorate in clinical psychology from the Illinois School of Professional Psychology in Chicago, Illinois in 1998. Dr. Carroccia is a licensed clinical psychologist in Illinois who has extensive experience working with individuals with ADHD, as well as other conditions, including psychological trauma and maltreatment. For over twenty years, he has evaluated and treated hundreds of children, adolescents, and adults with ADHD. He works at a large not-for-profit health care system as a vice president of behavioral health care services. For many years prior to this he supervised doctoral interns and was the director of an accredited doctoral clinical psychology internship training program. Dr. Carroccia is the author of another ADHD*ology* book entitled *Treating ADHD/ADD in Children and Adolescents: Solutions for Parents and Clinicians.* He was also the editor of the clinical workbook *Treating Sexual Abuse and Trauma with Children, Adolescents, and Young Adults with Developmental Disabilities,* published by Charles C Thomas in 2017. He resides in the suburbs of Chicago with his wife and two sons. For more information about his books, please visit adhdology.com. ADHD*ology:* Assess, Address, Success.

EVALUATING ADHD IN CHILDREN AND ADOLESCENTS

A Comprehensive Diagnostic Screening System

An ADHD*ology* Book

By

GENE CARROCCIA, PSY.D.

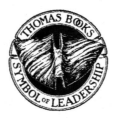

CHARLES C THOMAS • PUBLISHER, LTD.
Springfield • Illinois • U.S.A.

Published and Distributed Throughout the World by

CHARLES C THOMAS • PUBLISHER, LTD.
2600 South First Street
Springfield, Illinois 62704

ISBN 978-0-398-09320-4 (paper)
ISBN 978-0-398-09321-1 (ebook)

Library of Congress Catalog Card Number: 2019046287 (print)
2019046288 (ebook)

With THOMAS BOOKS *careful attention is given to all details of manufacturing
and design. It is the Publisher's desire to present books that are satisfactory as to their
physical qualities and artistic possibilities and appropriate for their particular use.*
THOMAS BOOKS *will be true to those laws of quality that assure a good name
and good will.*

Printed in the United States of America
MM-C-1

Library of Congress Cataloging-in-Publication Data

Names: Carroccia, Gene, author.
Title: Evaluating ADHD in children and adolescents: a comprehensive
    diagnostic screening system: an ADHDology book / By Gene Carroccia,
    PSY. D.
Description: Springfield, Illinois, USA: Charles C Thomas, Publisher,
    Ltd., [2020] | Includes bibliographical references and index.
Identifiers: LCCN 2019046287 (print) | LCCN 2019046288 (ebook) | ISBN
    9780398093204 (paperback) | ISBN 9780398093211 (ebook)
Subjects: LCSH: Attention-deficit-disordered children--Diagnosis--United
    States. | Attention-deficit-disordered children--Psychological
    testing--United States. | Attention-deficit disorder in
    adolescence--Diagnosis--United States. | Attention-deficit disorder in
    adolescence--Psychological testing--United States.
Classification: LCC RJ506.H9 C37 2020 (print) | LCC RJ506.H9 (ebook)
    DDC 618.92/8S89075--dc23
LC record available at https://lccn.loc.gov/2019046287
LC ebook record available at https://lccn.loc.gov/2019046288

This book is dedicated to Eugene C. Carroccia, M.D., my father and a clinician, who has given me tremendous support and assistance over the years. His keen editorial eye and contributions have made a great impact on my books, and I am eternally grateful.

INTRODUCTION

ADHD affects over six million children in the United States alone, and is a concerning societal problem. Despite its prevalence, clinicians may find it difficult to accurately diagnose ADHD and may not screen for and identify the numerous medical, sleep, psychological, trauma, neurodevelopmental, sensory processing, and fetal substance exposure conditions which can coexist and even worsen true ADHD, or cause ADHD-like presentations when it does not exist. ADHD commonly presents with other disorders. Research has found that as many as 67 to 80 percent of clinic-referred children (and 80 percent or more of clinic-referred adults) with ADHD have at least one other psychological disorder. Up to half have two or more other disorders (Pliszka, 2015), and 20 percent have three or more coexisting disorders (Spruyt & Gozal, 2011).

Unfortunately, the more conditions that exist, the more challenging it can be to provide effective diagnostic and treatment services. When children and teens have diagnostically complex presentations, they can baffle professionals and parents, and often do not receive the help they need. Their problems may worsen, and families can lose hope and continue to struggle. Untreated individuals can become dysfunctional adults who are less productive, unhappy, and experience significant difficulties in life.

However, these struggles can be replaced with successes. In clinical work, the diagnostic process should come first, and these findings should then direct the treatment. With comprehensive evaluations and appropriate referrals to other health care professionals, children and teens with ADHD and/or other conditions can enjoy better and more productive lives. This book provides three ways clinicians can provide more comprehensive and accurate ADHD evaluations so diagnostic accuracy and the appropriate treatments can be obtained. Part I of the book presents the ten-step ADHDology Evaluation Model for clinicians to learn to effectively conduct evaluations. Part II describes a number of medical, sleep, psychological, trauma, neurodevelopmental, sensory processing, and fetal substance exposure conditions, and how these can coexist with true ADHD, or cause ADHD-like presentations when it does not exist. It also informs readers how these conditions can resemble ADHD, and which specialists can further evaluate and treat these other conditions. Part III provides the Comprehensive Diagnostic ADHD Screening System (CDASS) checklists to help screen for and identify these conditions to better understand them and make additional necessary evaluation referrals.

Throughout this book the term "ADHD" is used. Some readers may say, "Some children have ADD and not ADHD. They aren't hyperactive or impulsive." The term "ADD," or Attention Deficit Disorder, describes a child or teen who has inattention problems without significant hyperactivity and impulsivity difficulties. However, for years the recognized, correct term for this disorder has been "ADHD - Predominantly Inattentive Presentation." Therefore, in this book the term ADHD will refer to all ADHD types, including ADHD with impulsivity and hyperactivity (Combined ADHD) and without these two difficulties (Inattentive ADHD). These conditions can present differently, have distinct brain signatures, and may require differing treatments. Those with Inattentive ADHD often have fewer behavioral problems. However, since Combined and Inattentive conditions share many similarities, unless stated otherwise, the information presented on ADHD should be applicable to all forms of ADHD.

Parents, educators, and interested others can read this book to better understand these complex topics, as well as assist clinicians with the ADHD diagnostic process. Finally, this book is not designed or intended to replace proper diagnostic services and treatment from licensed clinicians and behavioral health professionals, and is best used along with these professionals.

REFERENCES

Pliszka, S. (2015). Comorbid psychiatric disorders in children with ADHD. In R. Barkley (Ed.), *Attention deficit hyperactivity disorder: A handbook for diagnosis and treatment* (4th ed., pp 140–168). New York: Guilford Press.

Spruyt, K., & Gozal, D. (2011, April). Sleep disturbances in children with attention-deficit/hyperactivity disorder. *Expert Review of Neurotherapeutics, 11*(4), 565–577. doi: 10.1586/ern.11.7

ACKNOWLEDGMENTS

I would like to warmly thank a number of people that supported me on this long journey. My father, Eugene C. Carroccia, M.D., was encouraging and tirelessly contributed many essential editorial hours. Thanks so very much, Dad. I cannot express enough gratitude to my wife, Kirsten, for her intelligent perspectives, love, and endless patience during my weary hours of writing. My mother, Sharon Carroccia, LCSW, was warmly supportive of my efforts. Michael Thomas, publisher at Charles C Thomas Ltd., was also supportive and helpful with my questions. My good friends Albert Spicer, Psy.D. and Laura Spicer, Psy.D. contributed keen insights, moral support, and assistance with many parts of this process. I would like to share a hearty thanks to my colleagues Vanessa Houdek, Psy.D., Sara Skinner, Psy.D., Schaelyn McFadden, Psy.D., Jenna Berberich, Psy.D., Michael Ingersoll, Psy.D., and Huda Abuasi, Psy.D. for their support. Nancy Belmont, M.S. shared helpful information about speech pathology topics. I'd like to give a special thanks to John F. Smith, Ph.D. for his wisdom and friendship. Gregg Rzepczynski, J.D. and Susan Meade were generous with their perspectives. Finally, many thanks to Helen Minnis, M.D., Ph.D. for her endorsement and permission to share the important contributions she and her colleagues have made to the field.

CONTENTS

EVALUATING ADHD IN CHILDREN
AND ADOLESCENTS

Part I

HOW TO EVALUATE ADHD IN CHILDREN AND ADOLESCENTS WITH THE ADHD*OLOGY* EVALUATION MODEL

Chapter 1

THE ADHD EVALUATION AND
DIAGNOSTIC PROCESS FOR
CHILDREN AND ADOLESCENTS

INTRODUCTION

Attention-Deficit/Hyperactivity Disorder (ADHD) is a complex neurodevelopmental disorder that impacts different parts of the brain in various ways. But while it is widespread, ADHD is not a single, uniform condition. It has different causes, presentations, severity levels, and manifestations. Almost 10 percent of children and adolescents ages two to 17 in the United States have been diagnosed with this (Center for Disease Control and Prevention, 2018).

Since there has been greater awareness of ADHD, more children have been diagnosed with ADHD over the past several decades. Experts seem to disagree whether ADHD is overdiagnosed or incorrectly diagnosed. Inaccurate media reports may have contributed to public misperception that ADHD is overdiagnosed. In the 1960s and 1970s, only 20 percent of children believed to have true ADHD received treatment, while approximately 70 to 80 percent of children believed to have true ADHD are receiving treatment today (Smith, 2011).

ADHD can be determined through focused evaluations by outpatient mental health therapists, psychiatrists, neuropsychiatrists, primary care physicians, developmental pediatricians, neurologists, certain nurse practitioners, neuropsychologists, and school psychologists. While neurodevelopmental testing is often considered the most comprehensive and accurate approach to diagnose ADHD, it is not necessary in many cases. An effective ADHD evaluation consists of specific diagnostic tasks, screening for other possible conditions, presenting these findings to parents and relevant others, and providing appropriate referrals for other services, if indicated. ADHD evaluators need to know what ADHD looks like, but also need to appreciate individual presentations.

The terms psychological "evaluation" and "assessment" are used interchangeably by some professionals. However, in this book, the term "psychological assessment" will be used to refer to specially trained clinical psychologists called neuropsychologists who conduct a more extensive neuro-developmental testing process, also called neuropsychological and neurobehavioral testing. The term "evaluation" will be used to refer to the more basic ADHD diagnostic process used by outpatient clinicians who do not necessarily provide psychological testing. Typically, ADHD evaluations are less comprehensive and utilize clinical interviewing, several rating measures, and screenings for other conditions. "Evaluation" will also be used to describe other diagnostic examinations and services by non-behavioral health clinicians.

UNDERSTANDING ADHD

Clinicians who provide evaluations should firmly understand ADHD as a neurobehavioral condition and how it presents in children and adolescents. If clinicians do not accept ADHD as a brain-functioning condition or try to apply other psychological theories to explain the entire ADHD condition, diagnostic accuracy will be compromised. Clinicians like to diagnose what they know. If clinicians lack experience with ADHD and are more comfortable interpreting children's unwanted behaviors entirely as the result of attention-seeking, self-esteem, or anxiety issues, then they will be less effective evaluating ADHD. While other psychological perspectives can be important, they should not be solely used to interpret true ADHD.

To help clinicians and families better understand and appreciate ADHD, it is essential to know how it commonly presents and its impacts. Providers and parents should take the time to study informative ADHD books, research, and websites. One of the key components of ADHD treatment is a solid foundational understanding of the condition as a chronic neurobiological disability.

WHAT IS ATTENTION?

Attention can be defined as a set of complex neurocognitive processes that operate through a series of neural networks to provide self-regulation of sensory input, emotions, and motor output to achieve internal goals. Cognitive neuroscience provides three major conceptualizations of attention:

selective attention (the ability to focus on certain stimuli while ignoring others), executive attention (a number of processes involved in controlling behavior and thoughts), and sustained attention (the ability to remain focused during an extended time period) (Tannock & Brown, 2009). Mirsky described five core attention components that include focus/execute, sustain, stabilize, shift, and encode (Wilding, 2005). Attention can also be described as overt on-task behavior with appropriate fixation on an object or event. Inattention is frequent off-task behavior, including excessively disengaging from relevant stimuli (Tannock & Brown, 2009). Those with ADHD will have deficits in the core attention components, as well as in their visual and/or auditory attentional abilities.

TYPES OF ADHD DIAGNOSES

According to the Diagnostic and Statistical Manual of Mental Disorders–5, there are three main types of ADHD: Combined, Inattentive, and Predominantly Hyperactive/Impulsive. Most children and adolescents will have either the Combined or Inattentive ADHD. Combined ADHD is the most prevalent and accounts for 50 to 75 percent of all individuals with ADHD, Inattentive ADHD presents in about 20 to 30 percent, and the Hyperactive/Impulsive subtype is found in less than 15 percent of all individuals with ADHD (Spencer, Biederman, & Mick, 2007).

Combined ADHD causes problems with inattention, hyperactivity, and impulsivity. Children with this presentation are more disruptive, excessively active, messy, noisy, immature, and irresponsible than peers. The hyperactivity and impulsivity symptoms may decrease for some by adolescence or young adulthood, but the inattentiveness often remains.

Predominantly Hyperactive/Impulsive ADHD appears mostly in preschool or kindergarten age children who have not yet had to demonstrate longer attention spans required for first grade and beyond. Most of these evolve into Combined presentations as they reach first or later grades.

Inattentive ADHD causes problems mostly with attention and remaining adequately focused on tasks, with lesser to no hyperactivity, impulsivity, behavioral or defiance problems. This often emerges somewhat later in childhood than Combined ADHD (about ages eight to 12). They are more passive and apathetic, have greater depression and anxiety, and fewer social problems than those with Combined ADHD. Some teens and adults with this may previously have had hyperactive and impulsive symptoms that decreased over time (Barkley, 2013). However, those with the Inattentive presentation can still experience social problems often related to social reluctance or shyness. Children and teens with this also typically have deficits in processing speed, working memory, academic struggles, and often lack delinquent or aggressive behaviors (Johnson & Marlow, 2011). Finally, clinicians should ensure that those who present with poor attentional abilities have true Inattentive ADHD and not Concentration Deficit Disorder, which can closely mimic this type of ADHD. Please refer to Chapter 6 more information on this topic.

Provisional and rule out designations can be used by clinicians to indicate that they suspect or are considering ADHD, but this has not been fully evaluated and confirmed. A provisional designation is like a preliminary determination, and would indicate that the clinician is more confident, but has not fully confirmed ADHD. A rule out ADHD diagnosis indicates the clinician is considering this, but further exploration is needed.

Rule out and provisional qualifiers may be helpful while the diagnostic process is occurring and evaluations by other providers are being completed. Until the process is completed, determining if ADHD exists may be unclear. While DSM-5 criteria for ADHD states that impairment in two or more settings should occur (American Psychiatric Association, 2013), this may not always be observed, particularly for milder ADHD cases. Therefore, an ADHD diagnosis should not be dismissed in some situations (such as if a teacher does not report significant symptoms, but the parent does). Clinicians should explore other data, past history, and use their clinical experience and judgement. In these situations, other adults who know the child can complete ADHD measures. For those who do not meet full criteria for ADHD, clinicians should carefully explore if the child has other conditions that may be causing the ADHD-like symptoms.

When clinicians are finished evaluating and diagnosing ADHD, they need to clearly state which type of ADHD is present, as well as provide the severity level of mild, moderate, or severe, when possible. For ADHD conditions that do not fit in the ADHD types, are not better explained by other conditions, and are not rule out or provisional designations, clinicians can use the Other-Specified or Unspecified ADHD diagnoses (American Psychiatric Association, 2013). Although rule out, provisional, Unspecified, and Other Specified ADHD diagnoses are less precise, they may be helpful when clinicians lack clarity or information. However, these can also be misused or inappropriately linger. Some clinicians may use these without making the efforts to fully determine if ADHD and/or other conditions exist. When cases are diagnostically complex, these can be used while the diagnostic process continues. These designations should be updated after new data emerges.

Finally, when diagnostic uncertainty persists, other approaches can be used to determine if true ADHD exists. These include ADHD medication use for suspected Combined type, neurodevelopmental testing, use of QEEG testing, and the Walsh Biochemical Imbalances testing approach (all will be addressed later). Monitoring and extending the diagnostic window over time may also help to determine if ADHD exists.

THE ADHD EVALUATION PROCESS

Often clinicians can accurately diagnose ADHD without neurodevelopmental testing (Gualtieri & Johnson, 2005). A diagnosis for ADHD can often be determined from thorough clinical interview/s with parents and children or teens, meeting DSM symptom criteria, ADHD behavior rating and other measures, and identifying or ruling out other possible medical, sleep, psychological, and neurodevelopmental and sensory processing conditions. Even teacher measures are not absolutely critical, and parents can provide information about school functioning, grades, and school reports or documents. School observations can be helpful but will be impractical for most outpatient clinicians. Finally, while not required, self-report measures from children and teens may be helpful.

Diagnosing more straightforward ADHD can be quite accurate. However, determining more complex ADHD can be difficult or inconclusive because inattention, hyperactivity, and impulsivity are general symptoms that can have many different causes. Quick office visits or snap judgements should be avoided. Since the symptoms can be so general, ADHD can be a diagnosis of exclusion. The diagnostic process demands that a clinician become a psychological detective. Even neurodevelopmental testing, usually considered the highest diagnostic authority in determining ADHD, may be inconclusive or inaccurate at times.

When evaluating ADHD, it is essential to understand that ADHD often does not exist by itself, and coexisting conditions are common (Follan et al., 2011). The American Academy of Pediatrics' (2011) clinical practice guidelines state that ADHD evaluations should include examinations to explore other coexisting conditions. As many as 67 to 80 percent of clinic-referred children (and 80 percent or more of clinic-referred adults) with ADHD have at least one other psychological disorder, as many as 50 percent have two or more other disorders (Pliszka, 2015), and 20 percent have three or more coexisting conditions (Spruyt & Gozal, 2011). By using the Comprehensive Diagnostic ADHD Screening System (CDASS) checklists presented later in this book, clinicians can explore the many possible conditions that may coexist with true ADHD or may cause ADHD-like presentations.

The concept of differential diagnosis is central to this book. This is the process of distinguishing a disorder from possible others that may share the same or similar symptoms. The evaluator's job is to try to determine if the child or adolescent has true ADHD, other conditions that may coexist along with true ADHD, or if they have other disorders that cause ADHD-like symptoms when true ADHD does not exist. The initial ADHD evaluation process may generate more questions than answers, so other providers and further testing may be necessary. While this can be frustrating and difficult for clinicians and parents who would like straightforward answers, this is part of the process. If the child has multiple conditions that are correctly determined, this should help families and professionals better coordinate care and understand how the multiple conditions collectively impact the child.

For diagnostically complex presentations, specialized diagnostic services by other providers will be required. These may include psychological testing by clinical psychologists (to explore trauma, psychological conditions, and giftedness); neurodevelopmental assessments by neuropsychologists (for learning disorders, more complex ADHD, non-verbal learning disorder, intelligence levels, autism, processing speed and other issues); occupational therapy evaluations (for sensory processing and motor coordination conditions); speech-language evaluations (for speech deficits and expressive language issues); developmental or behavioral optometrist evaluations (for visual processing deficits); audiologist evaluations (for auditory processing deficits); Ears, Nose, and Throat (ENT) physician examinations (to explore sleep disordered breathing problems, allergies, and congestion); sleep studies (for sleep conditions); fetal alcohol spectrum disorder evaluations by neurodevelopmental specialists; neurologist examinations (for seizures, tic disorders, and head injuries); and medical examinations by developmental or primary care physicians (to rule out medical conditions). Neuropsychiatrists may be helpful for some conditions as well.

Finally, the accuracy of determining true ADHD may be improved by identifying the possible risk factors for ADHD (see this checklist in Chapter 13), as well as examining ADHD indicators that do not exclusively result from other conditions (see this checklist in Chapter 13).

THE ADHD*OLOGY* EVALUATION MODEL FOR CLINICIANS

1. Decide to Evaluate ADHD or Refer for Neurodevelopmental Testing and/or Other Providers

Depending on a child or teen's presentation, evaluators should determine whether they can provide an ADHD evaluation, or refer to a neuropsychologist and/or other professionals. This may or may not be able to be determined before services begin. When initially speaking on the phone to parents who request ADHD testing, evaluators may be able to ask about the child's difficulties to help decide if they should proceed with an evaluation. Most with suspected autism spectrum conditions, lower intelligence, learning disorders, sensory processing and motor disorders, or certain other conditions described later should probably first receive neurodevelopmental testing and/or other specialist evaluations because these other conditions can be challenging to accurately discriminate from ADHD. When children and teens have unclear diagnostic presentations with a large range of unclear or severe symptoms, neurodevelopmental assessments can be essential. As a general rule, clinicians and school staff (if permitted) should refer children and adolescents to neuropsychologists when they are unable to determine themselves if true ADHD is present. While ADHD evaluations are typically less accurate and conclusive with diagnostically complex cases, they may be helpful in generating referrals to other professionals.

During the initial phone contact with parents or at the very beginning of services, evaluators should explain their ADHD diagnostic process, and how this differs from neurodevelopmental assessments. Families should know that ADHD evaluations will require a number of diagnostic sessions, typically do not provide reports (but may provide letters to physicians), and can be less comprehensive and precise in their findings. Assessments will be more comprehensive and conclusive, provide reports and recommendations, are more expensive, and can be more difficult to obtain. Parents should be informed about these differences and given options to prevent later frustration if an evaluator provides inconclusive results, recommends additional testing, and doesn't proceed with treatment. Many parents may wish to start with an evaluation because they are easier to obtain and seek an assessment later if ADHD is undetermined.

Neurodevelopmental assessments, sometimes called neurobehavioral or neuropsychological testing, provide a battery of measures and neurocognitive tests. They include tests of attention (such as continuous performance tests and visual and auditory attention tests), executive functioning, memory, intelligence, and other psychological instruments. Some neuropsychologists may even include quantitative electroencephalography (QEEG) as part of the testing battery (described more in Chapter 2). Neuropsychological testing can use direct attentional tests that other clinicians do not use (Coles, 2001). Executive functions consist of a number of brain-functioning abilities, including cognitive flexibility, organization, planning, conceptual and abstract reasoning, self-monitoring, decision-making, self-control and response inhibition. A variable relationship exists between executive functions and ADHD. Not everyone with ADHD demonstrates deficiencies in executive functioning, and those with ADHD may differ greatly in these impairments (Mattfield et al., 2014).

An effective neurodevelopment assessment will provide a written report that presents the administered tests, fully determined diagnoses and "rule out" conditions, integrated findings to describe and explain the person's functioning and challenges, and recommendations for additional provider evaluations and treatment services. The report can be shared with other providers who work with the child as well as school staff. These reports can also be critical in assisting students to become eligible for 504 plans or Individual Education Programs (IEPs) from schools.

Neurodevelopmental testing is the best way to diagnose specific learning disorders. This testing can be important because reading, math, writing, and other academic problems can result from ADHD and/or specific learning disorders. Consequently, it can be difficult to determine in some cases why a person has learning problems without neuropsychological testing. To make matters more complicated, conservative estimates indicate that 25 to 40 percent of those with ADHD also have learning disorders (Tannock & Brown, 2009).

Unfortunately, there are several challenges with neurodevelopmental testing. First, it is expensive, typically costing about $1,000 to $3,500, or more. Private health insurance plans may not cover some or all of these testing services, and PPO plans tend to provide more coverage. Insurance companies may not approve neuropsychological testing if ADHD exists alone without complex presentations. Second, for most children and teens, this specialized testing will take time. It can take months from finding an available neuropsychologist to receiving the final report. Also, since there are far fewer neuropsychologists than other clinicians who evaluate ADHD, neuropsychologists may have longer waiting lists. Generally, more rural areas have fewer available providers. There are even fewer neuropsychologists who accept Medicaid. Larger health care and university hospital systems may have neuropsychologists who provide services and accept Medicaid, but the long waiting lists are common. Third, despite its more comprehensive approach, even these assessments can be inaccurate or inconclusive. Individuals may require additional testing over time, possibly from different neuropsychologists and/or other providers, to obtain multiple diagnostics perspectives. Utilizing multidisciplinary and trauma-informed approaches may improve accuracy. In the future, it is likely that ADHD will be diagnosed more precisely with brain imaging, genetic testing and other biomarkers. At this time, these tests are not routine or reliable in determining ADHD.

2. Explain the Evaluation Process

If an evaluation will occur, clinicians should explain the details about the process, including how many sessions this may require, what will occur, expectations about parental participation, and if a letter will be sent to the child's physician and/or school. Some families may want treatment quickly and can become frustrated by the extended diagnostic process if they do not understand and agree to this.

3. The Clinical Diagnostic ADHD Interview

Clinicians should first conduct a thorough initial clinical diagnostic interview. It is important to have the primary caretaker attend most to all interview sessions. Both parents can be helpful, but parents who spend less time with children may be less knowledgeable and report fewer difficulties. The clinical interview may take one to three sessions. These sessions should focus on obtaining the child and family history and exploring functioning in all areas of the child's life, such as developmental milestones, social functioning, behavioral issues at home and school, and academic performance. Clinicians should also ask about previously diagnosed medical and psychological conditions and any prior testing or treatment services, in or outside of the school. If any reports exist, they should be examined. Identified conditions that may impact ADHD-like symptoms should be further explored.

As part of the interview process, the DSM criteria and the ADHD CDASS checklists in Chapter 13 can be used as initial screeners. Positive screening results can indicate that ADHD may be present, and the evaluation process should proceed. During the interview, clinicians should carefully review the ADHD-like symptoms, exploring where they occur, when they began, and if they have intensified. Evaluators should also obtain information regarding the grades and what academic and behavioral problems occurred for each year, starting with the most recent. They can also ask for specific teacher comments from each year, as well as what learning, homework, and behavioral difficulties occurred.

During interviews, evaluators should be diligent, and explore if there are any other explanations for ADHD-like symptoms. They should inquire if there have been family, social, personal (such as sexual orientation or gender struggles) or other stressors or changes that could have caused the symptoms. If stressors exist, evaluators should try to determine if the child has these with or without true ADHD. ADHD can easily cause anxiety, stress, depression, and self-esteem difficulties from academic underachievement, learning difficulties, homework problems, conflicts with parents and teachers, behavioral difficulties, social problems with peers, and disappointments.

During the diagnostic process, it can be helpful to speak with children and adolescents without the parents present. This will give them an opportunity to discuss their struggles and potentially upsetting family, social, or personal issues that may be causing ADHD-like symptoms, or may be contributing to true ADHD. There are a range of traumatic, dysfunctional, and difficult situations that may cause or compound psychological conditions, including domestic violence, highly negative or toxic relationships with parents or step-parents, divorce, parental separation, parental substance abuse, various forms of abuse, and other family stressors and struggles. Clinicians should specifically ask children and adolescents if they have experienced or witnessed physical or sexual abuse involving family members or others in or outside of the home. Any additional experiences of psychological trauma should be explored. While this can be difficult for clinicians, it is a critical part of the interview process and a key mode of obtaining trauma information. Clinicians should prepare families for their mandated state requirements to report child abuse and neglect at the very start of clinical services, and before the diagnostic process begins.

Additionally, when alone, the child or teen may disclose or further discuss academic or learning problems, alcohol and drug use or experimentation, peer issues, bullying, or any other troubling topics. These should be explored as to their impact, when they started, how frequently they occur, and their severity. Children and teens with true ADHD have higher rates of family discord, social problems with parents and peers, academic difficulties, and substance use. Therefore, it is critical to try to determine if these issues are causing ADHD-like symptoms due to anxiety, depression, and other factors, or if they coexist with and/or result from true ADHD. Obtaining a timeline of when the ADHD symptoms started and when these other difficulties began can assist with this task. True ADHD seems more likely if ADHD symptoms occurred earlier in life before these other difficulties began.

During the ADHD evaluation, when possible, clinicians should attempt to obtain information from a variety of sources for a better understanding of the child's individuality, cultural dimensions, functioning, strengths, and challenges. Additional family members can be invited to evaluation sessions, and/or parents can give behavioral rating forms to other adults who know the child well. Also, when evaluating potential anxiety, depression, traumas, or other conditions, particularly in younger children, it may be difficult for some to articulate the content of their thoughts and feelings. Clinicians should proceed slowly and patiently during sessions, and review these topics several times if necessary to explore their internal experiences and triggers to symptoms.

Behavioral observations can be helpful during the evaluation process. However, the child or teen may or may not demonstrate ADHD symptoms in the clinician's office. Information about a child's ADHD-like behavior is best obtained from parents, teachers, and adults who spend the most time with them, and not from brief contacts with professionals. Some with ADHD can display no symptoms during office sessions, while their parents insist they have significant problems at home or school. Children and teens with ADHD can demonstrate fluctuating symptoms and their expression will be influenced by settings and other factors. Those who do not understand this will incorrectly expect that symptoms will appear in all settings.

Because genetic transmission is the most common way that ADHD occurs, evaluations should include asking if the child's parents or other family members have or had ADHD symptoms. This includes both sets of grandparents, aunts and uncles, and siblings. As a quick screener, DSM ADHD symptoms can be read aloud to parents to explore if they or family members had these during their childhood or still experience these currently. Because males are two to three times as likely to have ADHD as females, male relatives more often report symptoms. While clinicians will not be evaluating or diagnosing parents or other family members, positive reports can be helpful because these can increase the child's likelihood of having true ADHD.

4. The Use of ADHD and Other Measures

The use of standardized rating scales and measures from multiple sources is an important component of an evidence-based evaluation of children and teens with ADHD. Clinicians with advanced professional degrees can purchase psychological measures from special psychological testing publishers. These measures are critical to ADHD evaluations and are relatively simple to use. Interested clinicians may be able to obtain additional training to use measures more effectively. Rating forms can be very helpful in determining if unwanted symptoms and behaviors are at statistically significant levels above the expected age-based norms. The American Academy of Pediatrics guidelines recommend that ADHD measures are given to parents and teachers as part of the ADHD evaluation process. Other adults who have regular contact with the child can also complete ADHD rating measures, including daycare workers, close family and friends, and other school staff.

To obtain teacher ratings, clinicians can give the measures to parents, who should then give these to teacher/s or a school social worker who can distribute these to teachers. Parents can write notes or emails to request their completion by a certain date. Clinicians can also contact the teachers to distribute measures, but this may take time and a release of information will be required. For children in middle school and high school, ADHD measures should be given to teachers of core subjects. Teachers who know the student well and have frequent contact will be most important. While giving measures to all or most teachers can be more time consuming to score, it can provide teachers' perspectives to help to identify impairments for each class.

Mothers, fathers, and teachers can sometimes report conflicting and confusing information with their rating measures. One study found that mothers reported greater ADHD and oppositional defiant disorder (ODD) symptoms and externalizing problems for their children than fathers, and parents (particularly mothers) often gave more severe ratings of behavioral problems than teachers. Research indicates that estimates of parent-teacher agreements have low, but statistically significant correlations. Additionally, ratings between mothers and fathers in measures tend to be more similar than between parents and teachers (Langberg et al., 2010).

Rating discrepancies among mothers, fathers, and teachers can be challenging to interpret. One solution for discrepant parent ratings is to identify which parent spends the most time with the child and weigh that more heavily. Despite differing results or if only one parent reports significant difficulties, when other supporting data exists, an ADHD diagnosis can still be made (Langberg et al., 2010). Additionally, if clinicians question the accuracy or validity of ratings by parents or teachers, they may refer to the measure's validity scales to see whether the rater has an overly negative or positive response style. Additionally, when measures are given to two parents or family members, clinicians should inform them to complete their ratings separately. They can compare their results afterwards, but they should provide their own independent ratings.

Listed below are psychological measures for parents, children and adolescents, and teachers to complete. At a minimum, parents and teachers should complete two different ADHD rating scales and one broadband measure each, while children and teens can complete one self-report broadband measure, and possibly an ADHD self-report measure.

Broadband measures inquire about a range of symptoms across different conditions and can be quite helpful or even essential. Significant elevations in broadband measures may indicate that depression, anxiety, social problems, and other issues are secondary results of ADHD and/or other conditions, primary difficulties when no true ADHD exists, or that true ADHD and these issues coexist. While not critical, it can be helpful to provide problematic behavior and executive functioning measures to parents and teachers as well. The more measures obtained, the more information and perspectives clinicians will receive. Clinicians will have to decide how many and which measures they will utilize during their evaluations. As a general rule, it is better to provide more measures for more diagnostically complex or unclear presentations.

Self-report measures completed by children and adolescents during ADHD evaluations can be challenging. Self-report broadband measures will be important to gain their views on a range of symptoms. Some will be more honest about their depression, anxiety, or other struggles in these measures compared to verbal reporting during interviews. However, self-report ADHD measures may not be helpful. It is common for children and adolescents to have lesser self-awareness and report fewer ADHD symptoms than parents or teachers. While adolescents and older children should be given self-report ADHD measures, they may not be accurate, but can indicate if they experience ADHD difficulties and this may help with their acceptance of the diagnosis.

There are a number of ADHD and psychological measures available. Those presented below are not intended to be a definitive list, but options for consideration.

Parent/Caregiver Measures for Children and Adolescents

Parent ADHD Symptoms and Behaviors Measures:
- ADHD Rating Scale–5 for Children and Adolescents, Home Version: Child or Adolescent for ages 5–17
- Vanderbilt ADHD Parent Rating Scale for ages 6–12
- Connors 3–Parents Short or Parents Full-length for ages 6–18

Parent Problematic Behaviors Measures:
- Home Situations Questionnaire (HSQ) for ages 4–11
- Child and Adolescent Disruptive Behavior Inventory (CADBI), Parent Version

Parent Broadband Measures:
- Behavior Assessment System for Children–3 (BASC-3)–Parent Rating Scales–Preschool, Child, and Adolescent versions
- Child Behavior Checklist (CBCL), two versions for ages $1^{1}/_{2}$–5 or 6–18

Parent Executive Functioning Measures:
- Behavioral Rating Inventory for Executive Functioning (BRIEF2)–Parent Form for ages 5–18
- Comprehensive Executive Function Inventory (CEFI)–Parent Response
- Barkley Deficits in Executive Functioning Scale–Children and Adolescents (BEDFS-CA) Long Form

Self-Report Measures for Children and Adolescents

Self-Report ADHD Symptoms and Behaviors Measures:
- ADHD Rating Scale–5 for Children and Adolescents, Home Version
- Connors 3–Self-Report Short or Full-length for ages 8–18

Self-Report Broadband Measures:
- Behavior Assessment System for Children–3 (BASC-3)–Self-Report–Child or Adolescent versions
- Beck Youth Inventory II for ages 7–18
- Youth Self Report for Ages 11–18 (YSR)
- Other trauma, anxiety, and/or depression measures may also be used

Self-Report Executive Functioning Measure:
- Behavioral Rating Inventory for Executive Functioning (BRIEF2)–Self-Report Form for ages 11–18

Teacher Measures for Children and Adolescents

Teacher ADHD Symptoms and Behaviors Measures:
- ADHD Rating Scale–5 for Children and Adolescents, School Version: Child or Adolescent
- Vanderbilt ADHD Teacher Rating Scale for ages 6–12
- Connors 3–Teachers Short or Connors 3 Teachers Full-length for ages 6–18

Teacher Problematic Behaviors Measures:
- School Situations Questionnaire (SSQ) for ages 6–11
- Child and Adolescent Disruptive Behavior Inventory (CADBI), Teacher Version

Teacher Broadband Measures:
- Behavior Assessment System for Children–3 (BASC-3)–Teacher Rating Scales (TRS)–Preschool, Child, and Adolescent versions
- Caregiver-Teacher Report Form for Ages $1^{1}/_{2}$–5 (C-TRF)
- Teacher's Report Form for Ages 6–18 (TRF)

Teacher Executive Functioning Measures:
- Behavioral Rating Inventory for Executive Functioning (BRIEF2)–Teacher Form for ages 5–18
- Comprehensive Executive Function Inventory (CEFI)–Teacher Response

5. Screen for Other Possible Conditions

Use of the CDASS

The ADHD*ology* Comprehensive Diagnostic ADHD Screening System (CDASS) presents many conditions and their screening checklists to help improve the accuracy of diagnosing ADHD and identify other potential conditions. The CDASS checklist "ADHD Indicators" in Chapter 13 can help improve diagnostic precision by identifying a significant pattern of ADHD symptoms. The CDASS checklist "Risk Factors Associated with ADHD" in Chapter 13 can also contribute to the determination process. The checklists in Chapter 14 can help explore the potential presence of medical, sleep, psychological, trauma, neurodevelopmental, sensory processing, and fetal substance exposure conditions which can cause ADHD-like presentations when ADHD doesn't exist, or may coexist with and even worsen true ADHD. Once identified, these conditions will need to be evaluated further. Part II of this book presents the condition descriptions, as well as their evaluation and treatment information, and Part III presents the CDASS checklists for the conditions.

When ADHD-like and other symptoms exist, evaluators should create a timeline of all symptoms. If the other difficulties occurred first and then the ADHD-like symptoms emerged, this may suggest that true ADHD does not exist. While this may not be accurate because ADHD can develop after other conditions emerge, it can help distinguish secondary ADHD-like effects from other disorders. Conversely, true ADHD seems more likely if ADHD symptoms occurred earlier in life before these other difficulties began. Also, successful identification and treatment of other conditions should reduce or eliminate ADHD-like symptoms which may help to determine if true ADHD exists.

Vision and Hearing Evaluations

As a general rule, as part of an ADHD evaluation, all parents should obtain comprehensive vision and hearing tests for any child or adolescent suspected of having ADHD, academic, and behavioral difficulties because undetected hearing and/or vision deficits can cause ADHD-like and scholastic difficulties. While many parents may say that their children received these exams in school, these quick screenings are not comprehensive and may not detect milder, moderate, or other types of vision and hearing difficulties.

Learning Disorders

Many children and teens with true ADHD experience learning challenges, academic underperformance, and lower grades. However, learning difficulties can also result from learning disorders (LD) of reading, mathematics, and written expression, as well as visual and auditory sensory processing disorders, expressive language disorders, and certain other conditions. Unfortunately, all of these can appear similar to ADHD. A challenge during evaluations is to determine if a child or teen with academic or learning problems has true ADHD, learning disorder/s without true ADHD, true ADHD with learning disorder/s, other neurodevelopmental conditions listed above, or other causes. ADHD and LDs can commonly coexist. Determining the presence of LDs can be difficult because only psychological testing can identify these. The CDASS checklists for learning disorders and other conditions can help screen for these, but are not meant to be a substitute for neuropsychological testing or other evaluations.

Visual and Auditory Sensory Processing Disorders

Children and teens who experience reading, math, handwriting, and/or fine motor difficulties may have a visual processing disorder (VPD). VPD is when the eyes work adequately, but the communication between the brain and eyes are not working properly and visual information is not interpreted correctly. Any child or teen with significant learning and academic problems should receive a VPD evaluation. Similarly, auditory processing disorders (APD) can closely mimic ADHD-like symptoms and cause significant academic problems, even when no hearing problems exist. APD typically occurs when hearing is normal, but the communication between the brain and ears is not working properly. As a result, spoken information and other sounds are not interpreted correctly, and focusing and behavioral difficulties can result. Developmental or behavioral optometrists can test for vision problems and visual processing disorders, while certain audiologists and occupational therapists (OT) can evaluate auditory processing disorders. Even neurodevelopmental testing may not adequately identify these two conditions. While APD impairs the ability to understand language, a receptive language disorder can also cause these difficulties. Speech therapists diagnose and treat receptive language deficits, and may be able to differentiate between these similar conditions. Using the CDASS checklist may help to determine if referrals are needed. A developmental optometrist can explore VPD and will probably be less expensive than neuropsychological testing for learning disorders. If an optometrist does not determine a VPD, then neuropsychological testing could evaluate for learning disorders and may screen for APD as well.

Sleep Problems and Conditions

The screening and review of sleeping problems is vital in ADHD evaluations. It can be diagnostically challenging to determine whether sleep problems are causing the ADHD-like symptoms or coexists with true ADHD, especially since because children and teens with ADHD have significantly more sleeping problems than those without ADHD. Any sleep conditions that impact a child's amount and/or quality of sleep should be explored carefully because it can increase the severity of true ADHD or cause ADHD-like symptoms.

Referrals to Occupational Therapists for Higher Levels of Hyperactivity in Young Children

Children, particularly under age six or seven, with high levels of hyperactivity and motor activity should be referred to an occupational therapist (OT). The OT should determine if sensory processing disorders are present, particularly vestibular sensory processing disorder, proprioceptive sensory processing disorder, vestibular intolerance to movement, and vestibular underresponsivity conditions (these are addressed in Chapter 7). These sensory processing conditions can closely mimic ADHD and can be very difficult to differentiate from ADHD, even with measures. Thus, an OT evaluation is often necessary.

Physicians to Rule Out Possible Medical Conditions

As part of a standard ADHD evaluation, children and teens should be seen by their primary care physician to rule out certain medical conditions that may cause ADHD-like behaviors. If these conditions exist, clinicians can consult with physicians to discuss the possible impact on ADHD-like presentations. Clinicians also can write a letter to the primary care physician with their evaluation findings, and suggest specific medical conditions be explored (see these below). A copy of this letter can be given to the parents as well so they may discuss this with the physician. Hopefully, physicians will not be reluctant to explore these medical conditions as a routine part of ADHD evaluations. Although only a minority of children and teens have undetected medical conditions that can cause ADHD-like difficulties, ruling these out is part of a comprehensive diagnostic approach. If medical conditions are identified, physicians and evaluators will have to determine to what degree these are causing ADHD-like symptoms when true ADHD does not exist, or if they coexist with true ADHD. These conditions include:

- Vision difficulties
- Hearing difficulties
- Hypoglycemia
- Asthma or other breathing concerns
- Allergy and related medication use
- Diabetes
- Anemia
- Thyroid disorders

- Toxic heavy metals exposure (such as lead, mercury, cadmium)
- Deficiencies in iron, zinc, magnesium, B vitamins (including B6, and not just B12 which is the easiest to test for) and D vitamin
- Additionally, discuss the possibility of:
  - food allergies and sensitivities
  - seizures
  - conditions causing chronic pain or bodily discomfort
  - head injuries

6. Obtain School Information

In addition to completed teacher measures, it can be helpful to obtain any additional school information about the child's functioning by obtaining report cards (particularly teacher comments and patterns of grades), notes to parents, school testing reports, and 504 or IEP documents. However, most school information will be obtained from parents during clinical interviews, including teacher comments, school behavioral incidents and complaints, and subject grades for each school year. While not necessary or commonly done, evaluators can also call teachers or school social workers for their input.

7. Obtain Prior Behavioral Health Diagnostic and Treatment Information

If these exist, clinicians should speak with or obtain diagnostic and treatment records from past or current behavioral health providers, including psychotherapists, prior psychological testing reports, psychiatrists, and psychiatric hospitalizations. Obtaining prior treatment records is also a good risk management approach, particularly if there have been suicidal or serious aggressive behaviors. Prior evaluation and psychological testing reports can offer baselines to compare current behaviors. However, prior mental health providers may or may not have been diagnostically accurate in these reports.

8. Synthesize and Formulate Findings

The evaluator should now review all of the interview, measures, and other clinical data to determine if true ADHD will be fully diagnosed, if it will be given a provisional or rule out designation, or if it is not present. Other fully diagnosed, provisional, or rule out conditions should be determined as well. If other possible conditions may exist, clinicians should determine if ADHD will be diagnosed or if other providers' services are required for further diagnostic clarification before a full ADHD diagnosis is given. The child's strengths as well as cultural factors and issues should be appreciated and incorporated in these diagnostic formulations as well. When ADHD is diagnosed, it is important to conceptualize how each child or teen manifests this and/or other conditions, how the disorder/s impact them, and then communicate this to families in the next step. If ADHD or ADHD-like presentations result from prenatal substance exposure, head injuries, and/or early pathogenic care, the presentation and treatment responses may differ somewhat.

9. Review ADHD Evaluation Results and Recommendations with Family

This step involves reviewing and discussing the findings with the family. This includes results of the measures, the determined diagnoses and/or provisional or suspected rule out conditions, the child's strengths and challenges, any relevant and impacting cultural issues or factors, referrals to other providers for additional evaluations (and treatment) for potential other suspected conditions, treatment recommendations, suggested psychotherapy approaches, and suggestions about obtaining school services within a 504 Plan or Individualized Education Program. Finally, depending on the results, the evaluator may or may not proceed with providing treatment.

10. Write Letters to Child's Primary Care Physician, Other Providers, and School

This final step involves writing clinical letters to document and share the evaluation's results and recommendations with the child's other providers and school (if this is desired by the family and release of information forms are obtained). More information about these letters will be addressed in the next chapter.

TREATMENT OF ADHD

After ADHD is effectively evaluated, the six phase ADHD*ology* Treatment Approach presents a comprehensive long-term framework to help guide parents, educators, and clinicians to address, manage, and positively transform ADHD at home and school. This is discussed in the ADHD*ology* book *Treating ADHD/ADD in Children and Adolescents: Solutions for Parents and Clinicians,* published by Charles C Thomas Publisher, LTD.

1. **Evaluate ADHD and Other Coexisting Conditions**
   a. Obtain a comprehensive ADHD evaluation or neurodevelopmental assessment
   b. Explore other possible coexisting medical, sleep, neurodevelopmental, sensory processing, and psychological conditions
   c. If other conditions are suspected or detected, obtain additional evaluations and treatment from appropriate providers
2. **Education About ADHD**
   a. Receive accurate information about ADHD
   b. Learn about grieving issues concerning ADHD to move toward acceptance
3. **Address and Manage ADHD at Home**
   a. Learn and use effective behavior management perspectives andn-methods, and maximize parental effectiveness at home
   b. Utilize additional services and management approaches to address various ADHD challenges
   c. Address sleep problems
4. **Address and Manage ADHD School Issues**
   a. Address homework and school behavioral problems through the use of the notebook systems
   b. Obtain 504 Plans or Individual Education Plans at school
   c. Utilize additional ways to address and manage school issues
5. **Medication Treatment for ADHD**
6. **Additional and Alternative ADHD Approaches and Treatment**
   a. Utilize additional approaches including diets, fish oil supplements, increasing sleep, increasing physical activity, green time, limiting screen time and video games, and mind-body therapies
   b. Utilize alternative treatments including neurofeedback, correcting vitamin and mineral deficiencies, Walsh's Biochemical Imbalances Approach and Advanced Nutrient Therapy, Brain Gym® and Bal-A-Vis-X

REFERENCES

American Academy of Pediatrics (2011, November). Clinical practice guideline–ADHD: Clinical practice guideline for the diagnosis, evaluation, and treatment of attention-deficit/hyperactivity disorder in children and adolescents. *Pediatrics, 128*(5).

American Psychiatric Association. (2013). *Diagnostic and statistical manual of mental disorders* (5th ed.). Washington, DC: Author.

Barkley, R. (2013). *Taking charge of ADHD* (3rd ed.). New York: Guilford Press.

Center for Disease Control and Prevention (2018, March 20). *Data & statistics (for ADHD)*. Retrieved from www.cdc.gov/ncbddd/adhd/data.html

Coles, C. D. (2001). Fetal alcohol exposure and attention: Moving beyond ADHD. *Alcohol Research & Health, 25*(3), 199-203. Retrieved from http://pubs.niaaa .nih.gov/publications/arh25-3/199-203.pdf

Follan, M., Anderson, S., Huline-Dickens, S., Lidstone, E., Young, D., Brown, G., & Minnis, H. (2011). Discrimination between attention deficit hyperactivity disorder and reactive attachment disorder in school age children. *Research in Developmental Disabilities, 32*(2011), 520–526.

Gualtieri, C. T., & Johnson, L. G. (2005, November). ADHD: Is objective diagnosis possible? *Psychiatry, 2*(11), 44–52.

Johnson, S., & Marlow, N. (2011). Preterm birth and childhood psychiatric disorders. Pediatric *Research, 69*, 11R–18R. Retrieved from http://www.nature.com/pr /jounral/v69/n5-2/full/pr9201188a.html

Langberg, J., Epstein, J., Simon, J., Loren, R., Arnold, L., Hechtman, L., & Wigal, T. (2010, March). Parental ratings on ADHD symptom-specific and broadband externalizing ratings of child behavior. *Journal of Emotional and Behavioral Disorders, 18*(1), 41–50. Retrieved from http://www.ncbi.nlm.nih.gov/pmc/articles/PMC3117618/

Mattfield, A. T., Gabrieli, J. D. E., Biederman, J., Spencer, T., Brown, A., Kotte, A., Kagan, E., & Whitfield-Gabrieli, S. (2014). Brain differences between persistent and remitted attention deficit hyperactivity disorder. *Brain, 137*(9), 2423–2428. doi:10.1093/brain/awu137

Pliszka, S. (2015). Comorbid psychiatric disorders in children with ADHD. In R. Barkley (Ed.), *Attention deficit hyperactivity disorder: A handbook for diagnosis and treatment* (4th ed., pp. 140–168). New York: Guilford Press.

Smith, B.L. (2011, July-August). ADHD among preschoolers. *Monitor on Psychology, 42*(7), 50–52.

Spencer, T. J., Biederman, J., & Mick, E. (2007 July). Attention-deficit/hyperactivity disorder: Diagnosis, lifespan, comorbidities, and neurobiology. *The Journal of Pediatric Psychology, 32*(6), 631–642.

Spruyt, K., & Gozal, D. (2011, April). Sleep disturbances in children with attention-deficit/hyperactivity disorder. *Expert Review of Neurotherapeutics, 11*(4), 565–577.

Tannock, R., & Brown, T. E. (2009). ADHD with language and/or learning disorders in children and adolescents. In T. E. Brown (Ed.), *ADHD comorbidities: Handbook for ADHD complications in children and adults* (pp. 189–231). Arlington, VA: American Psychiatric Publishing.

Wilding, J. (2005, November). Is attention impaired in ADHD? *British Journal of Developmental Psychology, 23*(4), 487–505.

Chapter 2

ADDITIONAL ADHD
EVALUATION CONSIDERATIONS

EVALUATING ADHD IN PRESCHOOL AGE CHILDREN

The ADHD evaluation process for preschool age children can be challenging because it can be normal for young children to demonstrate developmentally appropriate ADHD-like behaviors. By four years of age, up to 40 percent of children may have concerning difficulties with inattention. Research reported over 72 percent of preschoolers were described as hyperactive. While early identification of ADHD can be helpful, it is often difficult to accurately diagnose ADHD in children under four due to the behavioral similarities in neurotypical children (Mahone & Schneider, 2012).

ADHD is the most commonly diagnosed psychological condition in the preschool years (Mahone & Schneider, 2012). Parents of children with Combined ADHD typically notice traits between ages two to four (Kelly, Pressman, & Greenhill, 2009). But by six years of age, many with ADHD-like traits improve within three to six months on their own. Fifty percent of younger children diagnosed with ADHD will have ADHD by later childhood or early adolescence. Preschool children with inattentiveness and hyperactivity for at least a year are much more likely to have ADHD through childhood and adolescent years. Thus, the severity of early ADHD symptoms and how long they last during early childhood can suggest who are most likely to have persisting ADHD (Barkley, 2013). Some younger children with hyperactivity and impulsivity may not manifest significant inattentive symptoms before first or later grades, and may be initially diagnosed with Predominately Hyperactive/Impulsive ADHD. However, as they become older and their inattention becomes problematic, many will be diagnosed with Combined ADHD.

The process of evaluating younger children for ADHD is similar to the diagnostic work involved with older children. But despite diligent diagnostic efforts, it can be difficult to definitely state if a child has true ADHD for children younger than six, and particularly those under four. Since younger children can outgrow some or all ADHD symptoms before age six, a conservative approach is to delay a diagnosis, take more time to monitor and evaluate ADHD, and explain to parents that additional time is needed for a clearer determination. For these children younger than six and one-half or seven who have ADHD-like symptoms, "provisional" or "rule out" qualifiers to the ADHD diagnosis permit more time to see if the symptoms persist. Provisional or rule out diagnoses may also be helpful during the evaluation process and if other provider referrals are necessary for diagnostic clarity. If there is the "wait and see" period without a clear diagnosis, clinicians can still provide behavioral management treatment. Additionally, medications may be attempted for severe behavioral difficulties.

As a general rule, if ADHD symptoms persist beyond ages six and one-half to seven, then the condition is more likely to continue and there can be more confidence that true ADHD exists. However, other factors can contribute to the likelihood that true ADHD will persist in younger children, including an increased number and more severe symptoms, early symptoms, and the number of risk factors (particularly the presence of family members with ADHD; see Chapter 3).

Temperament has been used as an alternate explanation for ADHD-like difficulties in some younger children. It is the children's behavioral style and the way they react to and experience their environments, and can also worsenen or improve by the setting. Some have proposed that children diagnosed with ADHD may actually have difficulties based on having a poor fit between the environment and their temperament. When ADHD-like behaviors exist for young children at only one setting, they may have a poor temperamental fit rather than true ADHD. Also, unhealthy environments, dysfunctional families, inadequate schools, and innate difficulties (such as neurodevelopmental disorders) can influence a child's adaptability (Lougy, DeRuvo, & Rosenthal, 2007) and may contribute to ADHD-like difficulties. Young children with temperaments of negative moods, demandingness, high intensity, low adaptability, overactivity and inattention are at greater risk for ADHD in later childhood (Barkley, 2013).

CHANGES IN ADHD AS CHILDREN BECOME OLDER

Younger children with impulsivity and hyperactivity difficulties can demonstrate self-management problems when they begin school. For those without true ADHD, their initial school difficulties can be due to a developmental lag, and they may need one or two years to mature. However, for those with true ADHD, the self-regulation difficulties remain and intensify with age (Brown, 2009). Combined ADHD that persists seems particularly likely when there is greater parent-child conflict, maternal negativity and directiveness, and defiant behaviors (Barkley, 2015, March 19a). Individuals with Inattentive ADHD tend to demonstrate attention problems later, and so this is often diagnosed in later childhood or adolescence (Dendy, 2006). Some may not demonstrate significant ADHD difficulties until middle or high school when they switch class rooms, have multiple teachers, and higher levels of organizational demands. Additionally, some teens may not clearly demonstrate ADHD difficulties until high school because their parents have heavily managed their lives (Brown, 2009).

For those with true ADHD, inattention often remains during middle childhood into early adolescence, while hyperactivity and impulsivity can decline (Barkley, 2015, March 19a). Seventy to eighty percent of children diagnosed with Combined and Inattentive ADHD in childhood will continue to have symptoms by their teen years (Dendy, 2006). Some can learn to compensate for their challenges by puberty, and so it may appear that the ADHD is gone. However, with close examination, the symptoms exist and they may benefit from treatment. While rates can vary, as children with ADHD grow older, between 60 to 70 percent will have symptoms that continue into adulthood. While 30 to 40 percent of diagnosed children will not have the full condition by adulthood, some may still suffer from residual ADHD traits (Hallowell & Ratey, 2005). Although it is possible some children can outgrow the disorder completely, at least some symptoms tend to remain through adulthood for most.

As children become older, their manifestations of ADHD and related difficulties can change. Some learn to manage it better than others, and some may seem less impacted by it, particularly those with milder versions. Sometimes parents lack awareness and understanding of how ADHD changes over time, and this can cause problems. Families who have effectively managed ADHD during a child's younger years can be blindsided by adolescent ADHD challenges they do not understand. Medication use, school situations, coexisting conditions, and family environments will also evolve over time, and these changes can impact social, academic, home, and occupational functioning in different ways. Frequently, parents will obtain only one evaluation or comprehensive assessment for their children with ADHD. However, because the condition changes over time, multiple evaluations and assessments can be helpful to track, understand, and treat these evolutions. Also, evaluations or assessments for older teens may be needed to assist with new challenges, including college entrance testing and/or college accommodations.

DIAGNOSTICALLY COMPLEX PRESENTATIONS

Some children and adolescents have complicated clinical presentations with symptoms and functioning difficulties that often arise from various undetected medical, sleep, neurodevelopmental, fetal substance exposure, sensory processing, and psychological conditions. These may create ADHD-like difficulties or coexist with true ADHD. They are puzzling because their conditions or blends of symptoms and conditions create misunderstandings and confusion. Obviously, the more diagnostically complex, the more difficult it will be to accurately diagnose, understand, and treat the problems. This ambiguity and lack of effective treatment can persist for years, while all continue to suffer and struggle. Children and teens with these challenges require more referrals to other providers, as well as more frequent evaluations. Additionally, the term "diagnostically complex" can be used to educate parents and other providers about these challenging presentations.

There are several reasons why families do not receive adequate diagnostic identification and treatment for these complex presentations. The first is that these disorders are often comorbid and can be difficult to distinguish from each other (Gillberg Neuropsychiatry Centre, 2013). Second, some families do not seek out health care services at all or do not go outside the school for services. Third, some clinicians may be unaware of these other conditions or may be too hesitant to address them. Fourth, with younger children, sometimes not enough time has elapsed to track the difficulties to obtain a clear understanding. Fifth, specialists may not communicate adequately with other providers about their findings and treatment, and so their approaches are not adequately coordinated into comprehensive care. Finally, there are not enough qualified and accessible health care specialists and integrated multidisciplinary programs. This can be due to rural limitations, health care insurance restrictions (such as limited Medicaid providers and approval for specialized services), and an overall lack of child specialists, even in metropolitan locations.

One way to address diagnostically complex cases is to extend and expand the diagnostic process with more evaluations from other providers and more frequent evaluations over time. One of the main goals for clinicians evaluating ADHD should be to identify other possible conditions and to make referrals to the correct specialists. Unfortunately, determining these other conditions can be challenging, expensive, and time consuming. Because this process requires parents to be persistent and visit multiple providers, clinicians should help parents understand its importance and encourage and support them. Additionally, with complex presentations, professionals should consider conditions that tend to be confusing, such as fetal alcohol spectrum disorders, sensory processing conditions, and nonverbal learning disorders. Lastly, while a smaller percentage of those with true ADHD do not respond to stimulants, a lack of response or partial response may suggest other undetected conditions.

There are additional diagnostic options to consider for unclear presentations, and these are further addressed in this book. They include utilizing neurodevelopmental assessments, ADHD medication use, QEEG testing from neurofeedback providers, and special blood and urine testing with the Walsh Biochemical Imbalances approach. Hopefully, in the future, more advanced and precise brain imaging, genetic testing, and other neurobiological diagnostic approaches will be available to address complex cases.

THE ESSENCE PERSPECTIVE

Early Symptomatic Syndromes Eliciting Neurodevelopmental Clinical Examinations (ESSENCE) refers to a group of early childhood neurodevelopmental disorders that share overlapping symptoms with other conditions, creating diagnostic complexity and requiring multiple providers. Gillberg (2010) has stated that ESSENCE refers to children who present in clinical settings with symptoms before age five that impact the multiple areas of attention, activity, behavior, communication and language, general development, motor coordination, social functioning, mood, and sleep. They also share genes and environmental risk factors. ESSENCE disorders include ADHD, autism spectrum disorder, early onset bipolar disorder, Tourette syndrome, dyspraxia, intellectual and developmental disabilities, specific language impairment, behavior phenotype syndromes, neurological and seizure disorders with significant cognitive and/or behavioral problems (Gillberg Neuropsychiatry Centre, 2013), and attachment disorders (Pritchett et al., 2013). Unfortunately, many of these children will only see one provider when they require multiple professionals. Significant difficulties in at least one ESSENCE domain before age five often indicates that major problems will likely occur in the same or overlapping domains later, so early intervention is vital (Gillberg, 2010).

DIFFERENCES IN ADHD PRESENTATIONS

Any person on any day can demonstrate inattention, fidgeting, disorganization, procrastination, forgetfulness, impatience, and other ADHD-like traits. However, true ADHD will cause impairments and symptoms that persist over time. True ADHD exists on a continuum of mild, moderate, or severe symptoms from young children to the elderly. The severity of these symptoms will determine the amount of problems they will experience in their lives. Compared to the general population, ADHD exists on the more extreme end of a continuum of inattention, impulsivity, and excessive activity levels. Those with true ADHD will demonstrate symptoms for at least six months that cause impairment and distress by age 12. Some can have very mild or borderline ADHD, where treatment may not be sought or even considered. For milder ADHD, there may be minor impairment only at school or home. A child or teen can have one or two significant ADHD-like symptoms but may not have the required six or more inattention symptoms, and/or six or more hyperactive and impulsive symptoms to qualify for a full ADHD condition.

ADHD impairments may occur in various settings outside the home, but some may demonstrate lesser or no symptoms in activities they enjoy. Similarly, those with ADHD can exhibit different behaviors with different adults. If parents require expectations that children do not like (such as completing homework and chores), then they can be more defiant and argumentative. Because mothers typically interact more with children, children and teens with ADHD can exhibit consistently worse behaviors with mothers than fathers (Barkley, 2015, March 19b). For adults they like or who have fewer demands (including fathers, grandparents, or some teachers), they can be more compliant and demonstrate fewer or no behavioral problems. Without appreciating this, some evaluators can incorrectly perceive frustrated and complaining mothers as a large part of the problem.

Sometimes parents experience ADHD problems only at home, while there are minimal to none at school. Conversely, parents can report no problems at home, while there are poor academic performance and/or school behavioral difficulties. Because teacher reports are not always accessible and parents can convey basic school information, a diagnosis based on parents' reports will lead to a diagnosis 90 percent of the time. However, the best indication of ADHD can be obtained by counting the symptoms endorsed on parent and teacher measures (Barkley, 2015, March 19a).

Children and adolescents with milder ADHD, higher levels of intelligence and ADHD, and those with supportive environments at home or school may not demonstrate difficulties for some time. This can be particularly true for some younger children and Inattentive types. Those with Inattentive ADHD tend to have fewer behavioral difficulties and may only exhibit academic issues. However, as the child becomes older and life demands more of them, the ADHD tends to increasingly impair them. ADHD will also affect children and teens differently depending upon their families. This includes how healthy the home environment is, how supportive and understanding the parents are, if the parents regularly interact with the school and monitor school services, if medication is given, and if parents consistently utilize long-term ADHD management approaches.

LEVELS OF INTEREST AND ADHD

Children and teens with ADHD can excel at tasks and activities they like, as well as those that are new or stimulating. Some parents, teachers, or providers may incorrectly believe children do not have ADHD because they can sustain focus on things they enjoy. If a child with ADHD loves horses, they may be able to read and maintain their attention on this topic for hours. However, if they dislike doing chores or homework, they will struggle to complete these perceived boring tasks. Similarly, those with ADHD often love screen media, and can play video games, watch fast paced shows, or do internet activities for hours. Generally, if a person enjoys something, adrenaline will temporarily override the ADHD brain-functioning limitations to permit sustained focus.

LESSER SELF-AWARENESS AND ADHD

Children and adults with ADHD often have lower self-awareness and self-monitoring abilities. They may deny or minimize having any problems or ADHD-related difficulties. This can be confusing to others, who may be frustrated that they do not acknowledge their problems and have not changed their behaviors. These children or teens may unintentionally offer inaccurate or minimal information about their difficulties during ADHD evaluations. They can be sincerely unaware of how others perceive them and unaware of their own negative behavior. Consequently, their self-reports on ADHD measures may not be as helpful, particularly for younger children, while their self-report measures for depression, anxiety, or trauma may be more accurate. However, if children or teens demonstrate low awareness of their ADHD, this can be important to address during the evaluation results discussion. Finally, individuals with Inattentive ADHD conditions tend to have somewhat more self-awareness than those with Combined ADHD.

CULTURE AND ADHD

ADHD exists all over the world and is not a culturally-based construct only in North America (Polanczyk et al., 2007). A review of 50 studies across the planet suggested that ADHD rates in children are similar in the United

States and many other countries (Dwivedi & Banhatti, 2005). Like other conditions, ADHD will exist with the many dimensions of each person's cultures which can impact its expression and how it is perceived and addressed by others. The clinician's awareness of these cultural components will be important during ADHD evaluations and treatments.

One dimension involves socioeconomic factors. A disproportionate number of ethnic minority families live in significantly stressful and toxic environments with fewer economic, health, housing, and academic resources. Unfortunately, these factors can make children more vulnerable to ADHD (Dwivedi & Banhatti, 2005). Additionally, because parent and teacher rating scales are essential in the ADHD evaluation process, cultural biases will be inherent in the diagnostic process (Fox, Regan, & Bernard, 2014). However, if neuroimaging or other neurobiological markers are used to objectively measure ADHD, this could reduce subjective evaluation components and lessen differences among cultural groups (Dwivedi & Banhatti, 2005).

Another related concept is understanding how different cultures perceive and address ADHD (Curatolo, D'Agati, & Moavero, 2010). One study found that Chinese and Indonesian clinicians reported significantly higher scores for disruptive hyperactive behaviors than those in Japan and the United States (Dwivedi & Banhatti, 2005). Israeli schools have had great tolerance for high activity levels, and this has created challenges in distinguishing higher activity from disorders. In China, there are strong national pressures for children to achieve while remaining on-task for long hours in highly structured classrooms. Individualized educational plans are not used in their schools. Chinese herbal treatments have been used as much or more than ADHD medications. Other barriers in China have included the great stigma for psychological disorders and a tremendous lack of trained, available medical and mental health providers. They also have strong governmental limitations on stimulant medications (Hinshaw et al., 2011).

Within the United States, one large study found that children and teens diagnosed with ADHD in the western states had the lowest rates. It was also found to be more prevalent in African-American and Caucasian children compared to other races (Visser et al., 2014).

While the predominant cultural view of ADHD in the United States is that it has a neurobiological basis, some other countries do not share this view. In Brazil, many clinicians have psychoanalytic views of ADHD which believe that behavioral problems do not result from neurobiological disorders. Some indigenous children from the Amazon regions were found to have ADHD also (Hinshaw et al., 2011).

Cultural beliefs and acculturation levels will affect parents' perceptions about behavioral health and treatment as well. While each family is unique, these cultural issues can include the roles of spirituality, gender, respect, individualism versus collectivism, and help-seeking behaviors. The views of parents and clinicians may differ and this can have important therapeutic alliance and treatment implications. Clinicians should therefore ask specific questions to provide culturally competent clinical services (Fox, Regan, & Bernard, 2014). Evaluators should ask parents if they believe there are relevant cultural issues present, and they can include these factors in their diagnostic conceptualizations.

DETERMINING ADHD BY MEDICATION

While not the best way to distinguish ADHD, this approach can sometimes be helpful for families who are desperate for relief. At times a clear diagnosis of ADHD may not exist, but stimulant medications are attempted. If there is an improvement, this can suggest that true Combined ADHD exists. Some authors have stated that this is not a valid diagnostic approach because most children and adults, whether they have true ADHD or not, will improve their attentional levels on these medications. Studies have demonstrated that stimulants, including caffeine, can enhance concentration, alertness, and mental clarity. As a result, for those with only inattention difficulties, stimulant responses may not clearly indicate if true Inattentive ADHD exists. Also, 20 to 30 percent of children with true ADHD may not respond positively to medications. As a result, if prescribing physicians and families do not observe a positive response to ADHD medication, some may falsely believe that ADHD does not exist (Garber, Garber, & Spizman, 1996). To improve accuracy, families can try a number of ADHD medications at sufficient doses to determine if they are effective. Furthermore, most with true Combined ADHD should experience improvements with hyperactivity, impulsivity, and even ODD behaviors when they are on effective ADHD stimulants and doses. Therefore, this diagnosing through stimulants approach can be effective for some with true Combined ADHD. Finally, this approach will be less precise for children five and younger because stimulant medications can be less effective for them.

THE USE OF QEEG TESTS

Electroencephalography (EEG) or Quantitative EEG (QEEG) tests are administered by neurofeedback providers. As stated previously, these can be helpful with diagnostically complex cases. They can help indicate or confirm if a child or adolescent has true Combined or Inattentive ADHD and/or a range of other conditions, including sensory processing deficits, seizures, mood or anxiety conditions, sleep difficulties, and neurodevelopmental conditions. QEEG tests are brain maps that explore brain wave frequencies and other aspects of brain functioning. QEEGs are typically done at the beginning of neurofeedback treatment to create baselines, but QEEGs can be used as diagnostic tests to help suggest if true ADHD exists or not. Insurance plans often do not cover this testing, but some plans may. QEEGs can be used with children starting at about age five and can cost about $400 and up. Some neuropsychologists combine QEEG and neuropsychological testing to improve their accuracy of diagnosing ADHD.

While not definitive by itself, some believe that QEEG tests can be up to 90 percent accurate in detecting ADHD (Hallowell & Ratey, 2005). However, its accuracy can vary and the use of QEEGs is not a standard of care yet for diagnosing ADHD. Some neurofeedback providers do not believe QEEGs should be used for definitive diagnostic purposes. Some critics say these can give inaccurate or imprecise results, and they are far less than 90 percent accurate. Additionally, certified and experienced neurofeedback providers are limited in many areas, so access may be challenging. However, due to some difficulties in diagnosing ADHD, this may be a helpful approach.

ADHD EVALUATION RESULTS IN LETTERS

Once clinicians have completed the ADHD evaluation, the results should be documented in a report or letter. Some ADHD evaluators prefer to write letters to the child's primary care physician, and then give copies to the parent, other providers, and school. It is important to share evaluation findings with other providers for several reasons, especially since research has shown that better care and outcomes are achieved when mental health providers partner with primary care physicians (Novotney, 2015). To share information with others, clinicians must obtain a signed release of information form. However, the letter can be given to the parent, and they can distribute this to others without a release form.

ADHD evaluation letters should clearly state what difficulties exist, strengths, diagnostic formulations and findings, and recommendations. Letters should include what psychological conditions are fully diagnosed, what suspected conditions are rule outs and not able to be fully determined and why, referrals to other specific providers for additional evaluations and services, proposed treatment plans, and recommendations to schools to conduct case studies to determine if official school plans will be provided. Concerns with diagnostically complex presentations should be clearly discussed.

If the evaluation was completed by a psychotherapist, the letter should also state if that individual will provide therapy or if therapy will be suspended until additional evaluations occur.

Letters should assist physicians, other providers, and the family to better understand the child and to help obtain appropriate additional referrals and care. The evaluation letter can also be documentation for physicians that an evaluation occurred, and can be useful if medication is prescribed. Additionally, sending letters about diagnostic findings and treatment approaches to physicians may be expected by some health insurance companies as part of best practices, and can also be helpful from risk management perspectives.

Copies of these letters may be given to parents in most cases so they have written details of the evaluation findings, and parents should keep a copy for their records. Parents can be encouraged to bring a copy of this letter to other providers as well. This will be particularly helpful in diagnostically complex cases when others are needed to contribute to the diagnostic process. Finally, a copy of the letter can be given to the child's school as documentation of their diagnoses. These letters can support parental requests for the school to conduct a psychoeducation evaluation to determine eligibility for a 504 Plan or Individual Education Program.

REFERENCES

Barkley, R. (2013). *Taking charge of ADHD* (3rd ed.). New York: Guilford Press.

Barkley, R. (2015, March 19a). *ADHD: Nature, course, outcomes, and comorbidity.* Retrieved from www.continuingedcourses.net/active/courses/course003.php

Barkley, R. (2015, March 19b). *ADHD in children: Diagnosis and assessment.* Retrieved from www.continuingedcourses.net/active/courses/course004.php

Brown, T. E. (2009). Developmental complexities of attentional disorders. In T. E. Brown (Ed.), *ADHD comorbidities: Handbook for ADHD complications in children and adults* (pp. 3–22). Arlington, VA: American Psychiatric Publishing.

Curatolo, P., D'Agati, E., & Moavero, R. (2010). The neurobiological basis of ADHD. *Italian Journal of Pediatrics, 36*(1), 79. doi: 10.1186/1824-7288-36-79

Dendy, C. Z. (2006). *Teenagers with ADD and ADHD: A guide for parents and professionals* (2nd ed.). Bethesda, MD: Woodbine House.

Dwivedi, K. N., & Banhatti, R. G. (2005). Attention deficit/hyperactivity disorder and ethnicity. *Archives of Disease in Childhood; 90(Suppl I),* i10–i12.

Fox, F., Regan, F., & Bernard, S. (2014). *ADHD and multicultural issues.* Retrieved from https://www.pdx.edu/multicultural-topics-communication-sciences-disorders/adhd-and-multicultural-issues

Garber, S. W., Garber, M. D., & Spizman, R. F. (1996). *Beyond Ritalin.* New York: Harper Perennial.

Gillberg, C. (2010, November- December). The essence in child psychiatry: Early symptomatic syndromes eliciting neurodevelopmental clinical examinations. *Research in Developmental Disabilities, 31*(6), 1543–1551. doi: 10.1016/j.ridd.2010 .06.002.

Gillberg Neuropsychiatry Centre. (2013, October 18). *ESSENCE.* Retrieved from http://gnc.gu.se/english/research/essence—early-symptomatic-syndromes-eliciting- neurodevelopmental-clinical-examinations-

Hallowell, E. D. & Ratey, J. J. (2005). *Delivered from distraction.* New York: Balantine.

Hinshaw, S. P., Scheffler, R. M., Fulton, B. D., Aase, H., Banaschewski, T., Cheng, W., Mattos, P... & Weiss, M.D. (2011, May). International variation in treatment procedures for ADHD: Social context and recent trends. *Psychiatric Services, 62*(5), 459–464.

Kelly, P., Pressman, A. W., & Greenhill, L. L. (2009). ADHD in Preschool Children. In T. E. Brown (Ed.), *ADHD Comorbidities: Handbook for ADHD complications in children and adults* (pp. 37–53). Arlington, VA: American Psychiatric Publishing.

Lougy, R. A., DeRuvo, S. L., & Rosenthal, D. (2007). *Teaching young children with ADHD.* Thousand Oak, CA: Corwin Press.

Mahone, E. M., & Schneider, H. E. (2012, December). Assessment of attention in preschoolers. *Neuropsychology Review, 22*(4), 361–383.

Novotney, A. (2015, October). In Brief. *Monitor on Psychology, 46*(9), 18.

Pritchett, R., Pritchett, J., Marshall, E., Davidson, C., & Minnis, H. (2013). Reactive attachment disorder in the general population: A hidden essence disorder. *The Scientific World Journal, 13,* Article ID 818157, 6 pages. Retrieved from https: //www.hindawi.com/journals/tswj/2013/818157/

Polanczyk, G., de Lima, M. S., Horta, B. L., Biederman, J., & Rohde, L. A. (2007). The worldwide prevalence of ADHD: A systematic review and metaregression analysis. *American Journal of Psychiatry, 164,* 942–948.

Visser, S. N., Danielson, M. L., Bitsko, R. H., Kogan, M. D., Ghandour, R. M., Perou, R., & Blumberg, S. J. (2014, January). Trends in the parent-report of health care provider diagnosed and medicated attention-deficit/hyperactivity disorder: United States, 2003–2011. *Journal of the American Academy of Child & Adolescent Psychiatry, 53*(1), 34–46.e2.

Part II

POSSIBLE CONDITIONS AND RISK FACTORS TO CONSIDER WHEN EVALUATING ADHD IN CHILDREN AND ADOLESCENTS

Chapter 3

RISK FACTORS ASSOCIATED WITH ADHD

ADHD has been correlated and associated with a number of predisposing influences and risk factors, including genetic and environmental factors, and deficiencies involving neural brain pathways, brain structures, and brain chemicals called neurotransmitters (Herbert & Esparham, 2017). However, even though heavily researched, the exact cause of ADHD is still unknown. ADHD is most frequently caused by a positive family history. It is considered one of the most heritable of all psychological disorders, with estimates of about 70 percent. The remaining 30 percent are likely the result of other environmental factors (see this checklist in Chapter 13) (Tarver, Daley, & Sayal, 2014). ADHD is considered a complex trait disorder affected by many susceptibility genes, with each gene contributing to the risk (Herbert & Esparham, 2017). The interaction of these multiple genetic and environmental factors appears to create a spectrum of neurodevelopmental vulnerability. The potential for ADHD rises as genetic and environmental risk factors increase (Curatolo, D'agassi, & Mover, 2010).

Family History of ADHD

Family history has been found to be the most significant predictor and risk factor for ADHD. Paternal history of antisocial behavior is also a strong predictor of ADHD (Mahone & Schneider, 2012). If one parent has ADHD, the odds of a child inheriting this can be 30 to 50 percent (Dendy, 2006; Hallowell & Ratey, 2005). If both parents have ADHD, the risk is 50 percent or greater. If a sibling has ADHD, there is 30 percent likelihood that other siblings will also have the condition (Hallowell & Ratey, 2005).

During the ADHD evaluation, clinicians should explore if other family members have diagnosed or undiagnosed ADHD. To screen for ADHD in other family members, clinicians can use DSM symptoms or the CDASS ADHD checklists to ask if these symptoms resemble difficulties in the child's mother, father, siblings, grandparents, uncles, aunts, or cousins. They can inquire whether family members had these challenges as a child, including academic, learning, reading, or behavioral problems. Clinicians can also explore potential adult ADHD issues, such as employment, substance abuse, relational, temper, behavioral, or financial difficulties. Family members may not have been formally diagnosed with ADHD, so this may be only an educated guess. Since ADHD is more frequent in males, fathers and male relatives are at greater risk of having this.

Premature Birth

Premature birth seems to increase the risk for ADHD due to neurobiological developmental difficulties (Mahone & Schneider, 2012). Normal pregnancies are about 40 weeks. Thirty-six weeks (before the beginning of the 37th week of pregnancy) can be used as a marker for a premature birth. Also, the greater the prematurity, the higher the risk. Children born preterm who develop ADHD seem to have a different clinical presentation from term children with ADHD. For children born preterm, the genders have equal frequencies of ADHD, are less likely to have coexisting conduct disorders, and have weaker associations to family and sociodemographic risks (Johnson & Marlow, 2011). Moderately preterm children have been found to exhibit slightly lower IQs and more emotional regulation, cognitive, attentional, and behavioral difficulties when compared to term children. Other studies found that inattention difficulties were observed in about one-third of very preterm children of 32 weeks or earlier by the time they reach school age, and in 15–25 percent of moderately preterm children. Another study showed that moderately preterm children born at 32 to 36 weeks had attentional problems at school age (Chu et al., 2012).

One important study of more than 1.1 million children's school records in Sweden found that the risk for developing ADHD during school years increased for children born a month or more before their due date, and then gradually rises with greater prematurity. They found that when compared to children born at 39 to 41 weeks, children born at 23 to 28 weeks gestation were over twice as likely to develop ADHD. Additionally, children born at 29 to 32 weeks had a 60 percent greater chance of developing ADHD, those born between 33 and 34 weeks had a 40 percent higher chance, children born between 35 to 36 weeks had a 30 percent greater chance, and those born from 37 to 38 weeks had a 10 percent greater chance (Lindstrom, Lindblad, & Hjern, 2011). A large population-based study of patients diagnosed with ADHD from Finnish nationwide registers reported the risk for ADHD by each week of fetal maturity, with greater odds of developing ADHD for each week of prematurity than reported in the Swedish study (Sucksdorff et al., 2015).

Post-Term Birth

Those born at 42 weeks or later have also been associated with higher risks for ADHD (Marroun et al., 2012).

High Birth Weight

Newborns with birth weights of more than 10 lbs. (over two standard deviations above the norm of 7 lbs. 8 ounces) were found to have a 20 percent higher risk of developing ADHD (Sucksdorff et al., 2015).

Low Birth Weight

Researchers have found that birthweights below about 5.5 pounds can increase the risk for ADHD (this is the low end of average birth weights). The lower the birth weight below average, the greater the risk of developing ADHD. Low birth weight is often associated with premature birth. These factors can be separate but often present together. ADHD is the most prevalent and researched neurodevelopmental condition for preterm and low birth weight populations (Johnson & Marlow, 2011; Mahone & Schneider, 2012).

Researchers who studied children ages six to 12 found those with both low birth weight (defined by less than 5.5 pounds) and moderate preterm birth (between 33- and 37-weeks gestational age) demonstrated more severe ADHD symptoms. The study also found that more severe Combined ADHD symptoms were significantly correlated with lower gestational age or shorter preterm duration. Lower birth body weight was associated with inattention, but not impulsivity or hyperactivity (Chu et al., 2012). A large study found that children born small for gestational age (5 lbs. or less) had an 80 percent greater risk of developing ADHD after an adjustment for confounders (Sucksdorff et al., 2015).

Additionally, children with ADHD who had very low birth weights (3.3 to 2.3 lbs.) and very preterm births exhibited greater risks for inattention than hyperactivity/impulsivity difficulties, and those with extremely low birth weight (2.2 lbs. or less) had greater prevalence of ADHD. Curiously, evidence has suggested that ADHD is caused differently in this group. They may have a purer and biologically determined form of ADHD. These children appear to have impaired brain growth, cognitive impairments, and structural abnormalities evident on MRIs (Johnson & Marlow, 2011).

Certain Pregnancy and Birth Complications

Some studies have not found a greater incidence of pregnancy or birth complications in children with ADHD compared to those without ADHD.

However, others studies have found a slightly higher prevalence of ADHD associated with unusually short or long labor, fetal distress, low forceps delivery, and toxemia/pre-eclampsia (pregnancy induced high blood pressure). Barkley (2013) stated the total number of pregnancy complications and/or repeated maternal infections increase the risk of ADHD, particularly with a premature delivery and low birth weight accompanied by bleeding in the brain. The types of infections and complications appear less important than the total number. Forceps use during delivery can damage the brain and may cause ADHD. Also, metabolic disorders of the pregnant mother (gestational diabetes, phenylketonuria) may result in ADHD-like presentations later in the child. Maternal anxiety, stress, and persistent stressful events have been associated with ADHD. Finally, prenatal drug and/or alcohol exposure can cause significant risks for ADHD, and these will be addressed in Chapter 8.

Situations Before, During, or Just After Birth that Cause Oxygen Deprivation (Ischemic-Hypoxic Conditions)

These events can negatively affect fetal brain development, may include significant functional and structural brain injuries, and often are not obvious at birth. They lead to less than optimal oxygen delivery and nutrient transport from the mother's blood to the fetus. One study examined medical records of many children ages five to 11, and found those with ischemic-hypoxic conditions had increased risks for ADHD, particularly those with neonatal respiratory distress syndrome. This syndrome occurs when infants do not receive adequate oxygen before, during, or after birth. Several reasons may be involved, including the umbilical cord wrapped around the neck. Neonatal respiratory distress syndrome was found to create a 47 percent higher risk of developing ADHD, preeclampsia caused a 34 percent higher risk, and birth asphyxia a 26 percent higher risk. Additionally, these associations were strongest in preterm births (Getahun et al., 2013). Finally, some prenatal drug exposure can also cause fetal oxygen restriction and thus impact fetal brain development (Minnes, Lang, & Singer, 2011).

Moderate to Severe Jaundice in Newborn Infants

While some studies have had conflicting results about the relationship between neonatal jaundice and the risk of developing ADHD, one study found ADHD was about 2.5 times higher when jaundice was present. It also found the risk of ADHD was significantly higher for boys as well as preterm and low-birth weight infants with jaundice (Wei et al., 2015).

Head Injury (Traumatic Brain Injury)

Depending on the severity, traumatic brain injuries (TBI) can cause a range of significant and life altering changes and impairments in personality, neuropsychological abilities, executive functioning, memory, impulse control, attention, mood, behavior, self-control, and frustration tolerance. TBIs can also impair sleep, which can then further cause attentional, mood, and other ADHD-like difficulties. TBIs and the accidents that cause them may also create posttraumatic stress.

More than 1.7 million TBIs occur each year. They are a massive public health issue and a leading cause of deaths and permanent disabilities, accounting for 30 percent of injury-related deaths in the United States. TBIs affect more men than women, and the most frequently impacted ages are birth to three, 15 to 19, and over 65. Mild TBI involves brief mental status change lasting less than 24 hours, or loss of consciousness for up to 30 minutes with normal MRI or CT imagining results. About 75 percent of TBIs are mild. Severe TBI involves an extended amnesia or unconsciousness period for more than 24 hours, but can have abnormal or normal imaging (McGuire et al., 2015).

ADHD may not be evident soon after brain injuries, but ADHD can occur up to six years after the event (Narad et al., 2018). Even minor falls, sports injuries or accidents without concussions or loss of consciousness can cause serious damage. Clinicians may need to ask parents about head injuries multiple times because they can often forget or minimize these. If additional head injuries occur over time, these can cause even more brain damage (Amen, 2013), and will further increase ADHD risks.

Because children and adults with ADHD have more accidents and injuries, it can be difficult to determine if head injuries caused ADHD, or did the injuries result from the ADHD. Clinicians can explore which came first by comparing when the injury occurred and when the ADHD symptoms were first noticed. Additionally, if a head injury is suspected, a SPECT scan can be more precise to show early damage, while CAT and MRI scans may not be as helpful and will only indicate late brain changes, such as atrophied or dead tissue (Amen, 2013). TBIs can also cause seizures for many as well.

The effects of the TBI itself, related sleep difficulties, and/or posttraumatic seizures can all cause or compound ADHD-like symptoms, so these factors will require evaluation and treatment. Neurologists can evaluate and treat head injuries, and may prescribe ADHD or other medications. Neuropsychologists can test to explore the impact of head injuries on functioning, posttraumatic stress and lifestyle changes, and can diagnose and treat TBI-related challenges. QEEG tests from neurofeedback providers can assist in identifying head injuries, and neurofeedback can provide significant improvements. TBI centers have specialists to assess and treat TBI difficulties. Finally, hyperbaric oxygen therapy (HBOT) can treat brain injuries by increasing the supply of medical grade oxygen to improve cerebral blood flow and brain tissue oxygenation.

Near Drowning Experience, Severe Smoke Inhalation, and Carbon Monoxide Poisoning

These events can disrupt the flow of blood and oxygen to the brain which may cause brain injury and an ADHD presentation.

Early Pathogenic Care

Early pathogenic care during first five years of life can cause ADHD or ADHD-like symptoms. Refer to this section in Chapter 11 for more information.

Single Parenthood, Lesser Maternal Education, and Lower Parental Socioeconomic Status

These factors produce a very small risk for ADHD (Barkley, 2013). Low maternal education is most likely a marker for a complex web of risk factors that is associated with social adversity, including family discord, relative poverty, and living in lower status housing areas (Lindstrom, Lindblad, & Hjern, 2011).

Childhood Neurotoxic Exposure

Since we live in an increasingly environmentally toxic world, certain neurotoxicant exposure can cause ADHD and ADHD-like difficulties for children. This is only an introduction, and further research is obviously needed. Aside from recent lead exposure, most other neurotoxins exposure can be difficult to determine, and these potential causes of ADHD may need to be long-term "rule outs." Unfortunately, challenges with identifying neurotoxic exposure may deter most families from exploring these. Maternal fetal substance exposure conditions are addressed in Chapter 8.

Behavioral, developmental, and learning disorders are on the rise. Their causes are complex and multidirectional. It is estimated that between 3 to 25 percent of child developmental defects result from neurotoxic environmental exposures, either singly or in combination with other environmental factors such as unhealthy maternal pregnant lifestyle choices (poor diet or substance use), maternal occupation (prenatal exposure to toxicants at work), and economic circumstances that expose children to toxicants (housing, water, other lifestyle exposures) (Koger, Schettler, & Weiss, 2005). Barkley (2013) reported that 25 to 35 percent of children with acquired ADHD develop this from toxins or other hazardous events.

Fetuses, babies, and young children are particularly vulnerable to environmental toxins, which can disrupt the development of their rapidly growing nervous, hormonal, and respiratory systems. Younger children often encounter higher levels of neurotoxins than adults because they spend more time on floors, put more things in their mouths, ingest more liquids (juice, fruit, water that increase exposure to pesticide contaminants), stir up and breathe more dust and residues, and have ten times the contact with dust as adults. Delayed neurotoxicity may occur when the effects of the exposure happen later in life (Koger, Schettler, & Weiss, 2005). Poverty can be another negative factor upon children's neurodevelopmental functioning because poor children are more likely to live in environments with greater exposure to pollution and industrial toxins (Lu, 2015).

The following are some but not all of the neurotoxins associated with ADHD, ADHD-like symptoms, and neurocognitive deficits. Most can also cause learning disorders.

Lead

Many research studies have found that lead exposure in children has been associated with higher rates of inattention and impulsivity (Braun et al., 2006). Lead exposure to pregnant mothers and younger children can be particularly damaging. According to the Centers for Disease Control and Prevention, children in over four million homes in the United States have been exposed to high lead levels. Lead is such a potent neurotoxin that almost any exposure can be damaging. Even low levels can increase risks of learning disorders and intellectual disabilities. Jacobson (2011) reported that postnatal lead exposure is the most extensively studied environmental toxin. The most consistent neurobehavioral effects from postnatal lead exposure are lower IQ scores, ADHD, and conduct difficulties.

According to the American Academy of Pediatrics' Clinical Practice Guidelines for ADHD diagnosis, lead exposure may predispose young children to ADHD, but very few of these young children will have elevated lead levels by school age. Thus, regular screenings of children for high lead levels may not aid in the diagnosis of ADHD. Yet, one study reported that about 21 percent of the children ages four to 15 with ADHD had elevated lead levels in their blood (Braun et al., 2006).

Unfortunately, lead is found in many homes. One of the most common forms of lead exposure occurs from lead-based paint from homes build before 1978. This toxic paint can chip, crack, and create dust that accumulates on and near windows, doors, stairs, porches, and in the surrounding soil. Lead can also be found in vinyl mini-blinds, some glazed pottery, fishing weights, refinishing furniture materials, stained glass solder, hunting ammunition, some candle wicks, and lead crystal.

Lead can also contaminate drinking water in homes from the water supply itself, the water service line that connects the water main to the home, solder in plumbing, and brass valves and faucets. In 1986, the United States required all solder to be lead-free. In 2014, the United States federal law, The Reduction of Lead in Drinking Water Act, created higher standards for all valves and faucets used for drinking water. However, some homes still have solder connecting pipes, values, and faucets that contain lead (Brush, 2017). While these laws have helped, lead contaminated drinking water continues to be a problem across rural and urban portions of the United States, including Chicago. A high number of residential homes, as well as some public schools, have had toxic lead levels in the drinking water. If there are concerns about lead contamination, families should examine their city's water supply report and obtain lead testing for their home's water (Brush, 2017).

Mercury

This is a highly toxic and naturally occurring metal and element found in certain larger fish (such as tuna, swordfish, orange roughy and shark), shellfish, certain amalgam dental fillings (which are often silver colored), fluorescent light bulbs, and glass thermometers. Consuming seafood is the most common mercury exposure. Mercury has a long history of causing neurocognitive deficits, including inattention, learning disabilities, motor dysfunction, memory difficulties, and visual impairments (Koger, Schettler, & Weiss, 2005). Mercury poisoning can cause changes in neurocognitive and emotional functioning, speech, vision, muscular abilities, headaches, and tremors.

Endocrine Disruptors

These chemicals negatively impact various hormones and can accumulate in hormone producing organs to cause many bodily and brain difficulties including ADHD-like symptoms and other neurodevelopmental problems (Lu, 2015). Endocrine disruptors have been found in common household cleaning products, personal care products (soap, shampoo, toothpaste, moisturizer), drinking water, vinyl items, canned foods, fish and meats (particularly those fed antibiotics, hormones, and other chemicals), fruits and vegetables exposed to routine herbicides and pesticides, house dust, plastics that leech into food and water, and office products. These chemicals are almost inescapable in daily life, their detection is extremely difficult, and they can be harmful even in low quantities.

Endocrine disruptors can negatively impact developing brains and reproductive organs, and affect how thyroid, estrogen, and androgen hormones are created and metabolized. They can be transmitted to fetuses prenatally and frequently present in higher concentrations in infants and young children. Hundreds of studies have explored how these chemicals impact animals' hormones, and human studies suggest their negative impact on children's learning and behavior. Some researchers blame the rise of neurodevelopmental disorders in children over the past two decades on the cumulative effect of endocrine disrupting chemicals (Lu, 2015).

The are many types of endocrine disruptors. While not a complete list, those presented below have been linked to ADHD.

Bisphenol A (BPA): This omnipresent chemical is used to make polycarbonate plastics found in food containers, liners in soda and soup cans, and cash register receipt paper. BPA appears to act like an estrogen and can alter thyroid, estrogen, and androgen transmission signals. One study found boys but not girls exposed to higher levels of BPA demonstrated more rule-breaking, aggression, and sleep problems (Lu, 2015).

Polybrominated Diphenyl Ethers (PBDEs): This chemical class lingers in fatty tissues and is a common flame retardant in many household products, including furniture, mattresses, electronics, clothing and plastics. One study found that higher prenatal exposures to PBDEs were correlated with lower IQs and increased hyperactivity at age five, although no effects at younger ages were observed. Another found that mothers with the highest levels of PBDEs in their urine were more likely to have children with decreased attention by age five, lesser fine motor skills, and lower verbal and total IQ scores (Lu, 2015).

Polychlorinated Biphenyls (PCBs): These are found in old fluorescent lighting fixtures and appliances from the mid-1970s or earlier and in foods such as fish caught in PCB contaminated lakes and rivers.

Certain Chemicals Used in the Home

In addition to common household chemicals with endocrine disruptors, cleaning products may contain alcohol, trichloroethylene, xylene, and other neurotoxins (Koger, Schettler, & Weiss, 2005). Therefore, checking labels can be helpful in identifying unwanted ingredients. Additionally, some children with ADHD have greater sensitivities to toxic chemicals in the home, school, or automobiles, which can worsen ADHD. Astute parents may notice changes in their child when exposed to certain offending products. A diary of these reactions can be helpful (Stevens, 2016).

Certain Pesticides and Lawn Chemicals

These include sprays that kill garden weeds, insects, or rodents. Pesticides like maneb and mancozeb contain manganese, and higher levels of manganese have been associated with ADHD (Koger, Schettler, & Weiss, 2005). In one study of boys eight to 15, pyrethroids, the most commonly used insecticide and an endocrine disruptor, was found in the urine of boys who were more than twice as likely to have impulsive and hyperactivity symptoms than controls. Previous studies have suggested that pyrethroids interfere with dopamine levels (Lu, 2015). Again, reading labels may be helpful.

Cadmium, Manganese, and Industrial Hazardous Toxins

Exposure to cadmium, a natural earth element used in making metals, and manganese, an essential trace element and naturally occurring in metals, have been associated with ADHD symptoms, learning disabilities, and other serious neurocognitive effects (Koger, Schettler, & Weiss, 2005). Cadmium and manganese can contaminate drinking water and air. Manganese is found in pesticides also. There are other common and less common neurotoxic industrial pollutants found in the air and water supplies which can cause ADHD-like and neurocognitive difficulties. Unfortunately, these will also be difficult to detect and stop exposure, unless the family moves away from these sources.

Neurotoxic Exposure Evaluation and Treatment

Many exposures can be subtle, gradual, and the effects may be delayed for years, making detection and/or removal of the source quite difficult (Koger, Schettler, & Weiss, 2005). The more constant toxin exposure sources in the air, water, and frequently consumed foods or beverages can be even more difficult to determine. Yet some toxins are easier to identify, test, and treat than others. Detective work by parents and the use of symptom diaries to help monitor when reactions occur may be critical for identification. Evaluators should explore if symptoms worsen after exposure to pesticides, lawn chemicals, household chemicals, or other potential known toxins. There may be neurocognitive and medical symptoms which are suspicious or atypical, perhaps providing clues of exposure.

Lead, certain heavy metals, and some toxins can be more easily tested through urinalysis. However, lead testing will only yield positive results if there is current and ongoing lead poisoning. If lead exposure was only in the past, despite damage that may have occurred, current lead testing results will be negative. While lead testing is more common, testing for other heavy metals and neurotoxins is not routine. Stevens (2016) stated that the chances of mercury, cadmium, and other neurochemical exposures causing ADHD traits seems to be low, while lead exposure creates higher risks. However, due to genetics and other risk factors, children may have a range of sensitivities and vulnerabilities for various neurotoxic exposures. Clinicians can suggest that parents ask pediatricians for blood tests for some toxic metals, such as mercury and lead. While less common, hair analyses can also be used to detect these and other heavy metals.

Once again, endocrine disruptors detection and treatment will probably be difficult. Some can be more sensitive to the different endocrine disruptors than others. Removal of the offending source will be very challenging because they are ubiquitous. One way to reduce exposure is to commit to eating more organic and fresh foods, and purchase products that are vinyl free, organic, stored in glass, and more "natural" versions of products (although even "natural" versions can still have toxicity). This can be a major lifestyle change and many families may be unwilling or lack conviction to do this.

Removal of all impacting toxin sources will be important for treatment. While perhaps not easy to do, families can web search the safety levels of their air and drinking water near their homes or schools. They can explore if there are local polluting factories which may be emitting neurotoxins, as well as testing their home drinking water. Chelation therapies may be used to remove some heavy metals and neurotoxins, but their effectiveness has been controversial.

Heavy metals and toxic substances are two of the biochemical factors addressed by Dr. William Walsh in his Walsh Biochemical Imbalances approach. When individuals have heavy-metal overload, toxic levels of pesticides, or other organic chemicals exposure, he advocates a three-part approach. This involves determining and avoidance of additional toxic exposures, biochemical treatment to hasten the toxicin's exit from the body, and correction of the underlying chemical imbalances to minimize future vulnerabilities to the toxin (Walsh Research Institute, 2005-2016b).

Certain Mineral and Vitamin Deficiencies

Despite some inconsistent findings, researchers have demonstrated that some vitamin and mineral deficiencies have been associated with ADHD symptoms. Some of the most common are zinc, magnesium, iron, B vitamins (particularly B6) and D vitamin. For more information on iron deficiency, refer to the "anemia" section in Chapter 4. Unless there is specific testing for these deficiencies, it will be difficult to determine if low levels exist.

Evaluation and Treatment

Primary care physicians can request testing to determine if the child or teen has these deficiencies or imbalances. Iron, vitamin D, and vitamin B12 are routine tests that can be easily ordered. When requesting vitamin D, a 25(OH)D test should be requested because this is the most accurate. Besides vitamin B12, testing for the rest of the B vitamins may be more challenging and can require other practitioners. While controversial and less common, zinc and magnesium deficiencies can be tested with blood levels (Laake & Compart, 2013). However, Stevens (2016) shared that some experts believe that blood testing for magnesium does not provide accurate results or guidance. Additionally, it can be helpful to obtain micronutrient testing to explore a wide range of vitamin, mineral, and nutrient imbalances and deficits. If pediatricians do not support this approach, this testing can be obtained from other providers, such as dietitians and naturopaths. After deficiencies are determined, supplementation can be considered, and qualified health professionals should supervise this approach.

Walsh Biochemical Imbalances

William Walsh, Ph.D., based on the pioneering research of Carl Pfeiffer, MD, Ph.D., has created decades of research that indicate there are specific biochemical imbalances that can cause ADHD, ODD, violent behaviors, learning disorders, bipolar disorder, autism, and other conditions. Walsh and others who use this approach stress the importance of understanding that each person has their own unique genetic differences and biochemistry that may include potential deficits or excesses of certain chemical factors. Biochemical individuality explains why some psychiatric medications work for some people, but not for others. Walsh (2014) has a large chemical database of over 10,000 individuals with behavioral disorders and 5,600 people with ADHD. He stated that with specialized testing and nutrient treatment for these underlying biochemical conditions (either deficiencies or excesses), children and adolescents can dramatically improve.

Walsh shared that children with Inattentive ADHD often have deficiencies in folic acid, vitamin B-12, zinc, and choline, and can improve their attentional abilities after taking these supplements. For individuals with predominantly hyperactive and impulsive difficulties, Walsh stated that they often have a metal metabolism disorder that involves excessive copper levels and zinc deficiency. This imbalance in metals is associated with low dopamine and elevated norepinephrine and adrenalin activity. While stimulant medications for ADHD can elevate dopamine activity, Walsh's nutrient approach can balance copper and zinc levels with similar results. Those with

Combined ADHD often have multiple chemical imbalances, and specialized testing is required to determine these. Many of these individuals have a seriously elevated copper/zinc ratio, but they may also have a methylation disorder, toxic overload, pyrrole disorder, or other imbalances (Walsh, 2014).

Evaluation and Treatment

The Walsh Biochemical Imbalances Approach and Advanced Nutrient Therapy requires specific blood and urine testing to determine if certain imbalances exist. This approach is an alternative one, with few labs and providers offering these services. However, the lab testing, consultation services, and treatment can be done remotely by some clinicians. After testing is completed, individualized compounds of nutrient therapies of vitamins, minerals, and amino acids based on the testing results are created by special pharmacies to correct the imbalances and neurotransmitter activity. For children with ADHD, this can take up to three months to achieve the full effects. The disadvantages of this approach are these services are typically not covered by health insurance, fewer provides are available, and treatment will take longer than stimulant medications to be effective. The advantages are no side effects and it can specifically target the biochemical imbalances to create potentially effective to highly effective results. Furthermore, these providers state that many can reduce or eliminate psychiatric medications with these nutrient therapies (W. J. Walsh, personal communication, October 19, 2014). For more information and provider referrals, visit the non-profit Walsh Research Institute at www .walshinstitute.org.

Exposure to Artificial Food Colorings, Preservatives, Flavors, and Additives in Foods and Beverages

Although controversial, since the 1970s, some clinicians and researchers have expressed concerns about the impact of artificial colorings and additives in foods and beverages for children. Symptoms for those with this sensitivity can include ADHD-like symptoms, sleep difficulties, and irritability (Stevens, 2016), as well as behavioral and aggressive problems. Barkley reported food additives and preservatives can cause a slight increase in inattentiveness and activity in only five percent or fewer children, and most are preschool age (Barkley, 2013). However, significant research has suggested that artificial additives and food coloring may interact with certain genetic factors to elicit ADHD symptoms in some individuals (Kleinman et al., 2011).

In one of the largest controlled trials, Bateman et al. (2004) conducted a population-based study that found artificial food coloring and sodium benzoate (a common food preservative) significantly caused hyperactivity in three-year-old children. Another large community-based study explored the effects of artificial food coloring and sodium benzoate on groups of three and eight or nine-year-old children. This study provided strong support that these food additives cause ADHD symptoms in the general population, as well as worsen symptoms in children with ADHD (McCann et al., 2007). This research seemed to influence the United Kingdom in 2009 and the European Union in 2010 to change their food regulations and restrict artificial food colorings (Kleinman et al., 2011). The European Parliament of the European Union passed legislation in 2010 that requires a warning notice on all foods that contain certain food dyes that state they "may have an adverse effect on activity and attention in children" (Kobylewski & Jacobson, 2010).

Evaluation and Treatment

The American Academy of Pediatrics has shared that eliminating food colorings and preservatives from the diets of children with ADHD is reasonable. To reduce exposure risks, families should avoid artificial coloring in foods and drinks, particularly red and yellow dyes (which are the majority of dyes), food additives such as aspartame and monosodium glutamate (MSG), and the preservatives sodium benzoate, sodium nitrate ("ADHD Diets," 2015), sodium nitrite, butylated hydroxyanisole (BHA), butylated hydroxytoluene (BHT), and calcium propionate (Stevens, 2016). Perhaps a smaller number of children with ADHD-like and behavioral difficulties may benefit from natural diets free from food additives, preservatives, and coloring. While these diets can be healthy, they may be difficult to maintain. However, until an elimination of all artificial additives is attempted, it will be unclear if a child has these sensitivities or not.

Skin tests for allergies and intolerances to food additives, dyes, and coloring have been unreliable, so elimination diets are necessary to identify specific negative responses (Millichap & Yee, 2012). Please refer to Chapter 4 for information on implementing elimination diets. Additionally, when using these, it is important to avoid all items with dyes, including foods, personal care products (toothpastes and shampoos), over-the-counter-drugs, and poster paints. Often one week of avoidance and then reintroduction of the suspected additive should indicate if sensitivity exists (Stevens, 2016). Finally, if food additives sensitivities exist, the removal of the offending foods, beverages, and products will be the only way to prevent recurrent negative reactions.

REFERENCES

Adamson, B., Letourneau, N., & Lebel, C. (2018, December 1). Prenatal maternal anxiety and children's brain structure and function: A systematic review of neuroimaging studies. *Journal of Affective Disorders, 241,* 117–126. https://doi.org /10.1016/j.jad.2018.08.029

ADHD diets. (2015). Retrieved from http://www.webmd.com/add-adhd/guide /adhd-diets

Amen, D. (2013). *Healing ADD* (revised edition). New York: Berkley Books.

Barkley, R. (2013). *Taking charge of ADHD* (3rd ed.). New York: Guilford Press.

Bateman, B., Warner, J. O., Hutchinson, E., Dean, T., Rowlandson, P., Gant, C., Grundy, J., Fitzgerald, C., & Stevenson, J. (2004). The effect of a double blind, placebo controlled, artificial food colourings and benzoate preservative challenge on hyperactivity in a general population sample of preschool children. *Archives of Disease in Childhood 89,* 506–511.

Braun, J. M., Kahn, R. S., Froehlich, T., Auinger, P., & Lanphear, B. P. (2006, December). Exposures to environmental toxicants and attention deficit hyperactivity disorder in U.S. children. *Environmental Health Perspectives, 114*(12), 1904–1909.

Brush, M. (2017, March 24). *Here's how to tell if you have lead pipes in your home.* Retrieved from https://www.alleghenyfront.org/heres-how-to-tell-if-you-have -lead-pipes-in-your-home/

Chu, S., Tsai, M., Hwang, F., Hsu, J., Huang, H. R., & Huang, Y. (2012). The relationship between attention deficit hyperactivity disorder and premature infants in Taiwanese: A case control study. *BioMed Central (BMC) Psychiatry, 12*(1), 1. Retrieved from https://www.ncbi.nlm.nih.gov/pmc/articles/PMC3411486/

Curatolo, P., D'Agati, E., & Moavero, R. (2010). The neurobiological basis of ADHD. *Italian Journal of Pediatrics, 36*(1), 79. doi: 10.1186/1824-7288-36-79

Dahmen, B., Putz, V., Herpertz-Dahlmann, B., & Konrad, K. (2012, September). Early pathogenic care and the development of ADHD-like symptoms. *Journal of Neural Transmission, 119*(9), 1023–1036. https://doi.org/10.1007/s00702-012 -0809-8

Dendy, C. Z. (2006). *Teenagers with ADD and ADHD: A guide for parents and professionals* (2nd ed.). Bethesda, MD: Woodbine House.

Getahun, D., Rhoads, G. G., Demissie, K., Lu, S., Quinn, V.P., Fassett, M. J., Wing, D. A., & Jacobsen, S. J. (2013, January). In utero exposure to ischemic-hypoxic conditions and attention-deficit/hyperactivity disorder. *Pediatrics, 131*(1), e53–e61. Retrieved from http://pediatrics.aappublications.org/content/pediatrics /early/2012/12/05/peds.2012-1298.full.pdf

Hallowell, E. D., & Ratey, J. J. (2005). *Delivered from distraction.* New York: Ballantine Books.

Herbert, A., & Esparham, A. (2017, April 25). Mind-body therapy for children with attention-deficit/hyperactivity disorder. *Children, 4*(5), 31. Retrieved from https://www.ncbi.nlm.nih.gov/pubmed/28441363

Jacobson, J. L. (2011, October 31). *Differential diagnosis of ARND: Other toxic exposures.* Presented at Recognizing Alcohol-Related Neurodevelopment Disorder (ARND) in Primary Health Care of Children Conference, Rockville, MD. Retrieved from http://www.niaaa.nih.gov/sites/default/files/ICFASD_ARND Program_D _508.pdf

Johnson, S., & Marlow, N. (2011). Preterm birth and childhood psychiatric disorders. *Pediatric Research, 69,* 11R–18R. Retrieved from http://www.nature.com/pr /jounral/v69/n5-2/full/pr9201188a.html

Kleinman, R. E., Brown, R.T., Cutter, G. R., DuPaul, G. J., & Clydesdale, F. M. (2011, June). A research model for investigating the effects of artificial food colorings on children with ADHD. *Pediatrics, 127*(6). doi: 10.1542/peds.2009-2206

Kobylewski, S., & Jacobson, M.F. (2010, June). Center for Science in the Public Interest. *Food dyes—A rainbow of risks.* Retrieved from https://cspinet.org/new /pdf/food-dyes-rainbow-of-risks.pdf

Koger, S. M., Schettler, T., & Weiss, B. (2005, April). Environmental toxicants and developmental disabilities. *American Psychologist, 60*(3), 234–255.

Laake, D. G., & Compart, P. J. (2013). *The ADHD and autism nutritional supplement handbook.* Beverly, MA: Fair Winds Press.

Lu, S. (2015, October). Chemical threats. *Monitor on Psychology, 46*(9), 63–68.

Lindstrom, K., Lindblad, F., & Hjern, A. (2011, May). Preterm birth and attention-deficit/hyperactivity disorder in schoolchildren. *Pediatrics, 127*(5), 858–865.

Mahone, E. M., & Schneider, H. E. (2012, December). Assessment of attention in preschoolers. *Neuropsychology Review, 22*(4): 361–383.

Marroun, H. E., Zeegers, M., Steegers, E.A., van der Ende, J., Schenk, J. J., Hofman, A.,...& Tiemeier, H. (2012, June 1). Post-term birth and the risk of behavioural and emotional problems in early childhood. *International Journal of Epidemiology, 41*(3), 773–781. http://doi.org/10.1093/ije/dys043

McGuire, L. S., Bregy, A., Sick, J., Dietrich, W. D., Bramlett, H. M., & Sick, T. (2015). Nonconvulsive seizures as secondary insults in experimental traumatic brain injury. In F. H. Kobeissy (Ed.), *Brain neurotrauma: Molecular, neuropsychological, and rehabilitation aspects* (chapter 12). Boca Raton, FL: CRC Press/Taylor & Francis.

McCann, D., Barrett, A., Cooper, A., Crumpler, D., Dalen, L., Grimshaw, K., & Stevenson, J. (2007). Food additives and hyperactive behaviour in 3-year old and 8/9-year old children in the community: A randomized, double-blinded, placebo-controlled trial. *Lancet, 370*(9598), 1560–1567. doi: 10.1016/S0140-6736 (07)61306-3

Millichap, J., & Yee, M. (2012, February). The diet factor in attention-deficit/hyper activity disorder. *Pediatrics, 129*(2), 330–337. doi:10.1542/peds.2011-2199

Minnes, S., Lang, A., & Singer, L. (2011, July). Prenatal tobacco, marijuana, stimulant, and opiate exposure: Outcomes and practice implications. *Addiction Science & Clinical Practice, 6*(1), 57–70.

Narad, M. E., Kennelly, B. S., Zhang, N., Wade, S. L., Yeates, K. O., Taylor, H. G... & Kuroski, B. (2018, May). Secondary attention-deficit/hyperactivity disorder in children and adolescents 5 to 10 years after traumatic brain injury. *JAMA Pediatrics, 172*(5), 437–443. doi: 10.1001/jamapediatrics.2017.5746

Ronald, A., Pennell, C. E., & Whitehouse, A. J. O. (2011, January 19). Prenatal maternal stress associated with ADHD and autistic traits in early childhood. *Frontiers in Psychology, 1,* 223. doi: 10.3389/fpsyg.2010.00223

Singh, A., Yeh, C. J., Verma, N., & Das, A. K. (2015, September 30). Overview of attention deficit hyperactivity disorder in young children. *Health Psychology Research, 3*(2), 2115. doi: 10.4081/hpr.2015.2115

Stevens, L. J. (2016). *Solving the puzzle of your ADD/ADHD child.* Springfield, IL: Charles C Thomas.

Sucksdorff, M., Lehtonen, L., Chudal, R., Suominen, A., Joelsson, P., Gissler, M., & Sourander, A. (2015, September). Preterm birth and fetal growth as risk factors of attention-deficit/hyperactivity disorder. *Pediatrics, Volume 136*(3), e599–e608.

Tarver, J., Daley, D., & Sayal, K. (2014, November). Attention-deficit hyperactivity disorder (ADHD): An updated review of the essential facts. *Child: Care, Health, and Development, 40*(6), 762–774.

Walsh, W. (2014). *Nutrient power.* New York: Skyhorse.

Walsh, W. (2015, November 15). *Advanced nutrient therapies for mental disorders.* Retrieved from www.walshinstitute.org/uploads/1/7/9/9/17997321/cam_london_keynote_dr_walsh_11_07_15_final.pdf

Walsh Research Institute. (2005-2016b). *Biochemical individuality and nutrition.* Retrieved from www.walshinstitute.org/biochemical-individuality-nutrition.html

Wei, C. C., Chang, C. H., Lin, C. L., Chang, S. N., Li, T. C., & Kao, C. H. (2015, April). Neonatal jaundice and increased risk of attention-deficit hyperactivity disorder: A population-based cohort study. *Journal of Child Psychology and Psychiatry, 56*(4), 460–467.

Chapter 4

MEDICAL CONDITIONS

While less common, the following medical conditions can cause ADHD-like symptoms or worsen true ADHD and should be considered during the ADHD evaluation process. If medical conditions have been diagnosed, clinicians should explore if parents are actively working with their physicians to manage these, and how consistent and effective treatments are. Clinicians and parents should discuss to what degree they believe the ADHD-like problems are currently caused by the medical conditions. Neuro-developmental testing may be able to help with this diagnostic discrimination process as well.

Vision Difficulties

Research has found that 5 percent of preschool children and 25 percent of school-age children have vision problems (Garber, Garber, & Spizman, 1996). Classroom learning depends 75 to 90 percent upon visual abilities (Kranowitz, 2005). Untreated vision problems can mimic ADHD symptoms and cause behavioral and learning difficulties. Children and teens with undetected vision problems may not know that their vision is abnormal, and thus may not complain.

Evaluation and Treatment

Children and adolescents suspected of having ADHD should receive comprehensive vision evaluations from a pediatric optometrist or ophthalmologist, and particularly for those who have academic, reading, or math difficulties. Clinicians may notice that when recommending a vision examination, some parents will say that their child passed a school vision test. However, these brief vision screenings can be inadequate and inaccurate in detecting a spectrum of conditions, such as milder to moderate and more complex vision problems, and farsightedness. Some children with blurry vision can still pass these quick screenings.

Optometrists differ from ophthalmologists. Ophthalmologists are medical doctors who specialize in eye conditions, diseases, and surgery, but do not provide visual processing testing or treatments. Optometrists are doctors of optometry who specialize in eye exams and care, do not provide surgeries, and typically address less complex conditions. Both provide eye exams, and diagnose and treat eye diseases. However, some pediatric optometrists, sometimes called developmental or behavioral optometrists, can test for vision problems as well as visual processing disorders. Consequently, they may be a good first option for comprehensive vision exams that include exploring visual processing deficits. It is important to distinguish between true vision problems and visual processing disorders because those with these processing deficits can pass standard vision exams. Visual processing disorders are addressed in Chapter 7. Finally, blurry vision can result from astigmatism, nearsightedness, and farsightedness, and these can be corrected with eyeglasses and/or surgery.

Hearing Difficulties

Estimates of hearing impairments in United States school-age children vary from 5 to 11 percent. Those with undetected hearing problems may not know that their hearing is abnormal or complain. Like eye exams in schools, typical hearing screenings in schools are not as accurate at identifying a range of hearing deficits. Conductive hearing loss is the most common type and is believed to be correctable. This can include ruptured ear drums, swimmer's ear, middle ear infections, and other sound-blocking difficulties. A large portion of undetected hearing loss in children is minimal sensorineural hearing loss, which occurs in 5 percent of children. Mild, minimal and unilateral hearing losses are not necessarily loudness problems, but clarity and distortion difficulties. A teachers' voice may be loud enough, but not clear. Children with these challenges will respond when called, but can confuse distinctive sounds needed for reading and language. Many classrooms are noisy and background noise often further garbles signals (Ulrich, 2004).

Failure to detect childhood acquired or congenital hearing loss can cause lasting deficits in language and speech development, academics, social and psychological functioning. Often congenital hearing loss is identifiable with infant screenings. The American Academy of Pediatrics recommends repeated hearing screenings at ages newborn, 4, 5, 6, 8, 10, 12, 15, and 18. Childhood risk factors for permanent congenital, delayed-onset, acquired, and/or progressive hearing loss include hearing concerns from parents, family history, five or more days of neonatal intensive care, in-utero infections, certain syndromes (including Waardenburg), neurodegenerative disorders, certain infectious diseases (especially meningitis), head trauma, damaging sound level exposures, nervous system trauma, toxic drugs, ear abnormalities, speech and language deficits, and global developmental delays (Harlor & Bower, 2009). Additionally, children may experience fluctuations in hearing due to congestion from allergies, colds, sinus, or ear infections.

Hearing problems can cause inattention, distractibility, forgetfulness, social problems, aggression, behavioral problems, higher energy levels, irritability, and stress-related difficulties interacting with others and communicating easily. These challenges can easily mimic ADHD. Ulrich (2004) shared that hearing deficits and ADHD can cause academic difficulties, inappropriate responses to questions, problems completing school assignments, trouble sustaining attention during lectures and oral instructions, impulsiveness, acting out, and lower self-esteem. Thirty-seven percent of children with hearing loss have failed at least one grade. Children with hearing loss can have a variety of learning problems, including reading, comprehension, vocabulary, word usage, and storytelling difficulties.

Evaluation and Treatment

As a standard practice as part of ADHD evaluations, children and teens should receive hearing examinations outside of the school. Schools and primary care physicians can perform limited hearing screenings, but these may be inadequate. Ears-Nose-Throat (ENT) or otolaryngologists are medical doctors who specialize in ear conditions and surgeries, but typically do not provide comprehensive hearing or auditory processing disorder evaluations. Audiologists specialize in the diagnosis and treatment of hearing loss, provide comprehensive hearing testing, and some can provide auditory processing deficits testing, which can easily resemble ADHD. It is particularly important to request audiology testing if the child is having suspected hearing problems, school performance concerns, atypical speech, or a delay in language development. Finally, those with hearing loss should also consider receiving speech and language evaluations.

Nasal Allergies and Related Medication Use

Nasal allergies (also called allergic rhinitis or hay fever) can be seasonal, environmental, or inhalant, and can result from pollens, animal dander, molds, or dust. Allergies are some of the most common chronic diseases, and are exaggerated immune reactions to substances that do not harm most people. Sleep difficulties can be common for children and teens with this due to coughing and congestion symptoms. Those with chronic nasal congestion may have poorer academic or sports performance, and lower energy levels. The severity and frequency of the symptoms usually determines the degree of impairment (Moon, 2013). Children with ADHD have higher rates of nasal allergies. Chronic and persistent nasal allergies can cause mouth breathing, which can lead to serious problems with abnormal facial growth and other difficulties (Fischman, Kuffler, & Bloch, 2015). Children and teens with allergies may have respiratory distress that contributes to poor quality of sleep and daytime fatigue, which can cause ADHD-like symptoms or worsen ADHD.

Evaluation and Treatment

If a child has allergies, determine how much this may cause ADHD-like symptoms, and if they improve after taking allergy medications. Oral antihistamines are often used for treatment; however, these can cause drowsiness, so nondrowsy medications should be considered during the day (Moon, 2013). If a child has allergies for only portions of the year, explore if the ADHD-like symptoms only exist or increase during allergy seasons. Primary care, ENT, or allergist physicians can further explore if allergies or allergy medications are causing ADHD-like symptoms. Mouth breathing may be associated with allergies and should treated if present.

Chronic Sinus Problems

While less common, these can cause breathing problems which may create irritability and ADHD-like presentations. Congestion can result from chronic colds, recurrent sinus infections, allergies, and other breathing problems related to sinus issues. Chronic sinus problems can also negatively impact hearing and the quality and amount of sleep, which can further worsen ADHD-like difficulties. Chronic sinus problems and congestion can contribute to enlarged adenoids, which may then cause sleep-disordered breathing and ADHD-like difficulties. Sinus problems, with or without allergies, can cause mouth breathing difficulties (see Chapter 5 for these topics). Jefferson (2010) reported that high and narrow mouth palatal vaults (the roof of the mouth) can cause compressed and narrow sinuses, which can create mouth breathing.

Evaluation and Treatment

ENT physicians and/or allergists/immunologists evaluate and treat these conditions. To clarify how sinus issues impact ADHD-like problems, determine when the sinus problems started, their severity and frequency now, and their occurrence with ADHD-like symptoms. This can also be further discussed with treating physicians. Orthodontists or oral surgeons can provide treatments if mouth palate or anatomic difficulties exist.

Asthma and Related Medication Use

Asthma is a growing chronic disease that impacts approximately five million children in the United States. It is an inflammation of the airway lining which causes muscle spasms surrounding the airways, making breathing more difficult. It can cause wheezing, coughing, and breathing difficulties. Asthma can cause coughs to worsen at night, after exercise, or exposure to allergens. It can cause frequent awakenings and poor-quality sleep (Moon, 2013).

Just prior to an asthma episode a child may have unusual tiredness, restlessness, irritability, or difficulty sitting still, all of which mimic ADHD. After taking short-acting or long-acting inhaled bronchodilator asthma medications, they may appear hyperactive and inattentive due to shakiness, dizziness, increased heart rates, trouble sleeping, or nervousness. Also, children with asthma may have poor sleep and daytime fatigue, which can contribute to ADHD-like symptoms. Asthma may result from allergies, and asthma symptoms may increase during higher allergy levels. One study found that children with asthma and ADHD were more likely to exhibit higher levels of anxiety, externalizing, and hyperactive/impulsive behaviors when compared to children with ADHD but no asthma (Borschuk, Rodweller, & Salorio, 2017).

Evaluation and Treatment

To distinguish between asthma, this medication, and true ADHD, monitor if the ADHD-like symptoms occur only just before asthma attacks or just after taking a short-acting inhaled asthma medication. The bronchodilator Theophylline may cause hyperactivity as a side-effect. Discerning the effects of long-acting bronchodilators may be more challenging. The child's physician can further explore these issues. Although primary care physicians can evaluate and treat asthma, a pulmonologist or allergist/immunologist referral may be necessary.

Enlarged Tonsils and Adenoids

Tonsils are a pair of lymph node tissues at the back of the throat that help fight infections. Adenoids are lymph glands behind the nose that prevent infections. When these are enlarged, ADHD-like symptoms can result due to air obstructions and breathing restrictions, causing sub-optimum oxygen delivery to the brain and body. Their surgical removal is common and may occur when they are often infected or enlarged. This surgery can produce significant improvements in nasal breathing, attention, behavior, academics, activity level, sleep, development, growth, and sleep-disordered breathing. ENT physicians treat these conditions. However, pediatricians and dentists can check for swollen tonsils too (Jefferson, 2010). Please refer to the sleep chapter for more information.

Diabetes

This is a disease involving problems with the body's ability to process blood sugar, or glucose. Type One diabetes that occurs before age five has been associated with increased risk of ADHD (Getahun et al., 2013). Borderline, mild, undetected, or untreated diabetes can cause inattention, lethargy, and lower levels of arousal. Blood sugar levels that are too high or low and/or fluctuate can negatively affect attentional abilities, as well as cause moodiness and irritability. For children with diabetes and allergies, allergy flare ups can increase blood sugar levels as well.

Evaluation and Treatment

Many parents will not know if their child was ever tested for diabetes. The child's physician may address this, or they can be referred to an endocrinologist. If the child or teen has been diagnosed with diabetes, explore if they are consistently taking their medicine and if their blood sugars are stable. If they are not consistent with daily treatment and/or blood sugars severely fluctuate, their physician should check if this may be causing ADHD-like symptoms. Long-term active monitoring and managing blood sugar levels will be a key part of stabilizing diabetes to address ADHD-like symptoms.

Hypoglycemia

Hypoglycemia and blood sugar (glucose) fluctuations are typically caused by other medical conditions, including diabetes and diabetes medication. Low blood sugar causes adrenalin to be released which may then produce agitation, aggression, acting out, anger, hostility, hyperactivity, lethargy, persistent tiredness, and inattention (Garber, Garber, & Spizman, 1996). The Walsh Research Institute has found that chronic low blood glucose levels don't generally cause behavior or attention disorders, but may be an aggravating factor (Walsh Research Institute, 2005-2016b). Many parents may not know if their child was ever tested for this, but pediatricians can easily evaluate and treat this condition.

Anemia and Iron Deficiency

Anemia is a condition of low red blood cells. While there are hundreds of types of anemia and several causes, the most common cause is iron deficiency. Iron deficiency anemia may be mild at first, but as the condition progresses, the symptoms worsen. It is more common in teenage girls. Some vegetarians and individuals who do not eat a healthy diet are also at risk, as well as those with blood dyscrasias (such as thalassemia, a genetic blood condition). Many parents do not know if their child was ever tested for anemia. Primary care physicians can order serum ferritin and complete blood count tests to evaluate this condition, and can often treat it with iron supplementation. However, this treatment should be supervised by a physician since excessive iron can be lethal. Children who had anemia in the past should receive testing to check their current iron levels.

Thyroid Disorders

Abnormal thyroid hormone levels can cause forgetfulness, inattention, confusion, lethargy, depression, and anxiety. Overactive thyroid levels (hyperthyroidism) can cause hyperactivity and inattentive symptoms. Underactive thyroid levels (hypothyroidism) can decrease brain activity and impair judgement, thinking, and self-control (Amen, 2013).

Evaluation and Treatment

Many parents will not know if their child was ever tested for this. The primary care physician can evaluate this with a thyroid panel blood test. Amen (2013) stated testing should evaluate thyroid stimulating hormones, free T3, free T4, and thyroid antibodies since many physicians will not routinely test for them.

Seizure Conditions

Seizures, particularly absence seizures (previously called petit mal seizures) and childhood absence epilepsy, can cause Inattentive ADHD-like presentations. Seizures are neurological events where an intense abnormal wave of electricity overwhelms the brain. Epilepsy is diagnosed when people have seizures more than once that do not have a specific cause, such as a result of illness, head trauma, or lack of oxygen. There are various types of seizures. Grand mal seizures are obvious because a person will shake intensely, fall to the ground, and sleep for hours. Absence seizures are less obvious, and are often misperceived as daydreaming or staring episodes. Seizures are not painful, but can be scary for children and others around them. Simple partial seizures can cause children to have a sudden overwhelming sense of terror. These children have no control over their actions and may do strange or inappropriate things that disturb others ("Seizures in Children," reviewed 2015). Partial seizures and epilepsy often have an aura or warning sensation and are longer than absence seizures (Sivaswamy, 2012). Complex partial seizures rarely occur more than several times per day or week, can last up to several minutes, and confusion often results. About one child in 4,300 to 8,300 under age 15 has absence epilepsy, with most children developing absence seizures between ages six and eight. The rates are higher in girls than boys, and it is unusual for these seizures to start after age 14. There are other seizures as well, such as temporal lobe seizures (Donner, 2010).

Absence seizures are one of the most common early childhood seizures. A typical experience is a child has daily blanking out episodes, does not respond to a teacher calling his or her name, blinks several times, and then returns to a normal state after 15 seconds. After weeks of this, the teacher may contact the parents, and the child is taken to see a pediatrician. Often, the parents state they have never witnessed these episodes (Sivaswamy, 2012). Absence seizures usually have no lasting effect on intelligence or other aspect of brain functioning. Other presentations for absence seizures include a sudden beginning, the child stops what they are doing, stares blankly, eyes roll upward, and has no reaction to others unless spoken to or touched. The seizure can last for ten seconds, and then the child can become alert or may have two to three seconds of confusion. Frequently the child will not even know a seizure occurred (Donner, 2010). Family history in first-degree relatives is another significant risk factor for epilepsy. Absence seizures can be distinguished from complex partial seizures because absence seizures are more frequent, briefer, and have fewer or no automatisms (unconscious behaviors like wandering, chewing, smacking of lips, or finger rubbing) (Olson, 2006).

Absence seizures can be typical or atypical. The staring spell is the typical presentation accompanied by brief unresponsiveness a number of times a day. Typical absence seizures can be induced in a physician's office by asking the child to breath quickly in and out. Children with absence seizures can also have generalized seizures (grand mal or tonic-clonic). Absence seizures may also include aspects of other types of seizures, such as twitching of the eyelids, mouth corners, or arms; the body or head may slump forward or objects in hands are dropped; movements of licking, swallowing, raising eyelids, or hand scratching. Atypical absence seizures are more difficult to define, with the staring phase being less clear. These often last between five to ten seconds, and can include twitching and confusion afterwards (Donner, 2010).

Seizure conditions can also result from more severe traumatic brain injuries (TBI), such as those with a penetrating head injury or extended unconsciousness (Olson, 2006). Posttraumatic epilepsy is defined as seizures that can recur up to a few years after the TBI, and often are not convulsive seizures. About 90 percent of people with TBIs experience seizures by the first or second year after the injury. Nonconvulsive seizures consist of absence seizures, nonmotor complex partial seizures, or simple partial seizures. Convulsive seizures are easier to detect and diagnose, while nonconvulsive seizures are more difficult, need continuous EEG monitoring, and frequently are not diagnosed or treated (McGuire et al., 2015).

Absence seizures with recurrent episodes that appear as staring, daydreaming, and inattention can resemble ADHD. Children can have frequent daily spells that may last up to 30 seconds, and these may impact their learning. Because these episodes are not intense and obvious, they commonly are not recognized for long periods or even years. By adolescence, many experience remission (Sivaswamy, 2012).

Children with epilepsy have higher rates of ADHD, with rates ranging between 12 to 57 percent (Falcone & Timmons-Mitchell, 2013). Yet the diagnosis of ADHD in children and teens with epilepsy can be controversial and complex. Various antiseizure medications can cause side effects that mimic ADHD symptoms. Also, some ADHD medications can increase the chance of seizures for those with epilepsy. Epilepsy can also coexist with other conditions, such as learning disorders, autism, developmental conditions, and intellectual disorders (Epilepsy Foundation of Western/Central Pennsylvania, n.d.).

It is unclear how seizures affect ADHD. Inattention may result from epilepsy medication, while the condition itself may produce certain ADHD-like difficulties. A number of studies have shared that ADHD symptoms sometimes begin before the first seizures, and even if the seizures are controlled, the ADHD may persist (Falcone & Timmons-Mitchell, 2013). For children with epilepsy and ADHD, attention difficulties are more common than impulsivity and hyperactivity. More research needs to be conducted to explore the long-term safety of stimulants for this population. One group of authors suggested that stimulant medication should be attempted if ADHD-like symptoms occur six or more months after the last epileptic seizure. Finally, EEG screening is not recommended to explore seizure conditions as part of ADHD evaluations, unless there are special indicators (Kattimani & Mahadevan, 2011).

Evaluation and Treatment

Neurologists are medical doctors who specializes in nervous system conditions including seizure conditions, but other physicians can address these disorders as well. An electroencephalogram (EEG) that records brain waves is essential in diagnosing absence seizures. Unfortunately, EEGs can be uncomfortable and time intensive. For children and teens with epilepsy, CT and MRI brain scans are seldom needed if the EEG and other features are typical. Family history of epilepsy is important to explore. Any moderate to severe head injury should be considered for seizure conditions as well.

Typical absence seizures are often well managed with antiepileptic drugs, but atypical seizures are not as easily treated. Childhood absence epilepsy seizures often cease from two to five years after they start, and medication may end or be phased out after the child has been seizure-free for two to three years (Donner, 2010).

When seizure conditions and ADHD coexist, it can be challenging to diagnose both conditions. If possible, clinicians can explore when the ADHD symptoms started and when the first seizure was detected. This may be difficult because absence seizures can persist for a long time before they are noticed. For those diagnosed with seizures who are on antiseizure medications and may also have ADHD, clinicians should explore if the seizure medications are causing the ADHD-like symptoms. Additionally, clinicians can also explore if the seizures are still occurring and are not being adequately managed by medication. A family may falsely believe that the seizures have stopped because antiseizure medication is used, yet they may still occur, especially the absence seizures. Additional EEGs, neuropsychological, and other testing may be necessary. Finally, QEEGs tests given by neurofeedback providers can screen for seizures and true ADHD.

Food Sensitivities and Allergies

In the United States, food allergies impact approximately 8 percent of children. The reactions tend to occur between minutes to several hours after exposure, and may include vomiting, swelling, coughing, hives, diarrhea, throat tightness, or loss of consciousness. Additional allergic reactions include ADHD-like symptoms, irritability, emotional responses, sleeping, and other difficulties. Zimmerman (1999) stated that allergic responses can trigger histamine to be released in the brain, which may then cause inattention and memory dysfunction. The most common children's food allergies are cow's milk and cheese, eggs, soybean, peanuts, tree nuts (pecans, walnuts), chocolate, shellfish, wheat (Moon, 2013), corn, and corn syrup. Specific food intolerances or sensitivities produce less severe reactions, and may affect brain functioning but not the more common immune responses (Millichap & Yee, 2012).

Curiously, some may crave the foods to which they are sensitive. Unfortunately, food allergies can be difficult to diagnose, and allergy blood and skin-testing can be unreliable and produce false positives. Food allergies and sensitivities may fluctuate daily as well. Refer to sensitivities to artificial food additives and colorings in Chapter 3 for more information on this topic.

Evaluation and Treatment

The National Academy of Child Development recommends that parents consider eliminating suspected food items from the diet to determine if food sensitivities and allergies exist. Elimination diets can be the best way to identify these, but can be difficult to use. These diets remove the suspected foods for two to four weeks and then slowly re-introduce each item every few days. During this time, it is helpful to eat a diet that is organic, lacks fruit or sugar-based drinks, and avoid processed foods with dyes or additives. As foods are reintroduced, children are carefully monitored for ADHD-like symptoms, mood or behavioral problems, runny nose, itchy eyes, red ears or cheeks, or other symptoms. There may be an immediate or delayed reaction. Another approach is to gradually remove items one at a time and notice if the ADHD-like symptoms reduce or cease. Careful journaling and observations are important in this process, and a positive family history of food allergies and sensitivities may be helpful. Many milk, egg, soy, and wheat allergies are eventually outgrown. There are no cures for food allergies and sensitivities, just avoidance of the offending foods. Physicians or other health care providers who specialize in this area may also be helpful.

Persistent/Recurrent Ear Infections

Middle ear infections (otitis media) are common and are the leading cause of pediatrician visits. They occur when bacteria or a virus infects the middle ear, and can linger and reoccur. While most heal on their own, repeated infections can lead to permanent hearing loss if left untreated. About 25 percent of children will experience recurrent ear infections. Bellis (2002) reported that some children with these infections experience speech and language delays or auditory processing deficits. Persistent and recurrent ear infections with fluid that occur for at least three months increase the risks for hearing loss. Symptoms include ear pain, hearing problems, fever, scratching or pulling ears, balance problems, seeping fluid from ear, comments that the ears feel funny or weird, as well as inattention and irritability. Infections can also cause intermittent or permanent hearing problems and/or language processing deficits that may appear as inattentiveness. Additionally, recurrent ear infections have been associated with learning problems, vestibular sensory processing deficits, and enlarged adenoids. As stated previously, adenoids can be related to mouth breathing and sleep apnea, both of which can cause ADHD-like symptoms. Finally, while certain older studies found a positive correlation between recurrent otitis media infections in early childhood with the presence and severity of hyperactivity (Hersher, 1978), other studies have found no association. At this time the connection seems unclear between middle ear infections and ADHD.

Evaluation

The greater number of and more severe ear infections the child has had, the greater the risk of hearing deficits, auditory processing difficulties, vestibular sensory processing deficits, language deficits, and/or enlarged adenoids. Those with histories of numerous chronic middle ear infections can be referred for hearing and auditory processing testing by an audiologist and an evaluation by an ENT physician.

Conditions Causing Chronic Bodily Pain or Discomfort

Children, and particularly younger ones, may experience hyperactivity, irritability, or other behavioral symptoms that result from chronic pain or discomfort from medical problems or sensory processing conditions. When children experience these, a chronic response can be excessive movements. Food digestion problems and sensitivities can cause inflammation and pain, which may also promote hyperactivity. Clinicians can explore if known medical or sensory processing conditions may be causing these symptoms, and if pain or discomfort occurs only when ADHD-like symptoms exist.

Primary care physicians should address these issues, and occupational therapists should evaluate sensory processing conditions.

Hunger, Food Insecurity, and Malnutrition

These can occur when a person does not receive enough food to meet their physiological needs. Children or teens who live in poverty, are homeless, neglected, or have other situations may not receive adequate quality and quantities of food. Chronic malnutrition or undernutrition in young and developing children can cause learning, academic, inattention, and ADHD-like difficulties. Children in poverty may experience hunger or lack consistent, healthy food during weekends or during nonschool periods because some may not receive the free meals they receive at school. Also, those with eating disorders may experience concentration difficulties. Clinicians working with children with economic challenges or homelessness backgrounds should consider this item when evaluating ADHD.

Other Prescription or Over-the-Counter Medication Use

While it is less common for medications to cause ADHD-like difficulties, some can produce unwanted side effects, particularly if they are taken over a long period. To determine which came first, ask when the ADHD-like symptoms started and when the medication began. Be aware that the underlying medical condition may be contributing to the ADHD-like symptoms as well. If the child or teen misses medication doses or does not take it consistently, parents can observe if the ADHD-like symptoms occur when not on the medication. Finally, the prescribing physician or pharmacist may be able to share if ADHD-like symptoms are possible side effects of the medication.

Other Medical Conditions

In theory, more stable and managed medical conditions should cause fewer difficulties, but some conditions may still create ADHD-like symptoms. Parents should be asked if they believe any identified medical conditions may cause or contribute to ADHD-like difficulties.

OTHER MEDICAL CONDITIONS ASSOCIATED WITH HIGHER RISKS OF ADHD OR ADHD-LIKE PRESENTATIONS

Phenylketonuria (PKU) is an inherited rare metabolic disease that causes a specific amino acid to accumulate in the body to potentially toxic levels. It can cause difficulty digesting foods, neurological damage, intellectual deficits, and ADHD-like symptoms. All infants at birth are routinely screened for PKU in the United States.

Children Who Suffered Stroke and particularly strokes affecting subcortical areas in the prefrontal-subcortical circuits can have higher rates of ADHD.

Meningitis, Encephalitis, or Other Brain Diseases, Infections, and Tumors

Meningitis is the inflammation of the meninges, the protective membranes covering the brain and spinal cord, caused by infections from bacteria, viruses, or other microorganisms. Encephalitis is the inflammation of the brain often caused by viruses, bacteria, or parasites. These and certain other brain diseases, infections, and tumors are associated with higher risks of ADHD, particularly when the basal ganglia is affected.

Lyme Disease

This has been associated with a number of neuropsychological symptoms, including ADHD. Lyme disease is believed to be one of the fastest growing infectious diseases in the United States, with more than 330,000 new cases occurring each year, across all states. It is caused by the bite of an infected, black legged deer tick that carries the Borrelia burgdorferi bacterium. A bull's eye rash may be an important clue to the tick bite. The antibodies can be hard to identify with traditional blood tests, so the disease can easily remain undetected and progress to mid or late-stage. Later stage presentations can produce serious neurological conditions, including seizures, autism, ADHD-like presentations, cognitive impairments (slow information processing, memory deficits, and word-finding difficulties), irritability, anxiety, depression, rage episodes, and rapid mood swings (Dalgliesh, 2013). Fortunately, many cases can be successfully treated with antibiotics if detected early.

Celiac Disease

This multisystemic autoimmune disorder has been associated with a number of central nervous system and ADHD symptoms. Celiac disease is a hereditary digestive condition that affects the small intestine lining and prevents it from properly absorbing nutrients. The condition prevents the digestion of gluten (found in wheat, rye, and barley). Those with celiac disease can have a number of medical and psychological problems, including ADHD, arthritis, Addison's disease, thyroid disease, diabetes, diarrhea, slowed growth, weight gain problems, learning disorders, depression, developmental delays, and other serious conditions. It is under-diagnosed in the general public but appears overrepresented in those with ADHD. One study of individuals with ADHD and celiac disease found that a gluten-free diet greatly improved their ADHD symptoms. The researcher suggested that it should be a part of ADHD symptom checklists (Niederhofer, 2011).

Leukemia, Head and Neck Cancer Treatments (chemotherapy and/or radiation) for these cancers can cause brain damage that creates ADHD symptoms. While those who received these may respond well to stimulants, the chance of positive responses is lower (Barkley, 2013).

Fragile X Syndrome is a genetic condition that frequently occurs with other conditions, including ADHD.

REFERENCES

Amen, D. (2013). *Healing ADD* (revised edition). New York: Berkley Books.

Barkley, R. (2013). *Taking charge of ADHD* (3rd ed.). New York: Guilford Press.

Bellis, T. J. (2002). *When the brain can't hear.* New York: Pocket Books.

Borschuk, A. P., Rodweller, C., & Salorio, C. F. (2017, May 1). The influence of comorbid asthma on the severity of symptoms in children with attention-deficit hyperactivity disorders. *Journal of Asthma, 1,* 1–7.

Dalgliesh, C. (2013). *The Sensory child gets organized.* New York: Touchstone.

Donner, E. J. (2010, February 4). *Absence seizures.* Retrieved from http://www.aboutkidshealth.ca/En/ResourceCentres/Epilepsy/UnderstandingEpilepsy Diagnosis/TypesofSeizures/Pages/Absence-Seizures.aspx

Epilepsy Foundation of Western/Central Pennsylvania. (n.d.). *Epilepsy and learning.* Retrieved on 02/13/17 from http://www.efwp.org/programs/Programs PSALearning.xml

Falcone, T., & Timmons-Mitchell, J. (2013). *Pediatric epilepsy and ADHD.* Retrieved from http://my.clevelandclinic.org/ccf/media/Files/Neurological-Institute/pediatric-epilepsy-and-adhd-fact-sheet.pdf?la=en

Fischman, S., Kuffler, D. P., & Bloch, C. (2015). Disordered sleep as a cause of attention deficit/hyperactivity disorder: Recognition and management. *Clinical Pediatrics, 54*(8), 713–722. doi: 10.1177/000992281458673

Garber, S. W., Garber, M. D., & Spizman, R.F. (1996). *Beyond ritalin.* New York: Harper Perennial.

Getahun, D., Rhoads, G. G., Demissie, K., Lu, S., Quinn, V. P., Fassett, M. J., Wing, D. A., & Jacobsen, S. J. (2013, January). In utero exposure to ischemic-hypoxic conditions and attention-deficit/hyperactivity disorder. *Pediatrics, 131*(1), e53–e61. Retrieved from http://pediatrics.aappublications.org/content /pediatrics/early/2012/12/05/peds.2012-1298.full.pdf

Harlor, A. D. B., & Bower, C. (2009, October). Clinical report—Hearing assessment in infants and children: Recommendations beyond neonatal screening. *Pediatrics, 124*(4), 1252–1263. doi: 10.1542/peds.2009-1997

Hersher, L. (1978, December). Minimal brain dysfunction and otitis media. *Perceptual and Motor Skills, 47*(3 Pt 1), 723–726. doi: 10.2466/pms.1978.47.3.723

Jefferson, Y. (2010, January/February). Mouth breathing: Adverse effects on facial growth, health, academics, and behavior. *General Dentistry, 58*(1), 18–25. Retrieved from https://www.ncbi.nlm.nih.gov/pubmed/20129889

Kattimani, S., & Mahadevan, S. (2011, January–March). Treating children with attention-deficit/hyperactivity disorder and comorbid epilepsy. *Annals of Indian Academy of Neurology, 14*(1), 9–11. doi: 10.4103/0972-2327.78042

Kranowitz, C. S. (2005). *The out-of-synch child.* New York: Penguin Group.

McGuire, L. S., Bregy, A., Sick, J., Dietrich, W. D., Bramlett, H. M., & Sick, T. (2015). Nonconvulsive seizures as secondary insults in experimental traumatic brain injury. In F. H. Kobeissy (Ed.), *Brain neurotrauma: Molecular, neuropsychological, and rehabilitation aspects* (chapter 12). Boca Raton, FL: CRC Press/Taylor & Francis.

Millichap, J., & Yee, M. (2012, February). The diet factor in attention-deficit/hyperactivity disorder. *Pediatrics, Volume 129*(2), 330–337. http:/pediatrics.aappublications.org/content/early/2012/01/04/peds.2011-2199

Moon, R.Y. (2013). *Sleep—What every parent needs to know.* Elk Grove Village, IL: American Academy of Pediatrics.

Niederhofer, H. (2011). Association of attention-deficit/hyperactivity disorder and celiac disease: A brief report. *The Primary Care Companion for CNS Disorders, 13*(3). Retrieved from https://www.ncbi.nlm.nih.gov/pmc/articles/PMC3184556/

Olson, D. (2006, November 01). *Differentiating epileptic seizures from other spells.* Retrieved from http://www.psychiatrictimes.com/articles/differentiating-epileptic-seizures-other-spells

Seizures in children. (reviewed 2015, January, 13). Reviewed by Roy Benaroch. Retrieved from www.webmd.com/epilepsy-in-children?

Sivaswamy, L. (2012, June 18). *Childhood absence epilepsy: 5 things pediatricians need to know.* Retrieved from http://www.psychiatrictimes.com/adhd/childhood-absence-epilepsy-5-things-pediatricians-need-know

Ulrich, M. (2004). *ADHD/ADD or hearing loss?* Retrieved from http://www.health articles.org/adhd_add_hearing_loss_071304.html

Walsh Research Institute. (2005-2016b). *Biochemical individuality and nutrition.* Retrieved from www.walshinstitute.org/biochemical-individuality-nutrition.html

Zimmerman, M. (1999). *The ADD Nutrition Solution.* New York: Henry Holt.

Chapter 5

SLEEP CONDITIONS

S leep difficulties are common for children and adolescents, with 25 to 67 percent experience some type of sleep problem during their lives (Cortese et al., 2006). Yet there is a lack of adequate detection of sleep disorders, and sleep problems are greatly underdiagnosed. One study found that some pediatricians did not screen for sleep problems because they assumed parents would report these and lack of time (Owens & Dalzell, 2005). Less than one in five pediatricians had any training in sleep disorders, and fewer than one in six felt confident to offer guidance about child sleep issues (Breus, 2013). Also, parents may not be aware of sleep problems because many children do not report them, and they can go undetected for years (Greene, 2014).

SLEEP DIFFICULTIES AND ADHD

The relationship between ADHD and sleep is complex and multifaceted. ADHD itself can cause sleep problems, sleep difficulties can cause ADHD-like symptoms, and ADHD and sleep conditions can coexist and exacerbate each other. The effects of disrupted, disordered or inadequate sleep can appear as behaviors and symptoms that are surprisingly like those of ADHD (Hvolby, 2015). In contrast to adults, some sleep-deprived younger children may not appear tired and instead exhibit disruptive behavior, inattention, hyperactivity, and impulsivity.

When sleep is impaired either acutely or chronically, there are brain and behavior changes. Collective evidence shows sleep plays a vital role in brain development and performance (Spruyt & Gozal, 2011). Inadequate sleep quantity and quality can limit the refreshing and deep delta wave sleep that children require. Disrupted sleep, reduced amount of sleep, or increased daytime sleepiness can cause or contribute to difficulties with attention, behavior, and mood. Researchers found that those with sleep conditions and

ADHD symptoms had improvements or an elimination of ADHD-like problems after treatment of their primary sleep disorder (Konofal, Lecendreux, & Cortese, 2010).

Sleep difficulties are common and stressful for families with ADHD. Between 25 to 50 percent of children and teens with ADHD are estimated to have sleep difficulties (Owens, 2009). The guess-estimated occurrence of sleep problems in children with ADHD is five times that of controls (Spruyt & Gozal, 2011). Parents of children with ADHD most commonly report bedtime resistance and delayed sleep onset (how long it takes to fall asleep), and also often report poor sleep quality, daytime sleepiness, and shortened sleep duration. Some may protest at bedtime due to expected trouble falling asleep. Older children and teens may lay in bed quietly for long periods, struggling to fall asleep while parents are unaware (Owens, 2009). Other sleep problems associated with ADHD include insomnia, greater nocturnal activity, restless sleep, parasomnias, nightmares, anxiety around bedtimes (Hvolby, 2015), periodic leg movement disorder, restless legs syndrome, and sleep-related breathing disorder (Silvestri et al., 2009).

Additionally, children with ADHD were found to have significantly higher night awakenings and sleep-disordered breathing. Many clinicians are unaware of sleep-disordered breathing (which includes snoring, chronic mouth breathing, and obstructive sleep apnea), and how this can cause significant ADHD-like, psychological and behavioral symptoms. Also, children and teens with ADHD can have greater variability in their sleep patterns, making evaluations and understandings of their sleep more confusing (Konofal, Lecendreux, & Cortese, 2010). Some children and teens have disturbed sleep due to stimulant use during the day, while these medications can calm others by reducing their ADHD symptoms at night and improving sleep. Research found sleep difficulties are more common in combined than inattentive ADHD types, while greater daytime sleepiness occurred more in inattentive types (Hvolby, 2015)

Researchers have reported the importance of screening for sleep problems in children and adolescents as a routine part of ADHD evaluations (Hvolby, 2015; Konofal, Lecendreux, & Cortese, 2010; Owens, 2009; Spruyt & Gozal, 2011). Unfortunately, however, many clinicians fail to do this. Exploring any medical conditions that may impair sleep, such as asthma and allergies, will be important as well. While it can be diagnostically challenging sometimes to determine whether sleep problems are causing the ADHD-like symptoms or coexist with true ADHD, this will be important to address during the evaluation process. Once identified, clinicians can treat sleep difficulties by improving sleep hygiene and should know when to refer to sleep centers and other professionals.

SLEEP-DISORDERED BREATHING (SDB): SNORING, MOUTH BREATHING, AND OBSTRUCTIVE SLEEP APNEA

Sleep-disordered breathing (SDB) is an umbrella term for a spectrum of breathing difficulties during sleep, including frequent or loud snoring, trouble breathing or loud noisy breathing, mouth breathing (during the day and/ or night), upper airway resistance syndrome, and obstructive sleep apnea. On the mildest side of the range is occasional snoring, and on the more severe end is obstructive sleep apnea. SDB is estimated to occur in 4 to 11 percent of school-aged children. Since SDB can have nonspecific and varied presentations, it is often underdetected (Bauer, Lee, & Campbell, 2016).

Since the 1990s, there is a large body of compelling literature that has found neurocognitive, executive functioning, memory, attention, learning, hyperactivity, and behavioral difficulties result from SDB. Research has consistently associated SDB-related neurocognitive deficits with poorer academic achievement across cultural contexts. Because academic underperformance is so prevalent with SDB, screening for SDB has been recommended in the assessment of children's learning problems (Galland et al., 2015). Indeed, SDB has been linked to a range of developmental and behavioral problems, including aggression (Breus, 2013). SDB can cause attentional, learning, and behavioral problems due to decreased oxygen and increased carbon dioxide levels in the prefrontal cortex, interrupting restorative aspects of sleep, and disrupting certain chemical and cellular balances in the brain and body (Chervin et al., 2006).

An important study found strong evidence that SDB causes serious ADHD-like, emotional, and social difficulties. It followed children from infancy, and by age four, those with SDB were found to be 20 to 40 percent more likely, and by age seven were 40 to 100 percent more likely to exhibit significant and diagnosis-worthy behavioral difficulties when compared to normally-breathing children. Their greatest difficulties were hyperactivity, conduct problems, emotional difficulties, and peer problems. The study suggested that if SDB symptoms occur by the first year of life, then an evaluation should be considered. Another study of third graders found that snoring was associated with a two to tenfold increase in hyperactivity, conduct, emotional and peer difficulties one year later. Other research of children ages two to 13 found that SDB symptoms predicted a four-fold increase in hyperactivity four years later (Bonuck et al., 2012).

SDB conditions can cause misdiagnoses of ADHD because many symptoms closely mimic ADHD. Fortunately, if SDB is detected and treated, then many or all symptoms may cease. Children can also have SDB and true ADHD, and treating the SDB may improve some ADHD difficulties. One researcher found 25 percent of all children with ADHD could eliminate their ADHD-like presentations if the SDB conditions were treated effectively (Fischman, Kuffler, & Bloch, 2015).

Snoring

Children who snore are at risk of not getting adequate sleep (Green, 2014), and have more behavioral and other difficulties. They have also been found to perform worse in tests of IQ, language, and spelling (O'Brien, n.d.). A number of studies have demonstrated how snoring worsens academic performance (Breus, 2005). Snoring has been found to be three times more common in children with ADHD (Owens & Mindell, 2005). Only 10 to 12 percent of children who regularly snore have no other health problems. Snoring in children can result from enlarged tonsils and adenoids, congestion, allergies, respiratory infection, or obstructive sleep apnea. Children with allergies may only snore during allergy seasons, or when they have a cold (O'Brien, n.d.). Some, but not all, who mouth breath snore.

Loud snoring can be particularly significant. Some families may joke about children snoring and do not understand its significance. In their clinical guidelines for the evaluation and management of obstructive sleep apnea, the American Academy of Pediatrics recommends that all children should be screened regularly for snoring to detect sleep-disordered breathing (Owens & Dalzell, 2005). Bruxism, or jaw clenching and teeth grinding during sleep, occurs at higher rates for those who snore (Idzikowski, 2013). Enuresis is positively correlated with snoring also (Fischman, Kuffler, & Bloch, 2015). Those who snore should be evaluated by an ENT physician and may also require a sleep study to determine if they have sleep apnea.

Mouth Breathing

Chronic open mouth breathing is a serious health condition that can be difficult to identify and treat. Many health care providers are unaware of its existence and the numerous health, behavioral, and learning difficulties it can cause. Numerous children with mouth breathing are misdiagnosed with ADHD (Jefferson, 2010). Mouth breathing can cause significant negative impact on growth (delays in weight and height) and craniofacial development causing vertical growth of the lower face or a long narrow "adenoid" face, posterior crossbite, anterior open bite, short upper lip, everted lower lip, lip incompetence, narrow palate, and tongue posture changes during speaking, resting, chewing, and swallowing. It can also create a range of neurobehavioral and learning difficulties, including impaired concentration, hyperactivity, sleep restlessness, irritability, and decreased school performance (Thome Pacheco et al., 2015, May/June). Mouth breathing can result from chronic airway restrictions, nasopharyngeal blockages, abnormal breathing, persistent sinus and/or allergy problems, sleep apnea, nasal obstructions, enlarged tonsils and/or adenoids, deviated nasal septum, chronic pacifier use, thumb sucking, obesity (Sinha & Guilleminault, 2010), hypertrophied turbinates, inflammatory diseases, and nasal architecture alterations (Thome Pacheco et. al., 2015, July/August).

Unbalanced facial musculature and skeletal changes can result from chronic mouth breathing, and this can cause changes to dental positioning, tongue, lips, jaws and palate. Some dentists and orthodontists may recognize the specific dental problems that suggest mouth breathing. Even when the causes of mouth breathing are corrected, it often continues from the acquired habit (Thome Pacheco et. al., 2015, July/August). As children with mouth breathing grow older and obtain secondary teeth, dental and bite issues and crossbites (malocclusion) can occur. Crossbites can be key indicators, and overlapping teeth that were removed due to lack of space can indicate a narrow airway and contribute to SDB (Sinha & Guilleminault, 2010). One study found that a deviated or swollen nasal septum was particularly prevalent in mouth breathing children. Another study found that children self-reported higher rates of sleeping with open mouths, headaches and dry mouth when waking, stuffy and runny nose, snoring, sneezing, and daytime sleepiness (Thome Pacheco et. al., 2015, May/June).

Hypoxia is a condition where the body does not receive adequate supplies of oxygen. Nasal obstruction can cause hypoxia, and mouth breathing could result from nasal obstruction. Mouth breathing may not be the most appropriate term because many have a combination of oral and nasal breathing. One group of researchers found the use of pulse oximetry, a small inexpensive device used to measure oxygen levels in the blood, could be effective in identifying suspected mouth breathers. It uses a finger meter that reads blood oxygen saturation within seconds. A reading below 95 percent could suggest hypoxia or lower than normal oxygen levels, and this could suggest nasal obstructions and/or mouth breathing. They found that those with mouth breathing had greater chances of being hypoxemic, and almost 30 percent had deep palatal vaults (high roof of the mouth) (Niaki, Chalipa, & Taghipoor, 2010).

Early detection and treatment for mouth breathing are critical because if not treated by later childhood to early adolescence, it can permanently cause a long narrow face. If mouth breathing is successfully treated, there can be significant improvements in ADHD-like symptoms, mood, academics, behavioral, and other difficulties.

Obstructive Sleep Apnea (OSA)

Obstructive Sleep apnea is a serious condition which causes episodes of stopping and starting breathing repeatedly during sleep. The episodes can occur up to hundreds of times each night, and the pauses in breathing during sleep cause oxygen levels to fall and can last seconds to one minute (O'Brien, n.d.). Those with sleep apnea may not receive optimal oxygen to the brain during sleep. Typically, children with sleep apnea snore loudly for a time, then become silent, then snort briefly, move about, and then resume snoring (Greene, 2014). OSA results from airway collapse and throat blockage. These repeated arousals to breathe can interfere with the child's quality of sleep, causing sleep deprivation, sleepiness, daytime restlessness, and hyperactivity. OSA can cause morning headaches; daytime sleepiness; mouth breathing; snoring; bedwetting; and academic, behavioral, and mood problems. About 20 to 40 percent of obese children have OSA, so childhood obesity should be addressed (O'Brien, n.d.). OSA is the most common type of childhood SDB (Garde et al., 2014).

OSA is estimated to occur in up to 5 percent of children ages two to 18, and peaks during the ages of two to eight when enlarged adenoids and tonsils occurs the most. OSA presents equally in both genders (Bauer, Lee, & Campbell, 2016). It can cause a number of ADHD-like difficulties, including restlessness, lowered academic performance, inattention, and oppositional behaviors (Greene, 2014), as well as aggressiveness, hyperactivity, and communication problems (Breus, 2013). OSA is associated with several serious conditions, including neurocognitive and behavioral conditions, and cardiovascular dysfunction such as pulmonary hypertension, ventricular remodeling, and endothelial dysfunction. Enlargement of the adenoids is a substantial contributor to the development of OSA in otherwise healthy children (Bhattacharjee et al., 2010). Additionally, up to 25 percent of children with ADHD may also have OSA (Foldvary-Schaefer, 2006).

Besides OSA, there are other, but less common, types of sleep apnea. Central sleep apnea occurs when the muscles that control breathing do not receive accurate brain signals. Complex sleep apnea syndrome occurs when there is both obstructive and central sleep apnea.

Sleep-Disordered Breathing Evaluation and Treatment

One of the easiest and most effective ways to screen for SDBs is to specifically ask parents about these symptoms, especially snoring. If present, an important first diagnostic step is a referral to an Ears, Nose, Throat (ENT or otolaryngologist) physician who should explore potential nasal obstructions. Nasal turbinates, or shelf-like structures on the inside walls of the nose, can become enlarged (sometimes from untreated allergies) and obstruct nasal airways. This condition can cause SDB from chronic nasal congestion, sinus difficulties, and airway blockages. A deviated or swollen septum can also cause nasal breathing problems and snoring. For those with chronic allergies, sinus and/or congestion problems and SDB, clinicians should explore if the SDB only occurs when these difficulties are present or are more severe. While this may be unclear, ENTs and allergy specialists can address this. Additionally, children and teens with SDBs can be misdiagnosed with ADHD due to sleep deprivation symptoms.

Medical conditions that may cause or contribute to SDB include asthma, allergies, gastroesophageal reflux, enlarged tonsils (Breus, 2005) and/or adenoids, as well as nasal passages problems. Undersized jaws can significantly reduce airways and can be genetically determined. A family history of OSA may assist in making this diagnosis because there is twice the risk if an immediate family member has this, and the risk increases if multiple family members have OSA (Fischman, Kuffler, & Bloch, 2015).

After specialists address these possible medical factors, a sleep study may be necessary. The gold standard for diagnosing SDB is polysomnography (PSG). This diagnostic test is commonly utilized within sleep studies to quantify sleep abnormalities and ventilatory difficulties. Sleep studies occur in a specialized sleep laboratory which requires an overnight stay. A PSG should be scheduled after children have been screened and found to have potential symptoms of OSA, including snoring. Unfortunately, PSGs are costly ($800 or more), and sleep centers may have waiting lists (Garde et al., 2014).

Described previously, finger pulse-oximeters are also used in sleep studies and may be a helpful screening approach to detect possible SDB and mouth breathing. Parents can check the child's meter readings during the day, and particularly while sleeping and just before arising in the morning. Readings below 95 percent are suggestive of suboptimal oxygen levels. They can cost between $30 to $80 online, and some are more accurate than others. While they can be adequate screeners, they are not definitive in detecting breathing and oxygen deficiencies because they do not measure the metabolism and delivery of oxygen to the brain. Thus, a normal reading could occur, even if SDB exists.

Another potentially more accurate and informative SDB screening tool is the Phone Oximeter. This is a mobile device that uses a microcontroller-based pulse oximeter connected to a smart phone. It utilizes a finger probe and can monitor vital signs with increased accuracy. The device measures blood oxygen saturation and pulse rate variability during sleep at home and over one or more evenings. One study found that it was an effective SDB screening tool used prior to PSG, and could help determine which children actually require PSGs. This tool is helpful because the identification of SDBs in children can be more difficult than in adults (Garde et al., 2014).

As mentioned, a common problem among children with sleeping problems is enlarged or inflamed tonsils and/or adenoids that chronically restrict airflow and reduce oxygen to the brain. Removal of these can correct the problems. Children who are scheduled for surgical adenoid and tonsil removals (adenotonsillectomy) frequently demonstrate mild to moderate SDB and ADHD-like difficulties (Chervin et al., 2006). One study showed half of the children had resolution of ADHD-like symptoms after surgery. Furthermore, the increased efforts of breathing and demands on the heart from airway obstruction require energy and can lower children's weight and height. Weight gain and increased growth hormone production can result after adenotonsillectomy (Sinha & Guilleminault, 2010).

In the past, ENTs would commonly recommend removal of tonsils and adenoids as the first treatment for childhood snoring or sleep apnea symptoms. But ENTs now seem more likely to recommend a sleep study first. If first diagnosed with sleep apnea, then tonsils and adenoids may be removed. These surgeries can be effective because SDB is considered a mechanical, structural, and neuromotor tone problem. Even children with relatively small tonsils or those at risk for SDB from obesity can benefit from the removal of tonsils and adenoids (Sinha & Guilleminault, 2010). Adeno-tonsillectomies for children with OSA has been associated with improvements of ADHD-like symptoms, academic performance, and neuropsychological behaviors (Hvolby, 2015). However, many children with OSA may have residual sleep apnea after the surgery (Bhattacharjee et al., 2010), so re-evaluation is important if symptoms persist after surgery. Adenoids can grow back, and so they may require a second operation. Children with greater risks of regrowth had the procedure at age four or younger, and have reflux symptoms.

The removal of tonsils and adenoids may not cure all SDB and related ADHD-like symptoms, particularly if there are other risk factors. Other corrective surgeries for SDB can include turbinectomy for obstructing or enlarged nasal turbinates, septoplasty procedures to address deviated nasal septa, corrective jaw surgeries, and/or other maxillomandibular procedures to open airways (Fischman, Kuffler, & Bloch, 2015). Weight loss and maintenance for obese children and teens can be an important treatment approach for SDB as well. Children with high arched palates can benefit from palate expanders from orthodontists to improve breathing (Sinha & Guilleminault, 2010).

If sleep apnea is diagnosed, a main treatment is the use of a continuous positive airway pressure (C-PAP) machine, which is connected to a mask that provides oxygen while sleeping to promote better breathing. This is the gold standard treatment and is used in children age ten and older. In addition, a combination of simple medications (such as Flonase) and behavioral treatments can be used to address sleep apnea in children and adolescents.

Chronic Mouth Breathing Evaluation and Treatment

This can be difficult to evaluate and treat. While parents can be the best reporters, some may be unaware of mouth breathing, and it can require weeks of monitoring during the day and night before they are aware of this. Even children may not know they are mouth breathing. While the prior information about evaluating and treating SDBs will apply to chronic mouth breathing, it can require additional diagnostic and treatment approaches. Multiple evaluations from different providers may be the best way to identify and treat this.

Treatment will consist of identifying the mechanical causes and correcting the habit of mouth breathing. The earlier the identification and treatment, the better to prevent facial changes and damage. ENTs can first explore if there are nasal or airway obstructions, including enlarged tonsils and adenoids or sinus and nasal problems (Sinha & Guilleminault, 2010). Sleep studies may be needed, especially if OSA is a consideration. Polysomnography, finger pulse-oximeters, and phone oximeters can be used in the evaluation. An allergy specialist may be required. Medications and/or surgery may be indicated. Myofunctional therapists can help through special orofacial exercises, but these providers are uncommon. Orthodontists experienced with treating mouth breathing can be quite helpful. They may be able to identify this from presentations of crooked teeth, cross bites, open bites, and narrow or high palate vaults. Orthodontia interventions may address the underlying cause, or treat the secondary results.

One study found the most common approaches orthodontists used for identifying mouth breathing were visual evaluation, questions for parents and child, and breathing tests. The visual evaluations include the child's ability to seal their lips, changes in their posture while standing, a long face, dark circles under the eyes, anterior open bite, gingivitis, and posterior crossbite. Using the mirror test plus either lip seal or water test is recommended to increase accuracy. The lip seal test involves completely sealing the child's mouth with tape and observing their reactions for three minutes. Those with mouth breathing will have more difficulty breathing. The mirror or fog test places a mirror under the child's nose and marking the steam area on the mirror with a marker after the second air exhalation. High nasal flow is about 60 mm of fog, which is normal nose breathing. Average nasal flow is 30 to 59 mm, and the lower end may suggest mouth breathing. Low nasal flow is under 30 mm and is most suggestive of mouth breathing. The water retention test asks the child to hold about one-half ounce of water in the mouth for three minutes. Those with mouth breathing will struggle to hold the water. However, about half in one study could pass the lip seal and water retention tests, indicating they had mouth breathing by habit only (Thome Pacheco et al., 2015, July/August).

After the causes are addressed, treatment should involve training the child to nose breathe only. Each day parents can seal the child's mouth with tape, and this should be increased daily until they can nose breathe for a minimum of two straight hours (Thome Pacheco et al., 2015, July/August). Some have suggested taping mouths at night during sleep, but this should first be discussed with physicians. Possible contraindications of night taping would be nasal congestion, allergies, or other breathing difficulties. Non-stick surgical tape that is available at drug stores may be good to use because it will not irritate skin. The child can also practice nose breathing by holding a small card or pen between their lips. Daily and consistent practice will be critical to reverse this breathing habit, and compliance may be challenging. To help with motivation, children and teens should be taught why mouth breathing is so unhealthy and important to change, and large daily rewards can be used for compliance.

ADDITIONAL SLEEP CONDITIONS

Increased Nocturnal Motor Activity

Research has confirmed that children with Combined ADHD can have hyperactivity that persists during their sleep, and have significantly more motor activity at night during their sleep with their arms and legs than neurotypical children. Increased nocturnal activity can cause sleep disruption, which can contribute to increased daytime ADHD-related difficulties (Konofal, Lecendreux, & Cortese, 2010). One study found that half of children with ADHD had complaints of motor restlessness that contributed to disturbed sleep (Silvestri et al., 2009).

Evaluation and Treatment

Children and teens may not be aware of their excessive nocturnal activity because they are sleeping, but parents or siblings may be. Since children and teens with Combined ADHD have greater movements when they sleep, it is important to distinguish this from the more serious periodic limb movement disorder (PLMD) and restless legs syndrome (RLS). Because they can be similar, those with increased nocturnal motor activity should be evaluated for these two potential conditions. If the excessive nighttime activity is ADHD related, medication may be a treatment option. Curiously, some research has shown that for some with ADHD, a late-afternoon dose of methylphenidate (Ritalin and Concerta) reduces nighttime activity and improves sleep quality (Konofal, Lecendreux, & Cortese, 2010). Finally, a sleep study may be needed.

Periodic Limb Movement Disorder (PLMD)

Most with this condition experience repetitive jerking motions, typically of the legs or upward flexing of the feet only during sleep, but these can occur during the day (although it is less common). The rhythmic and involuntary movements may occur about every 20 to 40 seconds in clusters of minutes or several hours. These can disrupt sleep, but most sleep through them and are not aware of the movements. Many will also have restless legs syndrome. The cause of PLMD is unknown, but it has been linked to low iron levels, diabetes, and kidney disease. As with other conditions, the sleep disruptions can cause daytime sleepiness, ADHD-like, academic, and/or behavioral problems (The Cleveland Clinic Foundation, n.d.). Researchers have found an increased prevalence of PLMD and restless legs syndrome in children with ADHD. One study found that 10 percent of children with ADHD also had PLMD (Konofal, Lecendreux, & Cortese, 2010).

Evaluation and Treatment

Children and teens with PLMD can be misdiagnosed with ADHD due to sleep deprivation symptoms. While more frequent and longer periods of movements can be more suggestive of PLMD, a neurologist should help with this diagnosis. For symptoms that occur only at night, identifying PLMD may be challenging because the family and child may not be aware of these. Those with Combined ADHD can have higher nocturnal activity, this will need to be distinguished from PLMD.

PLMD is evaluated with an overnight sleep study (polysomnography) which includes examination of heart rates, respirations, brain waves, and limb movements. An examination including urine and blood samples examining low iron levels, anemia, and metabolic disorders may be helpful. Treatment can involve correcting iron levels (and folic acid levels), avoiding caffeine, and taking medications to regulate the muscle movements, including dopaminergic agents, benzodiazepines, and particular anticonvulsants. Those with PLMD can also have restless legs syndrome, so this may require evaluation (The Cleveland Clinic Foundation, n.d.).

Restless Legs Syndrome (RLS)

Restless legs syndrome is another movement disorder that produces irresistible urges to move legs while awake or asleep, often accompanied by uncomfortable sensations. The urges to move typically occur in the evening near bedtime, but may happen when the legs have been inactive for longer periods, such as while sitting for several hours (The Cleveland Clinic Foundation, n.d.). While 2 percent of typical children and teens have RLS, studies found much higher rates in those with ADHD (Hvolby, 2015). RLS is a sleep disorder and neurological disease. The exact cause is unknown, but it can be inherited or caused by iron deficiency. It exists on a continuum from mild to severe, and appears to affect females more than males. Some medications and foods can worsen RLS, including antidepressants, antihistamines, chocolate, and caffeine (Martin, 2013). RLS has been studied less in children than adults, and it may manifest itself differently in children (Spruyt & Gozal, 2011). While RLS is similar to PLMD due to its excessive movements, they are different but may also coexist. RLS tends to cause individuals to remain awake, while PLMD often occurs after the person is asleep. Furthermore, restless legs can cause discomfort or unpleasant sensations in the legs while the person is trying to fall asleep.

Curiously, there seems to be an unclear connection between ADHD and RLS. They share some symptoms, and ADHD is more common in those with RLS (Martin, 2013). Additionally, RLS symptoms have been found to exacerbate ADHD for children who have both conditions, and vice versa, so identifying and treating RLS will be important (Konofal, Lecendreux, & Cortese, 2010). Children and teens who are hyperactive and fidgety as a result of RLS (and PLMD) can be misdiagnosed with ADHD.

Evaluation and Treatment

Identifying RLS can be challenging since there is no specific RLS test. Serum iron and ferritin levels should be checked for an iron deficiency (Martin, 2013). Magnesium deficiency may contribute to RLS as well, but determining this may be difficult because magnesium testing may not be accurate (Stevens, 2016). Pediatric sleep specialists or neurologists are often the main evaluators and treatment providers. While a sleep study is not required to diagnosis this condition, it can be helpful to rule out other sleep conditions.

Because growing pains and RLS can have similar symptoms of leg discomfort, RLS may be misinterpreted as this. The leg sensations and discomfort of RLS are chronic and lessen when the child moves, while growing pains' discomfort may persist and is not relieved by movement. Also growing pains can fluctuate, while RLS persists for years (Martin, 2013). Growing pains tend to affect preschool and older children before adolescence, can last for months to a few years, and are generally experienced in the leg muscles. These pains tend to occur in late afternoon and before bed, and can be intense enough to wake children from sleep.

Nighttime motor restlessness associated with ADHD and vestibular and proprioceptive sensory processing deficits can both be misdiagnosed as RLS. RLS, but not ADHD, can cause sensory experiences of leg and/or foot difficulties. Another diagnostic clue can be family history of RLS (Owens, 2009). Unfortunately, RLS is considered lifelong and is managed without cures. Treatments may involve iron supplementation for iron deficiency, massage therapy, ice packs, hot baths, and good sleep hygiene. In more serious cases, anticonvulsant medication may be used (Martin, 2013).

Insomnia and Sleep Initiation Difficulties

Insomnia estimates are between one to six percent in normally developing children. Short-term or brief insomnia can persist for up to three months and often results from specific stressors. Chronic insomnia occurs for more than three months at least three times per week, and can have complex causes. Sleep onset or initial insomnia is defined as trouble falling asleep after about 30 minutes after a person's head hits the pillow. Sleep maintenance insomnia (also called middle insomnia or nocturnal awakenings) is defined as waking in the middle of the sleep cycle, inability to fall back asleep, and difficulty remaining asleep. Early morning awakening (also called terminal insomnia or advanced sleep phase) occurs when a person awakens early (30 minutes or more) before they desire to wake and cannot fall back to sleep.

Delayed sleep phase disorder is a circadian-rhythm sleep disorder that can also cause sleep onset insomnia. With this condition, children and teens are on a later sleep routine than what is normally expected. When they are required to go to bed earlier than their typical time, they often will have trouble falling asleep.

Insomnia and sleep initiation problems can result from multiple factors, including bedtime resistance, increased instability of sleep onset, problems settling down before bed, increased sleep-onset problems, interruptions during bedtime routines, mood and anxiety disorders, inadequate parental limit setting and enforcement of consistent bedtime expectations, stimulant medication effects, poorer sleep quality, irregular sleep schedules, hectic family schedules, and other causes, including circadian rhythm issues (Spruyt & Gozal, 2011). Additional causes include chronic worrying, psychological trauma, SDBs, use of electronic screen devices before sleep, and medical conditions causing discomfort. Brief or longer-term stressors, including family or school difficulties, bullying or peer problems may also be involved. Finally, non-medicated children with ADHD can have multiple times the rate of insomnia due to increased arousal at bedtime and/or other factors.

Evaluation

Parents may not be aware of sleep difficulties, including how long it takes their child to fall asleep. Children may not be accurate reporters of their sleep problems or how long it takes them to fall asleep. Additionally, the time it takes a child to fall asleep may vary and fluctuate each night, so an average and/or range of time may be more accurate. Chronic insomnia can be misdiagnosed as ADHD because sleep deprivation can cause irritability, sleepiness, reduced attention, and executive functioning difficulties. Chronic insomnia can also cause depression and anxiety from worry and fears about anticipating sleep problems each night. There can be an overlap of symptoms with insomnia and inadequate sleep duration.

Inadequate Hours of Sleep/Chronic Inadequate Sleep Duration

In the United States, it is estimated that a third of children suffer from inadequate sleep, and rates are similar in many other countries as well ("Inadequate Sleep Leads to Behavioral Problems, Study Finds," 2009). Chronic inadequate sleep duration (also called partial sleep deprivation and insufficient sleep syndrome) occurs when individuals chronically obtain less than the necessary amount of sleep. It results from insomnia, going to bed too late and/or waking too early, disrupted and poor-quality sleep related to sleep disorders or medical conditions causing discomfort, resistance and other behavioral issues before bed, and family and environmental factors.

Chronic partial sleep deprivation in children and adolescents has been called an unrecognized epidemic. Most people do not appreciate how critical quality sleep is for brain development (Breus, 2005). The symptoms of sleep deprivation can easily resemble ADHD. While adults who receive inadequate amounts of sleep may be lethargic and distracted, children without adequate sleep can exhibit Combined ADHD-like symptoms, moodiness, and behavioral difficulties. Studies have demonstrated the relationship between insufficient sleep and ADHD-like presentations, with difficulties including decreased short-term memory, decreased attentional abilities, inconsistent performance, delayed response time, and irritability ("All About Sleep," 2011). Poor quality and fewer hours of sleep can cause problems with prefrontal cortical functioning, and executive functioning deficits of emotional regulation, working memory, and behavioral inhibition which can then produce significant academic and attentional deficits (Brown & Malow, 2016).

One study found that children with less than an average of 7.7 hours of sleep demonstrated ADHD-like symptoms when compared with children who slept longer, and short sleep duration was a statistically significant predictor of hyperactivity and impulsivity ("Inadequate Sleep," 2009). Another study of children ages two to 14 found that parents who reported their children as sleepy said they were also forgetful, excessively talkative, easily distracted, fidgety, and struggled to complete tasks. Also, partial sleep deprivation can accumulate over a week, and may not be evident the first day (Kurcinka, 2006).

Studies have demonstrated the negative impact of inadequate sleep on academics. One study found students with C to F grades had about 25 fewer minutes of sleep and went to bed about 40 minutes later than A and B students. For some students, even 20 fewer minutes of sleep can cause negative impact. Several studies reported that greater total sleep, earlier bedtimes, and later rising times during weekdays were associated with better grades (Breus, 2005). Other research reported when sleep duration is shorter, scholastic and neurocognitive performance decreases, but improves when optimized (Brown & Malow, 2016).

Teens can experience significant sleep duration deficits from increased demands in their social and academic roles, as well as hormonal changes. High schools start earlier, and sports activities, clubs, social events, phone and social media use, homework, and employment can cause later evenings. Thus, they go to bed later and awake earlier (Schwartz & Thomas, 2016). Additionally, delays in the body's clock or circadian rhythms during puberty and lowered sleep drive often contribute to bedtimes becoming increasingly later (Moon, 2013).

Adolescents require a minimum eight hours of sleep per night, and the average need is about nine hours. However, a majority of teens average only about seven hours of sleep per night. This deficiency can accumulate over the week, and cause teens to oversleep on weekends in desperate attempts to "catch up." Then on Sunday night, the difficulties begin again for another week. Adolescents may use caffeine drinks to try to overcome daytime sleepiness (Schwartz & Thomas, 2016). As adolescents grow older they experience lesser parental control and increased demands, so sleep often becomes a lower priority. Sleep deprived teens are at increased risk for impaired memory, negative moods, lowered motivation, drowsy driving and increased automobile accidents. Further, children and adolescents rarely complain about sleep problems. Parents may overestimate the amount of sleep they receive because they may be unaware of when children fall asleep or night awakenings (Breus, 2005).

Delayed Sleep-Phase Disorder

This is a type of circadian-rhythm sleep disorder that involves a misalignment of sleep timing with the daytime and nighttime cycle, ultimately causing disrupted sleep and impaired functioning. Circadian-rhythms can be called a person's biological clock, and this condition causes the internal clock to become dysregulated, with sleeping and waking occurring later than normal (usually two or more hours). This later cycle can cause initial insomnia and difficulty waking when the child or teen is forced to go to bed earlier than they desire. Individuals with this condition may be called night-owls, and may resent early mornings.

As people mature, sleep rhythms and biological clock patterns change. Many teens experience this condition, and this can be related to the changes of melatonin that occur in puberty and young adulthood (Moon, 2013). Sometimes it is difficult to determine if teens who prefer later bedtimes are driven by biological, genetic, or environmental factors (evenings with screen time use, excessive homework, or socializing), or combinations of all. Additionally, irregular sleep/wake circadian rhythm disorders seem to occur more in children with developmental disabilities (Brown & Malow, 2016).

Teens who increasingly desire to be independent may resist parents' demands to go to bed earlier. To improve this condition, teens should to be informed about the disorder, agree to manage it, and take responsibility for waking themselves in the morning (Moon, 2013). Unfortunately, this condition can create partial sleep deprivation as well as difficulties related to insufficient sleep. Repeated discussions about this topic may be necessary, and attractive rewards may be utilized for adherence to new sleep schedules.

Parasomnias

Defined as abnormal, unwanted, or disruptive experiences and conditions that occur before, during, or just after sleep, these include nocturnal enuresis (bedwetting), nightmares, sleep walking, sleep talking, sleep or night terrors (while sleeping the child screams, is highly upset, or may wander about but typically has no recall in the morning), bruxism (nighttime teeth grinding and clenching), sleep paralysis (a brief frightening experience of not being able to move or speak when falling asleep or waking), confusional arousals (child acts confused or strange when awakening), and rhythmic movement disorder (a childhood neurological condition with repeated involuntary body movements during or before sleep frequently involving the neck and head, with humming or sounds accompanying the movements). Spruyt and Gozal (2011) reported children with ADHD have more nightmares and more negative dream content.

Bruxism can be more common for those with ADHD. One study found it affected about 19 percent of children (Silvestri et al., 2009). It is often triggered by anxiety and stress, and many people experience this at some point in their lives. Children and teens who experience chronic bruxism can suffer from disrupted sleep and dental damage. Additionally, 75 percent of sufferers report daytime sleepiness, and it occurs at higher rates for those who snore. Individuals with other sleep disorders are at greater risk of developing bruxism. While it may fluctuate, sometimes with stress levels, it can be a chronic condition with no cures, only long-term management. There is some evidence that behavioral approaches are effective, including understanding the causes and trying to reverse the grinding habits. Abdominal deep breathing, and other stress reduction techniques before sleep, as well as improved sleep hygiene, can be helpful. Dentists can create mouthguards to minimize damage in some cases; however, children need to be old enough to use these and some dentists do not recommend this (Idzikowski, 2013). Magnesium deficiency can cause or contribute to bruxism, but determining this may be difficult (Stevens, 2016).

Nocturnal enuresis is a common sleep difficulty, and is considered problematic if the child is five or older and it occurs two or more times a week for at least several months. Children with ADHD experience almost three times the likelihood of having nocturnal enuresis. Curiously, many of the same regions of the brain involved with ADHD are also involved with bladder control (Kutsher, 2014). Enuresis is positively correlated with enlarged tonsils and adenoids and snoring. Children with OSA have higher rates of enuresis, and treating OSA may improve or eliminate it (Fischman, Kuffler, & Bloch, 2015). Magnesium deficiency can also be a cause or contributor, but again determining this may be difficult (Stevens, 2016). Treatment can include specific behavioral and/or medication approaches.

EVALUATION OF SLEEP DIFFICULTIES AND CONDITIONS

All children and adolescents with ADHD-like symptoms should be screened for sleep disorders and coexisting sleep problems with true ADHD. This should include exploring sleep difficulties with parents and children. A review of sleep schedules (times they go to sleep and wake up during school and nonschool days); sleep routines and habits (including naps); medication use; and psychological, neurodevelopmental, medical conditions that may impact sleep is needed (Schwartz & Thomas, 2016). Parents can utilize sleep diaries for two weeks or more to document and identify sleep durations, sleep quality issues, and sleep environment factors (Brown & Malow, 2016). Diaries can also record when parents notice mouth breathing and activity levels when checking the child periodically while sleeping. During the ADHD evaluation process, clinicians can also use sleep questionnaires and measures, as well as the CDASS sleep and other checklists.

Actigraphy is a device that resembles a wristwatch that can provide more objective sleep measures. It analyzes movements and determines sleep times, the amount of time to fall asleep, and wake times after sleep onsets. Persistent medical conditions that can impact sleep should be explored as well, including chronic pain, dermatological and gastrointestinal conditions, snoring, obstructive sleep apnea, pulmonary issues (coughs or asthma) (Brown & Malow, 2016), sinus and congestion difficulties, and allergies.

Clinicians should ask when the sleeping problems began and when the ADHD-like symptoms were first noticed. For ADHD-like symptoms that are secondary to primary sleep issues, there may be a discernable connection, but sometimes it may not be clear. For children or teens on ADHD stimulants, the potential impact of stimulants on insomnia at bedtime should be considered. For most with suspected sleep disorders and significant sleep problems, sleep studies can provide the greatest diagnostic accuracy. Sleep centers will also be essential for treating resistant sleeping problems that do not improve with sleep hygiene approaches from psychotherapists. Additionally, SDB should be confirmed by a polysomnograph, which is part of a sleep study.

TREATMENT OF SLEEP DIFFICULTIES AND CONDITIONS

Improving Sleep Hygiene

When sleep problems exist, behavioral interventions and sleep hygiene practices should be utilized as a first approach, whether medications are used or not. These approaches can be implemented while other sources of sleep problems are being addressed. Providing education about sleep problems to parents and children will be very important (Brown & Malow, 2016). The effectiveness of teaching basic healthy sleep hygiene should not be underestimated. Many families lack the positive routines that prevent sleeping difficulties, and are often unaware of what causes sleeping problems. Studies have suggested that the use of good sleep hygiene alone was effective in addressing sleep initiation problems in children with ADHD (Owens, 2009).

The following are effective sleep hygiene approaches. First, a regular and consistent sleep schedule is critical to help insure sufficient sleep is obtained. The child's bedtime and wake time should be the same each day, whether school is the next day or not. These established wake times permit sleepiness to increase by the evening so they are sleepy enough by bedtime. Naps should be avoided after age five or six because these can increase sleep onset difficulties ("Healthy Sleep Habits for Children," 2017).

The time to be in bed ready for sleep should be calculated by first determining the number of hours of sleep required, and then counting backwards from the time to awaken. For example, if 10 hours of sleep is needed and the time to awake is 6:30 am on school days, then 8:30 pm will be the sleep time with lights out in bed, not when starting to wind down. Parents should start with the middle time within the recommended range of sleep duration (see Chapter 14). They can then adjust this number to see if the child needs more or less sleep. If rushing in the morning is a challenge, parents can begin waking children earlier (Kurcinka, 2006). Parents should be aware that putting some children earlier to sleep can cause increased frustrations and delayed sleep onset if they are not ready for sleep. To address this, their sleep time should be gradually reduced over time (Brown & Malow, 2016).

For teens, the sleep schedule should not deviate more than two hours on any night, including weekends or nonschool nights. Younger children should have less deviation than two hours. Sleeping in on weekends should not occur, and this need should decrease if set sleep times are made a priority and maintained. An important goal will be to achieve the required number of hours of sleep each day (Schwartz & Thomas, 2016). Parents will need to be firmly committed to this goal.

Another important sleep hygiene approach is bedtime and sleep time. While bedtime is the relaxing wind down period in preparation for sleep, sleep time is when the lights are out and child is in bed (Kurcinka, 2006). Before sleep time there should be about 30 to 60 minutes of quiet and relaxing bedtime. While the amount may vary, bedtime should not be too brief. Activities can include bathroom hygiene, baths, showers, putting on pajamas, reading calming books without intense or scary themes, and listening to quiet music. Watching TV, computer use, and video gaming should not be part of bedtime. Stimulating or vigorous play should be avoided also. These activities do not need to occur exclusively in the bedroom, but they should end there for the last 10 to 15 minutes ("Healthy Sleep Habits for Children," 2017).

Some families are so busy that they do not have an adequate wind down period to help the child transition to sleep. They may be on the go and highly active all day, and then expect the child to suddenly shift gears and fall asleep quickly at night. Each child will differ in their time and specific activities they need to decompress before bed, so adjustments should be made. Relaxation exercises, deep breathing, or prayers can be used during bedtime as well. These wind down practices should be considered presleep rituals that help the child associate them with going to sleep.

Additional sleep hygiene approaches include having a light snack before bedtime, if hungry. These can include milk, a half turkey sandwich, low sugar cereal, or a banana. Heavy meals two hours prior to bed, as well as caffeinated drinks and foods (including chocolate) should be avoided. Regular exercise can help but should be finished at least three hours before bedtime because it can be stimulating. The bedroom should have a comfortable bed and temperature (not too hot and slightly cooler is better). It should be quiet and adequately dark (room darkening shades may help). Fans, white noise machines, or soothing sounds can be used. Additionally, beds should be for sleeping only to create a positive and strong association with sleep. There should be no phone or screen use, eating, or homework while in bed, day or night (Smith, Robinson, & Segal, 2018). Parents should not drag out saying goodnights, with interactions being consistent, warm, and brief. To maintain positive associations, bedrooms should not be used for punishments ("Healthy Sleep Habits for Children," 2017). A dim night-light is acceptable if children fear the dark, but shifting towards eliminating this with encouragement and rewards is best. Potentially upsetting discussions or arguments should be avoided before bed or in bedrooms as well.

TVs, any screen devices, and phones should be removed from bedrooms permanently. Screen devices can emit blue light that lowers melatonin which naturally promotes sleep. Also, there should be no screen use at least one hour before bed (or after studying to promote the best learning). Nothing should be watched that is stimulating, violent, or potentially upsetting at least two hours before bedtime. This includes news, arousing video games or social media, anxiety provoking videos, and intense dramas. Additionally, there should be no bright light during the wind down period, but bright light and opening windows after waking can be helpful, particularly for those with waking difficulties ("Sleep Tips," 2016).

Parents will need to become firm and consistent about managing phones and screen devices at bedtime. Parents should dismiss arguments that screens are necessary for "relaxing." They can explain there are new rules, and these devices are overstimulating and not helpful for sleep. Screen devices and phones can be earned as privileges, and are not rights. Parents may collect devices at bedtime, return them in the morning, and can keep them for one or more days if they do not comply. The wi-fi in the house can be turned off for the evening if children or teens struggle with compliance. Parents can also temporarily deactivate the child's or teen's cell service until they earn this privilege back.

The older the child, the more involvement they should have with these healthy sleep hygiene approaches. It will be important for them to understand this, and have an adequate partnership with parents. Multiple discussions may need to occur and specific bedtimes and sleep times should be clearly determined and written down. The use of regular and consistent rewards for cooperation can help increase compliance and motivation. One daily consequence can be earning a predetermined duration of screen time the next day for sleep time compliance, and no phone or screen time the following day for lack of cooperation. Other rewards and negative consequences can be utilized on a day-by-day basis.

This process of practicing healthy sleep hygiene practices will be a lifestyle change for the entire family. These will be difficult at first, but parents need to remain firm. Shifting towards earlier bedtimes may need to occur slowly, with a slightly earlier time every few days or week to increase sleep time to determine the optimal amount. Addressing insomnia and other sleep problems is imperative. Parents should not give up on this process prematurely, and should expect fluctuations in success until consistent progress is achieved.

Another approach to improving sleep involves ball blankets. These are blankets filled with loose plastic, weighted balls that provide light pressure across the body. They have been used effectively with children with ADHD and/or sensory processing disorders who have sleep difficulties (Hvolby, 2015). Lastly, neurofeedback treatment may be helpful for some sleep difficulties.

Addressing Insomnia

For children or teens with insomnia who lay in bed with excessive thinking or worrying, a worry journal can be helpful. This can be used to write down concerns, worries, frustrations, or anything they wish to unload from their minds that can be dealt with the next day. Creating a list of things for which they are grateful can be powerful as well, including things they were proud of that day and any acts of kindness ("Sleep Tips," 2016). If a journal is used, it should be finished about one hour before bedtime, and children should be taught that the purpose is to write worries down to forget them, and not to ruminate over these things again (as much as possible). Also, worry journals should be used outside the bedroom to maintain a positive association between the child's bedroom and sleep.

Some with insomnia may have greater anxiety levels, overachiever and perfectionistic traits. They may have negative expectations and beliefs about their sleep, such as "I know I will never fall asleep tonight," or "I will do terrible in school tomorrow because I'll be tired." This type of thinking can increase anxiety, prevent relaxation needed before sleep, and generate a "worry—not sleeping—worry more—remain awake" cycle that can continue for hours. When insomnia occurs, children and teens should not lay in bed more than 20 to 30 minutes if they cannot fall asleep. They should get out of bed and do some relaxing but somewhat boring activity like reading or listening to nonstimulating music, and not watch screens or use electronic devices. When they feel sleepy, children should get back in bed. If they can't sleep after 20 to 30 minutes, they can repeat this (Owens & Mindell, 2005).

For insomnia or chronic sleep difficulties related to mood or anxiety disorders and significant stressors, education about insomnia, and a competent psychotherapist should be obtained. The child or teen can be taught effective symptom management, coping, and relaxation skills to be used before and at bedtime, and parents can assist with this process. More extensive therapy and/or medications may be necessary for more severe cases. Finally, natural herbal teas and supplements may help with insomnia by increasing relaxation before bed. These include chamomile, lavender, catnip, lemon balm, and passion flower. Physicians should be consulted with their use.

Sleep Medications

Melatonin, a supplement in the United States and a prescription drug in some European countries, has been found to accelerate sleep onset in children with ADHD (Hvolby, 2015). It is believed to be safe when used for short periods. It can be used for children who have difficulties falling asleep and increasing time asleep, but it does not keep them asleep generally. However, the synthetic supplement version can cause side effects, including waking at night and nightmares (Moon, 2013). Melatonin is becoming increasingly popular for childhood sleep difficulties, even though the United States' Federal Drug Administration has not approved its use for sleep disorders. Experts agree that for circadian rhythm disorders and particularly delayed sleep phase disorder, it can be used along with regular pediatrician follow-up visits. One study of children ages six to 12 with ADHD and delayed sleep phase syndrome took 3 mg for those who weighed 88 lbs. or less, and 6mg for those that weighed more. They found that 65 percent of the children continued its use daily for 3.7 years, with no side effects or concerns. While it may be an appropriate treatment for insomnia and it seems to be well-tolerated, its long-term safety has not been established. It should not be used for those with immune conditions. While there are no clear guidelines for dosing, the Canadian Pediatric Society recommended 2.5 to 3.5 mg in children older than infants and 5 mg for teens. It should be given one half to one hour before bed (Janjua & Goldman, 2016). For children with ADHD taking stimulants, melatonin at bedtime shortened the time to fall asleep and enhanced sleep duration, but not daytime behavioral problems (Spruyt & Gozal, 2011).

The medications clonidine, guanfacine, trazodone, diphenhydramine, cyproheptadine, mirtazapine, and tricyclic antidepressants have been used to treat behaviors related to insomnia with mixed results (Spruyt & Gozal, 2011). Trazadone, antihistamines, mirtazapine, and hypnotic agents have been used off-label to treat children who have ADHD and insomnia, but their use is not part of clinical practice guidelines. Clonidine has been suggested to address stimulant associated sleep onset delay for those with ADHD (Hvolby, 2015).

Stimulant medications can cause insomnia and delayed sleepiness at night for some. If there are these concerns, parents should consult their prescribing physician, or obtain a second opinion from an experienced psychiatrist or sleep specialist. Curiously, some clinicians have reported that a small dose of methylphenidate taken before bed can help facilitate sleep. While this will not help all children and teens, robust clinical findings suggest it can help some (Konofal, Lecendreux, & Cortese, 2010). Finally, sleep problems that are more complicated, severe, or persistent may require treatment at a sleep center. This can involve working with sleep specialists, such as board-certified sleep medicine physicians and/or clinical psychologists experienced with sleep conditions.

REFERENCES

All About Sleep. (reviewed 2011, January). Reviewed by Gavin, M. L. Retrieved from http://kidshealth.org=KisHealth&lic=1&ps=107&cat_id=190&artticle...

American Academy of Pediatrics (2016, June 13). *American academy of pediatrics supports childhood sleep guidelines.* Retrieved from https://www.aap.org/en-us/about - the-aap/aap-press-room/pages/American-Academy-of-Pediatrics-Supports-Child hood-Sleep-Guidelines.aspx

Bauer, E. E., Lee, R., & Campbell, Y. N. (2016, December). Preoperative screening for sleep-disordered breathing in children: A systematic literature review. *Association of Perioperative Registered Nurses, 104*(6), 541–553.

Bhattacharjee, R., Khelrandish-Gozal, L., Spruyt, K., Mitchell, R. B., Promchiarak, J., Simakajornboon, N., & Brooks, L. J. (2010). Adenotonsillectomy outcomes in treatment of obstructive sleep apnea in children. *American Journal of Respiratory and Critical Care Medicine, 182,* 676–683.

Bonuck, K., Freedman, K., Chervin, R. D., & Xu, L. (2012, April). Sleep-disordered breathing in population-based cohort: Behavioral outcomes at 4 and 7 years. *Pediatrics, 129*(4): e857–e865. doi: 10.1542/peds.2011-1402

Breus, M. J. (2005). *Back to school, back to sleep.* Retrieved from www.webmd.com /sleep-disorders/features/fixing-sleep-problems-may-improve-child-grades-and -behavior

Breus, M. (2013, May 7). *ADHD or sleep disorder?* Retrieved from http:/blogs /webmd.com/sleep-disorders/2013/05/add-or-sleep-disorder.html

Brown, K. M., & Malow, B. A. (2016, May). Pediatric insomnia. *Contemporary Reviews in Sleep Medicine, CHEST, 149*(5): 1332–1339.

Chervin, R. D., Ruzicka, D. L., Giordani, B. J., Weatherly, R. A., Dillon, J. E., Hodges, E. K., Marcus, C. L., & Guire, K. E. (2006, April). Sleep-disordered

breathing, behavior, and cognition in children before and after adenotonsillectomy. *Pediatrics, 117*(4), e769–778. doi: 10.1542/peds.2005-1837

The Cleveland Clinic Foundation. (n.d.). *Periodic limb movement disorder.* Retrieved on
02/02/17 from http://my.clevelandclinic.org/childrens-hospital/health-info
/diseases-conditions/hic-Periodic-Limb-Movement-Disorder-in-Children-and
-Adolescents

Cortese, S., Konofal, E., Yateman, N., Mouren, M. C., & Lecendreux, M. (2006,
April). Sleep and alertness in children with attention-deficit/hyperactivity disorder: A systematic review of the literature. *Sleep, 29*(4), 504–511.

Fischman, S., Kuffler, D. P., & Bloch, C. (2015). Disordered sleep as a cause of atten-
tion-deficit/hyperactivity disorder: Recognition and management. *Clinical
Pediatrics, 54*(8), 713–722. doi: 10.1177/000992281458673

Foldvary-Schaefer, N. (2006). *Getting a good night's sleep.* Cleveland, OH: Cleveland
Clinic Press.

Galland, B., Spruyt, K., Dawes, P., McDowall, P. S., Elder, D., & Schaughency, E.
(2015, October). Sleep disordered breathing and academic performance: A
meta-analysis. *Pediatrics,136*(4), e934–e946. Retrieved from http://pediatrics
.aappublica tions.org/content/136/4/e934

Garde, A., Dehkordi, P., Karlen, W., Wensley, D., Ansermino, J. M., & Dumont, G.
A. (2014, November). Development of a screening tool for sleep disordered
breathing in children using the phone oximeter. *PloS One, 9*(11), e112959. doi:
10.1371/jounal.pone.0112959

Greene, A. (2014). *Dr. Alan Greene on sleep deprivation and ADD/ADHD.* Retrieved
from www.parents.com/parents/templates/story/printableStory.jsp?storyid=
/templatedata/hk/story/data/1524.xml&catref=prt1012

Healthy Sleep Habits for Children. (2017, June 1). Retrieved from https://my.cleve-
landclinic.org/health/articles/pediatric-healthy-sleep-habits

Hvolby, A. (2015, March). Associations of sleep disturbance with ADHD:
Implications for treatment. *Attention Deficit and Hyperactivity Disorders, 7*(1), 1–18.
doi: 10.1007/s12402-014-0151-0

Idzikowski, C. (2013). *Sound asleep.* London: Watkin.

Inadequate sleep leads to behavioral problems, study finds. (2009, April 28).
Retrieved from www.sciencedaily.com/releases/2009/04/090427131313.htm

Janjua, I., & Goldman, R. D. (2016, April). Sleep-related melatonin use in healthy
children. *Canadian Family Physician, 62*(4), 315–316.

Jefferson, Y. (2010, January/February). Mouth breathing: Adverse effects on facial
growth, health, academics, and behavior. *General Dentistry, 58*(1), 18–25.
Retrieved from https://www.ncbi.nlm.nih.gov/pubmed/20129889

Konofal, E., Lecendreux, M., & Cortese, S. (2010, August). Sleep and ADHD. *Sleep
Medicine, 11*(7), 652–658. doi: 10.1016/j-sleep.2010.02.012

Kurcinka, M. S. (2006). *Sleepless in America.* New York: HarperCollins.

Kutscher, M. L. (2014). *Kids in the syndrome mix of ADHD, LD, autism spectrum,
Tourettes, anxiety, and more!* (2nd ed.). London: Jessica Kingsley.

Martin, A. (2013, August 8). *How restless legs syndrome affects children.* Retrieved from
http://www.everydayhealth.com/sleep/0613/how-restless-legs-syndrome-affects
-children.aspx

Moon, R. Y. (2013). *Sleep—What every parent needs to know.* Elk Grove Village, IL: American Academy of Pediatrics.

Niaki, E.A., Chalipa, J., & Taghipoor, E. (2010). Evaluation of oxygen saturation by pulse-oximetry in mouth breathing patients. *Acta Medica Iranica, 48*(1), 9–11.

O'Brien, L. M. (n.d.). *Snoring in children.* Retrieved on 07/11/12 from ://www.peds forparents.com/articles/2785.shtml

Owens, J. A. (2009, May). A clinical overview of sleep and attention-deficit/hyper-activity disorder in children and adolescents. *Journal of the Canadian Academy of Child & Adolescent Psychiatry, 18*(2), 92–102.

Owens, J. A., & Dalzell, V. (2005, January). Use of the 'BEARS' sleep screening tool in a pediatric residents' community clinic: A pilot study. *Sleep Medicine, 6*(1), 63–69.

Owens, J. A., & Mindell, J. A. (2005). *Take charge of your child's sleep.* New York: Marlowe.

Schwartz, B. S., & Thomas, J. H. (2016, August 24). *Adolescent sleep issues: Why are they so tired?* Retrieved from http://www.chop.edu/news/adolescent-sleep-issues -why-are-they-so-tired

Silvestri, R., Gagliano, A., Arico, I., Calarese, T., Cedro, C., Bruni, O., & Brananti, P. (2009, June). Sleep disorders in children with Attention-deficit/hyperactivity disorder (ADHD) recorded overnight by video-polysomnography. *Sleep Medicine, 10*(10), 1132–1138. doi: 10.1016/j.sleep.2009.04.003

Sinha, D., & Guilleminault, C. (2010, February). Sleep disordered breathing in chil-dren. *Indian Journal of Medical Research, 131*(2), 311–320. doi: 10.3109/078538998 09029934

Sleep Tips For Your Family's Mental Health. (2016, November 4). Retrieved from https://www.healthychildren.org/English/healthy-living/sleep/Pages/Sleep-and -Mental-Health.aspx

Smith, M., Robinson, L., & Segal, R. (2018, July). *How to sleep better.* Retrieved from https://www.helpguide.org/articles/sleep/getting-better-sleep.htm

Spruyt, K., & Gozal, D. (2011, April). Sleep disturbances in children with attention-deficit/hyperactivity disorder. *Expert Review of Neurotherapeutics, 11*(4), 565–577. doi: 10.1586/ern.11.7

Stevens, L. J. (2016). *Solving the puzzle of your ADD/ADHD child.* Springfield, IL: Charles C Thomas.

Thome Pacheco, M. C., Casagrande, C. F., Teixeira, L. P., Finck, N. S., & Martins de Araujo, M. T. (2015, July/August). Guidelines proposal for clinical recogni-tion of mouth breathing children. *Dental Press Journal of Orthodontics, 20*(4), 39–44. Retrieved from https://www.ncbi.nlm.nih.gov/pmc/articles/PMC45 93528/

Thome Pacheco, M. C., Fiorott, B. S., Finck, N. S., & Martins de Araujo, M. T. (2015, May/June). Craniofacial changes and symptoms of sleep-disordered breathing in healthy children. *Dental Press Journal of Orthodontics, 20*(3), 80–87. Retrieved from http://dx.dol.org/10.1590/2176-9451.20.3.080-087.oar

Chapter 6

NEURODEVELOPMENTAL CONDITIONS

Neurodevelopmental conditions are quite prevalent. About one in six children in the United States have a developmental disability ranging from milder conditions of speech and language deficits to severe disorders such as autism, cerebral palsy, and intellectual disorders (Centers for Disease Control and Prevention, 2018, November).

LEARNING DISORDERS

Five to 15 percent of school-age children experience specific learning disorders (LD), with reading disorder being the most common. Those with LD have substantial and chronic problems with the task of reading, comprehension, and correctly using mathematical concepts and/or reasoning, spelling, and written expression. Their skills are significantly lower than their peers and not a result of hearing or vision impairments, motor disorders, neurological conditions, lack of education, or lack of the culture's predominant language. They typically demonstrate academic underperformance that is not commensurate with their cognitive abilities and intelligence levels. Their impairments should be determined from multiple sources, including psychological testing, educational evaluations, and standardized achievement testing (American Psychiatric Association, 2016). Reading, math, and writing skills deficits exist on a continuum from mild (some impairments) to severe (a full LD diagnose) (Drummond, 2005-2007). Those with more serious learning difficulties can have poor motivation and low interest in school work, causing avoidance or refusal to do classwork or homework. Consequently, they may also have secondary behavioral, frustration, depression, anxiety, and self-esteem problems.

LD diagnoses should not be given if the learning problems result from sensory processing difficulties, acquired brain damage, or overall lower intelligence levels. Environmental influences of larger families and lower socioeconomic status can negatively impact learning and language abilities due to less reading, fewer language games, and poorer preschool experiences (Parker, 2000). Injuries, illnesses, or other factors can impact hearing and auditory processing within the first three years, and therefore can have serious effects upon language and learning abilities (Bellis, 2002). Also, a LD diagnosis should not be given if the learning problems involve a language in which proficiency is lacking.

Visual and/or auditory processing disorders can cause significant reading and learning difficulties that may mimic a true learning disorder. These processing disorders can be particularly damaging when speech and language development occurs during early childhood due to their impact on reading abilities. Consequently, most children and teens with LD symptoms should first be screened or evaluated for these processing conditions. Other rule outs that may cause (or coexist with) persistent learning problems are significant depression or anxiety disorders, psychological trauma, nonverbal learning disorder, OCD, sleep-disordered breathing, fetal substance exposure, and neurotoxic exposures. Finally, LDs can be genetically transmitted, so family history is important.

Discriminating between LD and ADHD

There is a diagnostic challenge involving discerning LD from ADHD, particularly the inattentive type. Both of these can be misdiagnosed for the other, and can coexist. Each can cause school performance, reading, homework, writing, emotional and behavioral problems. Various studies found from 19 to 45 percent of children and teens with ADHD also have formal LDs (Weyandt & Gudmundsdottir, 2015), while in clinical samples, up to 70 percent of children with ADHD had a LD. Children with ADHD and LD can commonly experience motor problems and social difficulties as well (Tannock & Brown, 2009). Additionally, LDs and ADHD can cause slow processing speed deficits, such as moving, thinking, and reacting more slowly, memory difficulties, and taking longer to initiate and complete tasks (Braaten & Wolloughby, 2014).

To discern between true ADHD and LD, clinicians can explore if the child or teen has chronic and significant inattention difficulties separate from specific reading, math, and writing activities (such as at home and with non-scholastic activities). If the inattention only occurs during learning and academic tasks, then this would be more suggestive of LDs and not true ADHD.

The following are suggestive of specific LDs without true ADHD: below the seventh percentile in academic achievement; psychological testing indicating a significant discrepancy between IQ and achievement scores with a greater than 1 or 1.5 standard deviation; and attention problems that began in middle childhood and exist only with specific tasks involving reading, math, or writing. Also, a lack of hyperactivity, impulsivity, social aggression, and disruptive behaviors (Barkley, 2015, March 19b) would suggest Combined ADHD does not exist. The following information should also help in the diagnostic process.

Diagnosing Learning Disorders

If LDs are suspected, there are four diagnostic options to consider:

1. Obtain a visual processing evaluation from a behavioral or developmental optometrist, particularly if reading and handwriting difficulties exist. This could occur before psychological testing for LD because it is less expensive and time-consuming. While the CDASS checklist for visual processing problems can help to identify these concerns, this is not designed to replace a visual processing evaluation. Refer to Chapter 7 for more information on this topic.

2. Obtain a comprehensive neurodevelopment assessment to specifically test for LDs. This is the best way to determine if true LD, ADHD, or both exist.

3. A less precise way is to try ADHD medication and then monitor academic performance. While diagnosing from medication responses is not the best approach, many families have tried this because it is easier than obtaining testing. Stimulants can boost attention and executive functioning for most people with or without ADHD, so diagnosing Inattentive ADHD with medication responses may not be helpful. However, if hyperactivity, impulsivity, grades, and learning improve while on medication, then perhaps a LD is not present but Combined ADHD is. True LD can improve on stimulants, but often not as significantly as ADHD. If hyperactivity and impulsivity symptoms improve but not learning and grades, then perhaps true Combined ADHD and LD both exist. If there are no changes with medication use at sufficient dosages, then perhaps only LD exists. Approximately 15 percent of those with true ADHD do not respond to medication, so this should be considered. Finally, testing should be used to confirm LDs.

4. Refer the child to the school district for educational testing (hopefully from a school psychologist). However, schools do not typically use the term "learning disorder" and often do not provide comprehensive assessments. Consequently, these may be inaccurate or incomplete in their diagnostic work, and may not identify other relevant conditions and learning issues. Also, because school testing can be challenging to obtain, clinicians should assist parents in navigating the school system.

Finally, QEEQs from neurofeedback providers and special urine and blood tests with the Walsh Biochemical Approach may provide helpful diagnostic information.

Treatment for Learning Disorders

The sooner interventions are obtained, the better, even in preschool. Unfortunately, there are no cures and only long-term management approaches for learning disorders, except possibly neurofeedback and the Walsh's Advanced Nutrient Therapy. The main services involve official school plans, including accommodations with long-term, one-on-one, and specialized remediation tutoring services. Tutoring outside of the school should also be considered. Utilizing a disability approach can be helpful as well.

When persistent and significant LDs exist, three approaches should be taken. First, assessments should determine the source and nature of the learning problems. Second, targeted instruction should be provided to remediate with compensatory strategies and skill enhancements. Third, parents and teachers can accommodate the weaknesses and build upon strengths (Drummond, 2005– 2007).

School plans that provide remediation, compensatory strategies, and accommodations are essential for LD management. Accommodations should be implemented by classroom teachers, and can include reduced homework, calculator use, or extended time on tests. Compensatory strategies assist with learning-based strengths and weaknesses, and teachers should use them. Various approaches should be attempted until effective ones are discovered and utilized. Also, special education teachers can provide remediation tutoring and compensatory approaches and coordinate their work with classroom teachers. Teachers who do not understand LDs or coordinate their efforts with other services can cause great difficulties for students (Silver, 2006).

Tutors without specialized training in teaching those with LDs may not be effective. Experienced tutors should assess skill levels and address foundational reading, math, and writing deficits, and not just review difficulties with current class materials and homework. Without learning and mastering essential basic skills, progress may be unlikely. Even if a child has an IEP and individual tutoring at school, families should not assume that quality remedial instruction is being received. Parents need to monitor school plans to make sure they are actually being implementing.

Depending on the severity of the impairments, private specialized tutoring outside the school may be necessary. This can be a commitment of two or more sessions per week for one or more years. Fees can be expensive (about $45 to $65 per one-hour session, or more), and experienced tutors may be difficult to find. Franchise tutoring businesses or individuals may be utilized, including special education teachers at public schools who also work outside the school. Some schools, libraries, and churches may offer free tutoring before and after school, but nonspecialist tutors may not provide appropriate services for those with LDs. Some children who receive external tutoring may resent and resist this, but some tutoring businesses try to make it fun and engaging. Rewards for cooperation and good effort can help as well, such as earning screen time or phone privileges. Additionally, it can be very helpful for parents to commit time and attention with their children to provide extra assistance for learning, homework, and studying.

There are several other approaches to addressing LDs. While less common, educational therapy provides services usually outside of school that are more intensive and comprehensive than tutors. They can address complex school and learning difficulties that psychotherapists and neuropsychologists do not often address. These professionals have a variety of backgrounds, and typically work with children and teens with LDs, ADHD, and other neurodevelopmental conditions. Although different from tutors, they can provide tutoring, skills development and training, and scholastic case management. Educational therapists tend to utilize broader perspectives, and may coordinate and integrate information from other providers and school staff to create more effective learning plans and results. They usually work in private practices or learning centers, but most health insurance plans do not cover their services. Since they do not have state licensing requirements, their qualifications can vary and they may or may not have a master's degree, certifications, or training. Referrals for these therapists can be obtained from the child's providers or The Association of Educational Therapists (Clark, 2014-2018).

Neurofeedback treatment, which is a form of biofeedback and a powerful brain training approach, may permanently improve LDs, ADHD, and other conditions. There are different types, and its effectiveness can vary based on the provider and types used. Newer versions and combinations of neurofeedback types can maximize results. Walsh's Advanced Nutrient Therapy may be a helpful treatment for all LDs as well.

Since learning and motor conditions can affect more than academics, children with these challenges should be expected to perform chores and tasks at home that are based on their abilities. Although they may take longer, this can help develop confidence and a positive self-image. Parents should be creative in helping children find ways to complete tasks with which they struggle, such as using pictures or lists. As with other conditions, children with LDs should be specifically informed about their conditions and why they struggle. They should know they can have successful lives by learning to accept and manage their conditions while maximizing their talents and strengths (Silver, 2006). Finally, individual therapy can help children or adolescents with LDs or any other neurodevelopmental condition to accept the disability and address self-esteem deficits, coexisting conditions, or other difficulties.

Reading Learning Disorder

Also called dyslexia, this condition describes a range of significant and chronic reading problems. It is a language-based disability caused by a neurobiological condition that impairs the ability to properly sound out, pronounce, and comprehend words and text (Parker, 2000). It is not just letter reversals. There is substantial evidence of genetic transmission, and a male child has a 50 percent chance of acquiring this if a parent or sibling has it (Nicolson & Fawcett, 2008). Reading learning disorder is the most common and researched LD, affecting 5 to 10 percent of all school-age children with males more than females. Conservative estimates indicate that 25 to 40 percent of those with ADHD also have learning disorders (Tannock & Brown, 2009).

There are two types of reading LD difficulties: basic reading (difficulties understanding relationships between sounds, letters, and words) and reading comprehension (problems grasping meaning of words, phrases, sentences, and paragraphs). By the end of first grade or age seven, children should have basic reading skills. Tannock and Brown (2009) reported that the most reliable indicators of a true reading disorder are the failure to develop fluent and/or accurate word recognition and a deficit in spelling and decoding.

To be able to read, write, and spell, a person must be able to quickly decode, or correctly relate the letters to specific sounds (phonemes) for proper pronunciation. However, it does not necessarily include comprehension. Fluent readers can easily process the various phonemes that compose words. Those with dyslexia have difficulties sounding out or recognizing the smaller sounds that compose words. Their short-term memory for the individual sounds of words can be compromised and this can cause multiple attempts until they can pronounce the word correctly. They may also struggle with recalling how to pronounce words and the meaning of words, decreasing reading efficiency. Since the process of reading can be so difficult, those with dyslexia may give up and avoid reading, and fall further behind. In contrast, fluent readers can recall stored words more easily and improve their word recall by reading and using their words repeatedly, enhancing their skills, memory, and ease of reading. Skilled readers have greater phonemic awareness, which is the foundation of reading (Hurford, 1998).

Dyslexia exists on a continuum, but even borderline conditions require remedial services. Tests that assess reading achievement do not detect reading effort. Thus, a person with reading LD can pass these tests, but the tests may not indicate their fluency and other reading difficulties. Student may be so exhausted with the pronunciation of words that they do not understand the text. Reading retention difficulties may occur as well, where students struggle remembering, summarizing what is read, or associating the material to their own experiences (Kutscher, 2014). Children and teens with ADHD are also at higher risk for retention issues due to poorer working memories and slower processing speeds.

Children learn and read differently and at different rates, but by the end of third grade, most students should be able to read grade-appropriate material fluently with comprehension. The following are risk factors for developing reading difficulties: parents with histories of reading problems, speech or language delays and impairments (because language is critical for reading skills), hearing impairments, decreased or minimal reading skills acquired during preschool years (Drummond, 2005–2007), word-finding difficulties, problems learning color or letter names, difficulties remembering phone numbers or addresses, not sequencing syllables properly (such as "donimos" for "dominoes" or "aminals" or "animals"), difficulties following directions, lesser speech production, and peer relational difficulties (Parker, 2000). Many children with language delays and expressive and/or receptive language problems can also experience difficulties learning to read by first grade (Silver, 2006).

Children and adults with undiagnosed LD can experience poor achievement in school, low self-esteem, and employment limitations. Obviously, the earlier the learning conditions are detected and addressed, the better the chances of success. One study showed that 67 percent of young students identified as being at risk for reading problems achieved average to above average reading abilities when they received early services (Coordinated Campaign for Learning Disabilities, 1997). Without these services, deficient readers will fall further behind, and the reading impairments often become chronic. Eighty-eight percent of poor readers by the end of first grade will continue to have reading problems by the end of fourth grade without early and intensive services. Many children are not identified as having dyslexia until third grade or later, and this delay can impact reading abilities because the brain's wiring for reading decreases after third grade (Kutscher, 2014). Consequently, parents should not delay obtaining reading services or expect that children will "catch up" or "grow out of it."

Treatment

The most essential step is to receive specialized and individualized tutoring in a phonics-based approach to reading. It is critical to be able to sound out words; this cannot be bypassed, and whole language approaches do not help (Parker, 2000). Those with dyslexia need explicit instruction in phonics with bottom up learning by developing skills starting with small parts (letters and syllables associated with sounds) and working towards words (Hurford, 1998). Building an extensive reading vocabulary will be important as well.

An effective strategy to enhance reading comprehension skills is to preview what will be read. Teachers and parents can preview by summarizing the plot or essential points before the text is read by the child. Difficult or unfamiliar words should be reviewed before reading also (Parker, 2000).

Students with reading problems can prefer to subvocalize when reading, and reading aloud may help their recall and focus. Readers with poorer comprehension skills may focus more on pronouncing the words accurately, rather than understanding and focusing on the text's meaning. Similarly, students with ADHD with superior decoding skills who can read fluently may have difficulties maintaining concentration on their reading, which will lower their comprehension. Increasing active reader strategies can help, including pausing and asking questions, taking notes while reading, shortening the length of reading, and listing questions before reading to answer while reading (Parker, 2000).

For older students, the SQRRR (or SQ3R) method can enhance understanding of material, and increase more active reading involvement, particularly with textbooks (Hurford, 1998). It stands for *Survey* (briefly review first, scanning headings and chapters); *Question* (rephrase the headings into questions and ask what is the main idea); *Read; Recite* (restate the meaning of text); and *Review* (scan and check to see how much was recalled and understood) (Parker, 2000). To the reading challenged, initially SQ3R may seem tedious and will prolong reading. However, it can decrease reading time by increasing reading efficiency. Poorer readers may want to immediately begin reading without thinking about the task. The SQ3R requires readers to examine the entire text first, generate questions about what they will read, and attempt to answer these during the reading. This method helps readers absorb the meaning once instead of multiple, frustrated readings (Hurford, 1998). Finally, the use of laptop computers in class and for homework may assist.

Mathematics Learning Disorder

This condition, also called dyscalculia, is caused by a brain functioning condition that impairs the ability to perform arithmetic problems and comprehend math concepts. This LD often receives less attention than reading disorders, and parents may minimize the importance of having adequate math skills ("I was terrible in math as a child . . ."). (Garnett, 1998). Research has suggested that estimates of significant math deficiencies in school-age children range from 3 to 6 percent across the United States, Europe, Brazil, and Israel. Most mathematics LD studies report equal prevalence in the genders (Tannock & Brown, 2009). Other research has shown that 13 to 33 percent of those with ADHD also have math LDs (Barkley, 2015, March 19a).

Also, math deficiencies can be negatively impacted by coexisting reading disorders that affect math word problems, conceptual abilities, and challenges with memory, organization, and sequencing (Kemp, Smith, & Segal, 2012).

Written Expression Learning Disorder

This disability involves difficulty expressing thoughts in written or typed ways in a coherent manner. Their ability to communicate in writing is significantly below their age, educational experiences, and intelligence. It should not be diagnosed if an expressive language disorder exists, which is difficulty with spoken and written language. Written expression LD is different from dysgraphia (a handwriting condition) and reading LD, yet can coexist with either or both. Their written and typed work can be garbled, illogical, difficult to understand, and poorly organized. They may be excessively slow or avoidant of writing as well. These problems can also include spelling and grammatical errors. They can often print correctly and read well, but they struggle with expressing themselves in written or typed formats. A neuropsychologist or school psychologist could provide testing for this. Written expression problems may be a result of an expressive language disorder, reading learning disorder, or a visual processing disorder, so these conditions should be considered and explored.

OTHER NEURODEVELOPMENTAL CONDITIONS

Concentration Deficit Disorder (CDD)

This condition, also called sluggish cognitive tempo, appears similar to Inattentive ADHD and is often mistakenly diagnosed as this. Fewer clinicians seem to know about it. Some research has determined that while it frequently presents as Inattentive ADHD, it is really a separate disorder. An estimated 30 to 50 percent of individuals who appear to have Inattentive ADHD really have CDD (Barkley, 2010). In one survey, 59 percent of children who met criteria for ADHD (mostly the Inattentive type) also met criteria for CDD. They have few to no externalizing or ODD symptoms, but have greater depression and anxiety (Barkley, 2015). Because CDD is less researched and understood, it is more controversial. Some researchers believe that CDD is really Inattentive ADHD and not a separate condition. It has some relation to slow processing speed, but not everyone with CDD will have these deficits. CDD will impact children and teens more broadly than just processing speed (Braaten, 2014–2017).

Evaluation and Treatment

CDD is not in DSM-5. However, certain items have been utilized by researchers to detect this condition, which is important because it affects diagnosis and treatment. If at least 3 or more of the first 12 CDD checklist items in Chapter 14 are indicated with *Often,* this indicates clinical significance. If this is met, along with evidence of impairment in one or more life activities, then CDD could be diagnosed. While those with CDD may qualify for Inattentive ADHD, these checklist items are specific to CDD but not ADHD. Unhappiness, depression, anxiety, academic problems, and social problems tend to coexist with CDD (Barkley, 2015), so these and other conditions should be explored and treated if necessary. To help identify CDD, clinicians can also ask parents to complete the CBCL measure and teachers to complete the TRF measure (see Chapter 1) because they have normed sluggish cognitive tempo scales. Neuropsychologists aware of this condition will probably be the best qualified to diagnose it.

For treatment, fewer studies exist, and behavior management approaches seem helpful. While it is unclear if stimulants are effective, one study found the nonstimulant atomoxetine (Strattera) showed improvements (Barkley, 2015). Although somewhat different from ADHD, CDD can be treated with the ADHD*ology* Treatment Approach presented in Chapter one. Neurofeedback and Walsh's Advanced Nutrient Therapy may be helpful treatments as well.

Nonverbal Learning Disorder (NVLD)

This frequently undetected condition involves deficits within the right hemisphere of the brain. About one percent of the population has NVLD and it is equally prevalent in boys and girls. The term is a misnomer because it is not a specific LD. It does, however, impact lives more broadly than other LDs. Typically, due to superior verbal and rote memory abilities, their problems can be masked for years. Those with NVLD usually have many challenges, including behavioral, academic, social, motor, coordination, concentration, attention, and other neuropsychological deficits (Stewart, 2002).

This condition can coexist with true ADHD, but can also mimic it due to verbal impulsivity, excessive talking, attention, behavioral, distractibility, social, and handwriting difficulties. Academic problems with writing and math can become more evident in higher grades. Children and teens with NVLD are often odd, puzzling, and misdiagnosed. They often have good reading skills but experience writing and arithmetic problems, as well as decreased reading comprehension as they grow older. One of their greatest challenges can be frequent social problems with family and peers due to difficulties with understanding and interpreting nonverbal cues and information (Stewart, 2002).

Curiously, NVLD and Autism Spectrum Disorder-Level 1 (or ASD-1, formerly Asperger's disorder) have many similarities but are believed to differ in severity. These conditions can be conceptualized as existing on a continuum, with ASD-1 on one end and NVLD in the middle. Generally, the ASD-1 diagnosis is applied to children and adolescents with more severe social impairment and behavioral rigidity (Dinklage, n.d.). While these conditions can overlap with social skills, communication difficulties, and coordination problems, they do have differences. Unlike children and teens with ASD-1, most with NVLD typically have fewer difficulties with a limited range of interests, special skills or talents, and sensory processing issues. Additionally, individuals with Fetal Alcohol Spectrum Disorders can have NVLD-like symptoms.

Evaluation and Treatment

NVLD is not a DSM-5 condition, and at this time there are no official or standard criteria. While clinicians can use NVLD measures to screen for this condition, it should be determined by neuropsychological testing utilizing observations, history, and functioning (Dinklage, n.d.). The diagnostic discrimination between ADHD and NVLD can be challenging since their symptoms overlap, and ADHD and NVLD can coexist. Neuropsychologists should also distinguish between NVLD and ASD-1, and consider Fetal Alcohol Spectrum. Motor coordination problems should be assessed by occupational therapists because these children may have dyspraxia and/or sensory processing issues.

Treatment for NVLD can be more specialized, and like other neurodevelopmental conditions, it is managed and not cured. Key approaches include teaching self-observation, using language appropriately, and practicing taking someone else's perspective. A speech therapist may be needed to help them learn skills to become more socially engaged and appropriate with others, including conversational skills, looking another in the eyes when interacting, speaking clearly and with appropriate tone and volume, and choosing appropriate topics to discuss with others (Stewart, 2002). Individual or group therapies may assist with social skills, too. Occupational therapy may be helpful to address motor, coordination, and sensory issues. Family therapy can assist parents to better understand and manage the academic, organizational, and behavioral issues. As for any neurodevelopmental condition, individual therapy from experienced therapists can help address acceptance of the disability, self-esteem challenges, social problems, depression, and anxiety. Coexisting conditions should be addressed and treated as well. Psychiatric medications can be tried, but there are no specific medications for NVLD. Specialized school services, and accommodations, tutoring services, and/or educational therapy may all be helpful. Neurofeedback and Walsh's Advanced Nutrient Therapy may be helpful treatments as well.

Slow Processing Speed and Deficits

Processing speed is a brain function that determines how long it takes to perceive information, process it, and generate a response. Processing speed deficits cause individuals to move and react slower, think less quickly, experience memory difficulties, and take longer to initiate and complete tasks. Essentially, it is how long it takes to accomplish tasks and actions, and its impact can vary widely. Slower processing can be evident in verbal processing (or listening), visual processing, and motor speed. Boys are more affected than girls. Academic and social challenges, motor delays, and language impairments are more common with this condition. Slower processing speed is different from ADHD, but tends to coexist at a higher rate. One study of ages two to 20 with slow processing speed found 61 percent had ADHD (Braaten & Wolloughby, 2014).

While individuals can have processing speed difficulties without other conditions, it typically results from underlying disorders. The most common cause is ADHD, then LDs (including language-based and NVLD), and other neurodevelopmental conditions, such as autism spectrum disorders. One study found that of those with slow processing, 28 percent had a reading disorder, 20 percent had a math disorder, 20 percent had generalized anxiety disorder, 15 percent had autism, 6 percent had depression, and 15 percent had no other conditions. Children and teens can also experience transient processing speed deficits, and these usually result from anxiety, being worried or overwhelmed, depression, psychological stressors, or traumas (Braaten & Wolloughby, 2014). Transient presentations should have better prognoses. Processing speed weaknesses can occur in children and teens with above, below, or average intelligence abilities. However, these deficits will seem more apparent in those with average to above intelligence.

Concentration deficit disorder (CDD) has some overlap with slow processing speed, and most with CDD will have slow processing deficits. CDD will impact children and teens more broadly than just processing speed, and may cause lethargy, moving more slowly, and an overall mental fogginess or spacey presentation (Braaten, 2014–2017).

Evaluation and Treatment

Processing speed deficits can improve over time, but most will remain slower than peers, unless due to transient factors. Identifying the underlying conditions is paramount, and neurodevelopmental testing will be the best way (Braaten & Wolloughby, 2014). Diagnostically, it will be important to determine if the processing issues are primary or a result of depression, anxiety, traumas, or other stressors. As with other conditions, clinicians should try to identify which came first. Generally, slower processing not caused by depression, anxiety, or stressors will begin earlier in life and persist.

Treatment will require multiple approaches. It will be important to diagnose and address any underlying and coexisting conditions. If ADHD is the main source, ADHD medication may be a critical tool. If depression, anxiety, trauma, or stressors are the cause, treating these should facilitate improvement. Similar to treating ADHD, parents and children should understand the condition, and a disability perspective and management approach should be utilized at home and school. 504 or IEP school plans that provide accommodations and resources may be helpful or necessary. Family therapy and behavioral management approaches can be useful. Individual therapy may be important to treat associated depression, self-esteem, anxiety, trauma, bullying, and social skills difficulties. Lastly, neurofeedback and Walsh's Advanced Nutrient Therapy may be helpful treatments.

Dysgraphia

This is a handwriting disorder caused by a brain-functioning condition that affects the fine motor skills which impair the ability to print or write clearly, write properly within a space, or form letters correctly. The condition causes messy and slow handwriting (Somers, n.d.). Also called graphomotor skills dysfunction, it affects the neuromuscular systems of the hand and fingers to impair the mechanical skills required to produce written numbers, letters, and compositions. Handwriting is a complex skill that requires the integration of perceptual, cognitive, and visual-motor abilities to develop over time with practice. Handwriting styles tend to be established by about fourth grade, so handwriting difficulties after this time may be more chronic.

Like most conditions, dysgraphia exists on a continuum. It can commonly coexist with ADHD, and occurs more often in children and teens with ADHD-Combined than in Inattentive types. Those with dysgraphia can also have learning disorders, dyspraxia, deficient fine and/or gross motor skills. Several studies have found that children with Combined ADHD have handwriting difficulties involving irregular spatial arrangements, more unrecognizable letters, poor quality and inaccurate handwriting, faster and less efficient movements, inconsistent and variable writing size, and greater pen and pencil pressure when compared to peers. Another study found that the severity of the ADHD predicted worse handwriting outcomes (Langmaid et al., 2014).

Evaluation and Treatment

Some families may consider handwriting difficulties a low-level priority. However, it is best for clinicians to educate families that evaluations and treatments are available, particularly if the problems are significant. An experienced occupational therapist can assess dysgraphia, and some neuropsychologists may be able to evaluate this as well. Children with Combined ADHD can have gross and/or fine motor impairments that may impact handwriting. Handwriting problems can result from a visual processing disorder, dyspraxia, written expression learning disorder (Langmaid et al., 2014), as well as an immature symmetric tonic neck reflex (STNR), and these should be considered. Additionally, neurologists may be helpful if tremors or other neurological conditions exist.

For lesser handwriting difficulties not related to dyspraxia or other conditions, slowing down and holding the pencil position in a more traditional style can help, but can take time, patience, and practice. A special inexpensive pencil grip can be attached to pencils to help students hold a pencil in a better way. For those with more challenged fine motor abilities, occupational therapy services will be necessary. Additionally, special accommodations through 504 plans or IEPs, including school occupational therapy services and additional time for tests and assignments, may be needed. For significant handwriting problems, particularly for older students, tablets or laptop computers for written assignments at school and home may be an accommodation. Voice recognition software that types spoken words, and using graph and lined paper can be helpful. Finally, ADHD stimulant medications can improve dysgraphia for some. Neurofeedback may be helpful as well.

Speech and Articulation Deficits

Children and adolescents can have a range of speech and articulation problems. Articulation errors can be common in children up to age seven (Bellis, 2002). Speech problems and ADHD can coexist, and 10 to 54 percent of children with ADHD have been found to have speech impairments (Barkley, 2015, March 19a). Stuttering (or stammering) is a fluency disorder causing difficulty in the flow of speech and producing words and sounds smoothly due to pauses, prolonging sounds, or repetitions. Childhood apraxia of speech, also called verbal apraxia, is a motor speech disorder that causes difficulty with using the lips, tongue, jaw, and/or palate to create speech.

Verbal apraxia signs include a monotonous or flat voice, lack of speaking clearly, and speaking too loudly or softly. Children with speech deficits may also have articulation disorders which can include functional speech disorders, such as substituting /th/ for /s/ (or "lisping"). A phonological processing disorder is another speech condition involving the production of predictable pronunciation errors beyond the age when most children have stopped using them. Examples include production of the /w/ in place of /r/, or reduction of consonant clusters to a single consonant sound (such as the /sp/ in "spider" could be spoken as "pider" or the /pl/ in "plane" could be spoken as "pane").

Speech and articulation difficulties differ from expressive language problems. Speech deficits are caused by difficulties producing sounds and words adequately. Expressive language problems result from difficulties in expressing ideas in spoken language, while the ability to speak clearly is often not affected. However, speech problems and expressive language disorders can coexist, particularly with language delayed children. Family histories can increase the likelihood that these conditions exist.

Children and teens with speech problems have an increased risk for psychological and behavioral problems. This can be related to their difficulties expressing themselves and communicating adequately. They can have social problems, frustration, self-esteem, and behavioral difficulties. Also, pressured or rapid speech may result from ADHD hyperactivity. If this is impairing the child's ability to be understood and interact with others, then a speech evaluation referral should be made.

Evaluation and Treatment

Parents may not clearly recognize their child's speech deficits. Parents and peers tend to understand them better than others. Consequently, parents may report they do not hear the speech problems or minimize them, and this can affect their checklist responses. For most children, their speech should be understandable by age four, and most words should be spoken clearly and correctly by age seven. Clinicians should pay attention to their rate of speech (too fast or too slow), the volume (too soft or loud), articulation and clarity, and the quality of the speech. Clinicians often have a more objective ear, so if they cannot understand the child's speech (particularly over age 7), then a referral to a speech-language pathologist (or speech therapist) should occur.

A speech therapist outside the school district may provide the most objective evaluation, but school speech services may be the only option for some. The child should also receive a comprehensive hearing examination since hearing problems can affect speech and delays in language development. A speech therapist can also explore if the child has verbal apraxia. Additionally, it will be important to know if the child speaks other languages. If the child is struggling with speech in all languages, then this can suggest an underlying speech production condition. However, if the speech problems occur only in one language (particularly not their primary), then this may suggest a bilingual issue. If the child speaks another language, speech should be tested in the primary language.

Expressive Language Disorder

Children with this condition cannot communicate verbal or written thoughts at the same level as their peers. While they understand what they are trying to say, they struggle with creating sentences and expressing thoughts clearly in speech, sign language, writing, or typing. They can pronounce words properly, but will struggle with forming sentences coherently, using words and grammar properly, and may omit or substitute words incorrectly. They can understand speech adequately, have normal intelligence levels, and can understand complex spoken sentences. They tend to have smaller vocabularies and trouble organizing their sentences so others can easily understand them. They may point to things, rely on nonverbal gestures, or smile often to avoid using language. Some children may have difficulties with only more complicated ideas and thoughts, but are able to converse with more simple expressions (Davidson, n.d.). Injuries, illnesses, or other factors that impact hearing and auditory processing within the first three years of a child's life can have serious effects upon their language and learning abilities (Bellis, 2002). More than half of language and speech delays improve on their own for children under age three.

Symptoms vary drastically, exist on a continuum, and are based on the age of the child. There are two types of this disorder: developmental and acquired. Developmental expressive language disorders are much more common, have unknown causes, and appear when the child begins to talk. The acquired type typically occurs after a traumatic head injury or stroke. While the acquired type can occur at any age, it is more common in older individuals. Delays in language exist in 10 to 15 percent of children under three, and in 3 to 7 percent of school age children. This condition is two to five times more common in boys than girls (Davidson, n.d.).

Speech and articulation difficulties differ from expressive language problems. Speech deficits are caused by difficulties producing words and sounds adequately. Expressive language problems result from brain-functioning difficulties involving the expression of ideas, yet speech is typically clear. However, speech problems and expressive language disorders can coexist, and family histories for either or both are often present. Additionally, children can have expressive language problems and receptive language or auditory processing problems.

Those with this condition understand language better than they speak it. They also often experience difficulties with reading, writing, spelling, and other academic work. Children with more mild expressive language deficits may not show problems until school begins or when their school work is more advanced (Morales, 2012). Therefore, despite having adequate or higher intelligence, their academic performance may decrease over time, and they may be chronic underachievers. Due to their expression difficulties, these children and adolescents have more social problems. They are often reserved and withdrawn, and can become easily frustrated when communicating with others. When they are not understood they may even be aggressive, and can prefer to socialize with younger children. Due to their multiple challenges and stressors, they can experience self-esteem, depression, anxiety, and behavioral difficulties, particularly as they grow older and their problems continue.

Studies have found that up to half of preschoolers who received psychiatric services had undiagnosed language impairments (Beitchman et al., 2001). Speech and language disorders are frequent in children referred for psychological services, with estimates from 50 to 97 percent (Helland & Heimann, 2007). Expressive language disorder can cause ADHD-like symptoms that result from persistent frustration, social, academic, emotional and behavioral difficulties. However, 30 to 35 percent of those with ADHD have language disorders (Spruyt & Gozal, 2011), and 45 percent of children with ADHD also have some degree of language impairments. Also, children with language deficits and ADHD can have more academic problems than children with ADHD alone (Beitchman et al., 2001).

Evaluation and Treatment

A child suspected of having expressive language deficits should be referred to a speech-language pathologist. They may also require evaluations from other providers to determine if hearing deficits, auditory processing disorder, autistic spectrum, other neurodevelopmental conditions, or medical conditions exist. The speech therapist can determine if the child has apraxia of speech. If bilingual children struggle with verbal and written expression in multiple languages, this can suggest they have an underlying expressive language condition, as well as possible speech deficits. Treatment involves speech therapy with parents and teachers working together to integrate spoken language into the child's daily activities and play. With treatment, progress for the developmental type generally has a good prognosis, with most achieving normal expressive language abilities by high school.

The acquired form's prognosis will depend upon on the damage, and there is a range of recovery (Davidson, n.d.).

Receptive Language Disorder

This condition impairs the ability to understand language and is less common than expressive language disorder. Since auditory processing disorder (APD) can also cause these difficulties (see this condition in Chapter 7), receptive language disorder and APD can be difficult to differentiate. Speech and language pathologists diagnose and treat receptive language deficits, and may be able to help distinguish between these conditions, as will an audiologist. There is no checklist for this disorder due to its similarity to APD.

Tourette's Disorder and Tic Disorders

Tourette's disorder (TD) and tic disorders are conditions of the nervous system that cause the sudden repeated bodily movements, twitches, or vocal sounds that cannot be controlled. Tics are either motor or vocal. Motor tics are body movements, including blinking, shoulder shrugging, or arm jerking. Vocal tics involve sounds, and include humming, throat clearing, or yelling. Tics are also simple or complex. Simple tics involve just a few parts of the body, such as eye squinting or sniffing. Complex tics involve several different body parts and may involve patterns, such as head bobbing while arm jerking or jumping. Boys are affected three to five times more often than girls. TD typically occurs with other conditions (Centers for Disease Control and Prevention, 2014). In certain cases, symptoms can manifest up to six months after a streptococcal infection, or strep throat, often with mood fluctuations, severe anxiety, ODD, academic decline, sensory, eating and sleeping difficulties (called Pediatric Autoimmune Neuropsychiatric Disorders Associated with Streptococcal Infections or PANDAS) (PANDAS Network, 2017).

Those with TD have ADHD about 63 percent of the time (Centers for Disease Control and Prevention, 2015, August). For the diagnosis of Tourette's, motor and vocal tics must coexist, but persistent tic disorder requires either motor or vocal tics. TD symptoms usually begin between ages five to ten. Tics typically are worse during stressful or exciting times, and tend to improve when a person is calm or focused. The types and frequency of tics can change over time. Even though symptoms may fluctuate, the condition is chronic. In many cases, tics decrease during adolescence and early adulthood, sometimes disappear completely, yet may remain for life (Centers for Disease Control and Prevention, 2014).

Evaluation and Treatment

There is no single test for TD or tic disorders. Typically, neurologists or clinical neuropsychologists will diagnose these disorders. Although there are no cures, treatments are available to help manage the tics. Medication and behavioral treatments are available if tics cause stress, injury, pain, or interfere with school, work, or social functioning. However, many with TD have tics that do not interfere with their lives and do not need treatment (Centers for Disease Control and Prevention, 2014).

Giftedness

Giftedness is broadly defined as the ability to acquire and process information and solve problems faster than peers. It also describes children and teens with remarkable intelligence, talents, accomplishments, and creativity when compared to others their age. While giftedness is not a neurobehavioral disorder, children and teens who are gifted can have their own special challenges, including certain ADHD-like presentations. Additionally, some individuals can be gifted intellectually and/or be exceptionally talented in a certain area (such as reading, math, art, or music), while having significant weaknesses in other areas (Horowitz, n.d.). Giftedness can be defined in different ways, and school districts use various criteria for inclusion in gifted programs. In the past, an IQ score of 130 and above was the standard single criteria for schools, but some schools now use cutoff IQ scores of 120 or 125, along with other measures and criteria.

Because school work may be too easy and less stimulating, gifted children and teens risk being underchallenged academically and may become bored, frustrated, and exhibit behavioral problems. They can also display other ADHD-like traits, including social problems, inattention, oppositional tendencies, and struggles with criticism. Some may have high energy and difficulties with focusing or self-control. Others may act out in school because they are not able to express themselves adequately, as in strict classrooms or with teachers who don't engage them at their level. Gifted children and adolescents can have coexisting ADHD, learning disorders, autism spectrum disorders, and other conditions (National Association for Gifted Children and Supporting Emotional Needs of the Gifted, 2007). For some gifted children with true ADHD, their advanced abilities may mask their ADHD, while their attentional problems and impulsivity can lower their test scores and academic performance. Consequently, their ADHD and/or giftedness may not be detected. Alternatively, clinicians may pathologize gifted behavior because their drive, intensity, curiosity, perfectionism, and impatience can be mistaken for ADHD (Neihart, 2004).

Evaluation and Treatment

Children and teens with suspected giftedness can be referred to a clinical psychologist for an intellectual assessment. Clinicians should also explore if there are other coexisting disorders that may be masked or overshadowed by the giftedness. If possible, placement in accelerated learning environments should be considered. Accommodations for their strengths and weaknesses, as well as 504s or IEPs, may be necessary. Educating the child and family about giftedness can be highly therapeutic and may improve understandings of their quirky behaviors and personality issues.

Intellectual Disability

ADHD can occur in children and teens with borderline to mild intellectual disability (ID). In the general population, IDs occur at a rate of 7 to 10 percent, while ADHD has been found in 18 to 40 percent of children who have ID. Yet research has confirmed that the presence or absence of ADHD is not related to the underlying existence of the ID (Pliska, 2015). The upper IQ range for a mild ID would be a full-scale IQ score of about 65 to 75. However, the differentiation between ADHD and mild ID can be challenging because individuals with lower IQs can have ADHD-like symptoms. Those with mild IDs and below average IQs can have coexisting conditions (particularly conduct problems) and may struggle with school work, social problems, learning new skills, and other everyday tasks. These tasks may be difficult or overwhelming, and thus create boredom, frustration, and behavioral problems. They are often labeled as "slow learners" by schools. Children suspected of lower intelligence and ADHD should be referred to a clinical psychologist for testing to assess their intellectual functioning and determining ADHD. Stimulant medications have been found to work effectively for children and teens with ADHD and ID.

Autism Spectrum Disorder-Level 1
(ASD-1; Formerly Asperger's Syndrome)

Autism spectrum disorder (ASD) is a group of neurodevelopment disorders that cause social impairments, communication difficulties, as well as restrictive, repetitive, ritualistic, and stereotyped patterns of behavior. While ASDs are diagnosed by a common set of behaviors, they are complex and not well understood. Individuals can have ADHD and the mildest ASD, called ASD-Level 1 (formerly called Asperger's syndrome). ADHD is not typically diagnosed with more moderate to severe forms of autism. ASDs are present from infancy or early childhood. Although early diagnosis using standardized screening by age two is the goal, many are not detected until later in childhood, particularly those with higher functioning ASD. Children with ASD exist on a continuum of impairment and have a range of communication and behavioral difficulties. Those with severe conditions are greatly disabled and require extensive support for basic daily living activities (National Institute of Neurological Disorders and Stroke, 2015). About one in 59 children have ASD, and it is four times as prevalent in males than females (Centers for Disease Control and Prevention, 2018, November). Those who are female, African American, and Latino tend to be under-diagnosed with this condition.

ASD-1 is considered to be the mildest and highest functioning type of ASD. It is often not recognized before age five or six because language development is normal, but speech may be unusual. Individuals with ASD often have problems with socialization and communication that continue into adulthood (National Institute of Neurological Disorders & Stroke, 2015). ASD-1 is more common than lower functioning autism, and the symptoms range from mild to severe. Although children with ASD-1 share some similarities with more severe forms of autism, they typically have better functioning. In addition, individuals with ASD-1 generally have normal intelligence and near-normal language development, although they may develop problems communicating as they become older (Asperger's Syndrome, 2015).

Children with ASD-1 may have speech with a lack of rhythm, odd inflection, or monotone pitch. They often struggle with modulating their vocal volume, and may have to be reminded to speak softly in libraries or movie theaters. Unlike the withdrawal from the world seen in more severe autism, children with ASD-1 are isolated because of their poor social skills and narrow interests. These children will gather and share enormous factual information about their favorite subjects, but the conversations may seem like random collections of facts with no points or conclusions. They may approach others but can make normal conversation difficult by their eccentric behaviors and exclusive focus on narrow interests (National Institute of Neurological Disorders & Stroke, 2015). Many with ASD-1 are highly active in early childhood, but some may have delays with motor skills and can struggle with sports, bike riding, or catching a ball. They are often awkward and poorly coordinated, and can have a walk that appears either stilted or bouncy.

The newer diagnosis social (pragmatic) communication disorder (SCD) is related to ASD-1 because some children in the past who would have qualified for autism can now receive this disorder. While those with SCD have social communication difficulties similar to individuals with ASD-1, they lack the criteria of repetitive behaviors and/or restricted interests to qualify for a diagnosis of autism. Individuals with SCD can struggle with interacting with others in new situations and making socially appropriate "small talk" (Elder, 2018). Within the CDASS checklist for ASD-1 there is a section titled "Difficulties with Communication and Social Skills" that has symptoms applicable for both SCD and ASD-1.

Research has indicated that about 10 percent of those with ASD also have ADHD (Spruyt & Gozal, 2011). ASDs can share a number of ADHD-like symptoms, including difficulties with frustration tolerance, emotional outbursts, self-calming abilities, coordination and motor functioning, social skills, focusing, and impulsivity. Consequently, higher functioning ASD can be misdiagnosed as ADHD. Although speech development may be normal or somewhat delayed, difficulties can arise in the social use of language (Costello, n.d.). Other common coexisting conditions include tic, depressive, and anxiety disorders, OCD (National Institute of Neurological Disorders & Stroke, 2015), and sensory processing conditions.

Evaluation and Treatment

If ASD-1 is suspected, the child or adolescent should be referred for an autism neurodevelopmental assessment, and this provider would determine if ADHD is present too. Because ASD-1 and non-verbal learning disorders are so alike, there are similar items on both CDASS checklists, and experienced clinicians may be needed for differentiation. To be diagnosed with ASD-1, a child must have a combination of symptoms and significant social functioning challenges. Speech and occupational therapists should also evaluate impairments and need for these services. Occupational therapists can also assess and treat sensory processing conditions that commonly coexist with ASD.

A key aspect in differentiating between ADHD and ASD is to determine whether there are executive functioning problems or more fundamental developmental deficits. While children with ADHD can struggle socially, children with ADHD without autism have more typical social development, such as taking turns when playing with others, recognizing their name when called, imaginative play, appropriate facial expressions of emotions, humor, and empathy. Children with ADHD may not be able to persist with turn-taking play, but understand it. For children with autism, these traits can be missing and can be helpful indicators (Marner, n.d.).

After the diagnosis has been determined, typical treatments for ASD include behavioral modification and therapies provided by an experienced therapist or Board-Certified Behavioral Analyst (BCBA). However, this may be unnecessary for milder ASD-1. Other services include creating schedules and lists for structure, physical exercise, medical management by a developmental pediatrician, appropriate school services and accommodations, occupational therapy for sensory issues and motor/coordination issues, and speech therapy for speech and communication issues. Family therapy can be helpful to teach parents about ASD, help facilitate acceptance, and use behavioral management skills. While medication will not treat the condition itself, it may help with certain symptoms. The atypical neuroleptics Abilify, Seroquel, and Risperdal can be effective medications for the ASD symptoms of motor restlessness, sleep disturbances, and repetitive behaviors, but some do not require any psychiatric medications (Costello, n.d.).

For those with ASD-1 and ADHD, effective treatments can include ADHD medications, family therapy focused on parenting skills and behavior management skills, individual therapy to better understand and address social and coexisting issues, and any of the above stated ASD treatments (Costello, n.d.). Finally, neurofeedback and Walsh's Advanced Nutrient Therapy can be helpful treatments for autism spectrum disorders, with or without ADHD.

REFERENCES

American Psychiatric Association. (reviewed 2016, March). Reviewed by Parekh, Ranna. *What is specific learning disorder?* Retrieved from https://www.psychiatry.org/patients-families/specific-learning-disorder/what-is-specific-learning-disorder

Asperger's Syndrome. (reviewed 2015, May 12). Reviewed by Amita Shroff. Retrieved from www.webmed.com/brain/autism/mental-health-asperges-syndrome

Barkley, R. (2010). *Taking charge of adult ADHD.* New York: Guilford Press.

Barkley, R. (2015). Concentration deficit disorder (sluggish cognitive tempo). In R. Barkley (Ed.), *Attention deficit hyperactivity disorder: A handbook for diagnosis and treatment* (4th ed., pp. 435–454). New York: Guilford Press.

Barkley, R. (2015, March 19a). *ADHD: Nature, course, outcomes, and comorbidity.* Retrieved from www.continuingedcourses.net/active/courses/course003.php

Barkley, R. (2015, March 19b). *ADHD in Children: Diagnosis and assessment.* Retrieved from www.continuingedcourses.net/active/courses/course004.php

Beitchman, J. H., Wilson, B., Johnson, C. J., Atkinson, L., Young, A., Adalf, E., & Douglas. L. (2001). Fourteen-year follow-up of speech-language-impaired and control children: Psychiatric outcome. *Journal of the Academy of Child and Adolescent Psychiatry, 40,* 75–82.

Bellis, T. J. (2002). *When the brain can't hear.* New York: Pocket Books.

Boyse, K. (November 2012). *Non-Verbal learning disability (NLD or NVLD): Your child: University of Michigan health system.* Retrieved from http://www.med.umich.edu/yourchild/topics/nld.htm

Braaten, E. (2014-2017). *What's the difference between sluggish cognitive tempo and slow processing speed?* Retrieved from https://www.understood.org/en/learning-attention

-issues/child-learning-disabilities/information-processing-issues/whats-the-difference
-between-sluggish-cognitive-tempo-and-slow-processing-speed

Braaten, E., & Willoughby, B. (2014). *Bright kids who can't keep up.* New York: Guilford Press.

Centers for Disease Control and Prevention. (2014, August 8). *Facts about Tourette's Syndrome.* Retrieved from www.cdc.gov/ncbdd/tourette/facts.html

Centers for Disease Control and Prevention. (2015, August 10). *Other concerns & conditions* (related to Tourette syndrome). Retrieved from www.cdc.gov/ncbdd/tourette/otherconcerns.html

Centers for Disease Control and Prevention. (2018, November 15). *Autism spectrum disorder (ASD)–Data & statistics.* Retrieved from https://www.cdc.gov/ncbddd/autism/data.html

Clark, A. (2014–1018). *Educational therapy: What you need to know.* Retrieved from https://www.understood.org/en/learning-attentioin-issues/treatments-approaches/therapies/what-you-need-to-know-about-educational-therapy

Coordinated Campaign for Learning Disabilities. (1997). *Early warning signs of learning disabilities.* Retrieved from http://www.ldonline.org/artcle/226/

Costello, E. (n.d.). *Is it Asperger's Syndrome or ADHD?* Retrieved on 06/27/14 from http://www.additudemag.com/adhd/article/7952.html

Davidson, T. (n.d.). *Expressive language disorder.* Encyclopedia of Mental Disorders. Retrieved on 09/10/12 from http://www.minddisorders.com/Del-Fi/Expressive-language-disorder.html

Dinklage, D. (n.d.). *Aspergers disorder and non-verbal learning disabilities: How are these two disorders related to each other?* Retrieved on 09/05/14 from www.aane.org/asperger_resources/articles/miscellaneous/asperger_nonverbal_learnin...

Drummond, K. (2005–2007). *About reading disabilities, learning disabilities, and reading difficulties.* Retrieved from http://www.readingrockets.org/article/about-reading-disabilities-learning-disabilities-and-reading-difficulties

Elder, L. (2018, September 5). *Social communication disorder: Parents seek guidance.* Retrieved from https://www.autismspeaks.org/expert-opinion/social-communication-disorder-parents-seek-guidance-0

Garnett, K. (1998). *Math learning disabilities.* Retrieved from http://www.ldonline.org/article/Math_Learning_Disabilities

Helland, W., & Heimann, M. (2007). Assessment of pragmatic language impairment in children referred to psychiatric services: A pilot study of the children's communication checklist in a Norwegian sample. *Logopedics Phoniatrics Vocology, 32*(1), 23–30. https://doi.org/10.1080/14015430600712056

Horowitz, S. H. (n.d.). *Giftedness and learning disabilities.* Retrieved on 11/15/12 from www.ncld.org/types-learning-disabilities/adhd-related/giftedness/giftedness-learning-disabilities

Hurford, D. M. (1998). *To read or not to read.* New York: A Lisa Drew Book/Scribner.

Kemp, G., Smith, M., & Segal, J. (2012, July). *Learning disabilities in children.* Retrieved from http://www.helpguide.org/mental/learning_disabilities.htm

Kutscher, M. L. (2014). *Kids in the syndrome mix of ADHD, LD, autism spectrum, Tourettes, anxiety, and more!* (2nd ed.). London: Jessica Kingsley.

Langmaid, R. A., Papadopoulos, N., Johnson, B. P., Phillips, J. G., & Rinehart, N. J. (2014). Handwriting in children with ADHD. *Journal of Attention Disorders, 18*(6), 504-510.

Marner, K. (n.d.). *Is it ADHD or autism? Or both?* Retrieved on 06/27/14 from www.additudemag.com/adhd/article/10236.html

Morales, S. (2012). *Expressive language disorder.* Retrieved from http://www.child speech.net/u_iv_h.html

National Association for Gifted Children and Supporting Emotional Needs of the Gifted. (2007). *Is my child gifted?* Retrieved from www.sengifted.org/wp-content /uploads/2011/09/Is-my-child-gifted-brochure-2007.pdf

National Institute of Neurological Disorders and Stroke. (2015, November 03). *Asperger's syndrome fact sheet.* Retrieved from http://www.ninds.nih.gov/disorders /Asperger/detail_asperger.htm

Neihart, M. (2004). *Gifted children with attention deficit hyperactivity disorder.* Retrieved from www.ldonline.org/article/5631

Nicolson, R. I., & Fawcett, A. J. (2008). *Dyslexia, learning and the brain.* Cambridge, MA: MIT Press.

Non-Verbal Learning Disabilities. (2001-2002). Excerpted from the LDA of California and UC Davis M.I.N.D. Institute "Q.U.I.L.T.S." Calendar 2001–2002. Retrieved from www.ldaamerica.org/types-of-learning-disabilities/non-verbal -learning-disabilities/

PANDAS Network. (2017). *What is PANDAS?* Retrieved from https://www.pandas network.org/understanding-pandaspans/what-is-pandas/

Parker, H. (2000). *Problem solver guide for students with ADHD.* Plantation, FL: Specialty Press.

PsychCentral. (reviewed 2010, October 16). Reviewed by John M. Grohol. *Expressive language disorder.* Retrieved from http://psychcentral.com/disorders /sx41.htm

Silver, L. (2006). *The Misunderstood child: Understanding and coping with your child's learning disabilities* (4th ed.). New York: Three Rivers Press.

Somers, L. (n.d.). *Learning disabilities: Recognizing dysgraphia in children with ADHD.* Retrieved on 08/20/12 from http://www.additudemag.com/adhd/arti cle/print/725.html

Spruyt, K., & Gozal, D. (2011, April). Sleep disturbances in children with attention-deficit/hyperactivity disorder. *Expert Review of Neurotherapeutics, 11*(4), 565–577. doi: 10.1586/ern.11.7

Stewart, K. (2002). *Helping a child with nonverbal learning disorder or Asperger's syndrome.* Oakland, CA: New Harbinger.

Tanguay, P. (1998). *Nonverbal learning disorders: What to look for.* Retrieved on from http://www.ldonline.org/article/Nonverbal_Learning_Disorders%3A_What_To _Look_For

Tannock, R., & Brown, T. E. (2009). ADHD with language and/or learning disorders in children and adolescents. In T. E. Brown (Ed.), *ADHD comorbidities: Handbook for ADHD complications in children and adults* (pp. 189–231). Arlington, VA: American Psychiatric.

Tennessee Association for the Gifted. (n.d.). *The bright child vs. the gifted learner.* Retrieved on 09/05/14 from http://www.tag-tenn.org/comparison

Weyandt, L. L., & Gudmundsdottir, B. G. (2015). Developmental and neuropsychological deficits in children with ADHD (116–139). In R. Barkley (Ed.), *Attention deficit hyperactivity disorder: A handbook for diagnosis and treatment* (4th ed., pp. 116–138). New York: Guilford Press.

Chapter 7

SENSORY PROCESSING
AND MOTOR DISORDERS

OVERVIEW OF SENSORY PROCESSING DISORDERS

Sensory Processing Disorder (SPD), formerly known as Sensory Integration Dysfunction, is an umbrella term for children and adults who have neurological difficulties in the ways their brains receive, organize, and use sensory information. Those with SPD can misinterpret everyday sensory information and their responses become inappropriate. They can feel bombarded by this information, may seek out intense sensory experiences, or can be unaware of sensations that others perceive. They can also have sensory-motor symptoms of a weak body, coordination and other motor skills deficits. SPD affects 5 to 16 percent of children and symptoms will vary greatly depending on the sense affected and its severity ("What is SPD?", n.d.).

Miller, Nielsen, and Schoen (2012) stated there are three main types of sensory processing disorders:

1. *Sensory Modulation Problems* involve difficulties in regulating responses to sensations. There are three subtypes:
   A. *Sensory Underresponsivity* (or underprocessing sensory problems) is a condition where individuals are not sensitive enough and need more than normal sensory input.
   B. *Sensory Overresponsivity* (or overprocessing sensory problems) is a condition where individuals are too sensitive and overreact to sensory stimulation.
   C. *Sensory Seeking* is a condition where individuals intensely crave sensory experiences and process stimuli with interference (or "white noise").

2. *Sensory-Based Motor Problems* includes dypraxia and postural disorder, and involve positioning bodies in unusual ways, bodily weakness, awkwardness, difficulty in conceiving an action, problems planning and executing movements, and delays with gross and fine motor skills.
3. *Sensory Discrimination Problems* cause difficulties distinguishing one sensation from another, as well as distinguishing types or locations of sensory data. This includes position/movement and interoception (feelings from within the body that include pain, temperature, itch, sensual touch, muscular and visceral sensations, vasomotor activity, hunger, thirst, and 'air hunger').

While it is possible for a child to have only one type, a combination disorder of symptoms from two or three of the sensory modulation disorder subtypes is more likely. In one study, 34 percent of children with SPDs had two subtypes, and 25 percent had all three. Another study found that for children with sensory modulating, sensory-based motor, and sensory discrimination conditions, 30 percent had one, 43 percent had two, and 27 percent had all three (Miller, 2007). Additionally, clinicians should expect to see SPD combinations that do not fit neatly within the SPD conditions.

While the exact causes of SPDs have not been determined, research has suggested a number of potential factors ("What is SPD?", n.d.). These include nervous system disturbances, neurotransmitter and specific brain-functioning abnormalities, genetics, premature birth, birth traumas, heavy metal exposure, and inadequate care in orphanages. SPDs can occur on its own, or along with autism, ADHD, or other conditions. It presents on a continuum from mild to severe, and symptoms can fluctuate (Beil & Peske, 2009).

Sensory defensiveness occurs when children with sensory integration problems overreact to sensory stimulation due to their excessively aroused nervous systems. The sensory defensiveness causes unusual and difficult reactions. Children may become highly reactive, demanding, rigid, cry easily, distracted, inattentive, aggressive, irritable, avoidant, withdrawn, and intolerant of daily tasks. Additionally, they can experience disorganization, poor balance and coordination, struggles with transitions, problems calming down after physical activities, or desire excessive levels of activity ("Signs, Symptoms and Background Information on Sensory Integration," n.d.). Children with sensory defensiveness can also exhibit significant behavioral and ODD-like difficulties, as well as increased ADHD symptoms for those with true ADHD.

SPDs can also cause various eating difficulties, including strong aversions or desires for specific smells, textures, tastes, colors, appearances and temperatures of food, as well as oral-motor and fine motor feeding skill deficits. As result, only limited foods may be tolerated. Families with children or teens with these difficulties may thus experience daily battles with meals and nutritional limitations.

Some children with SPD can mask their problems by avoiding activities that could expose their deficits, and/or may gravitate to activities in which they excel. As a result, their SPD can be less obvious or is minimized for a time. Also, diagnosis and treatment can be delayed because SPD can resemble other conditions, including ADHD, and milder SPD conditions can be mistaken for personality quirks. Sometimes a child may be suffering from an immature sensory system and will outgrow the problems, while others will continue to experience difficulties through adulthood (Scherer, n.d.).

The difficulties those with SPDs experience can be highly frustrating, stressful, and draining. These challenges can cause these children to seem odd, unpredictable, controlling, emotional, and highly reactive or even explosive. Parents and teachers can be confused and overwhelmed by their range of behavioral and social difficulties. Also, they may not be able to articulate what they are experiencing or their problems. Older children can particularly struggle with feeling weird and different, which may drain their self-esteem and confidence. Further, they may experience secondary developmental issues from their reluctance to participate in normal activities and social experiences.

Since these conditions are confusing and unclear, it is essential that parents and clinicians understand SPD challenges and issues so they can best manage and treat them. Several excellent resource books for parents include *The Out-of-Sync Child* by Carol Stock Kranowitz, *Raising a Sensory Smart Child* by Lindsey Biel and Nancy Peske, and *Sensational Kids* by Lucy Jane Miller. Depending on which SPDs exist, the main treatments are occupational therapy (OT), vision therapy from behavioral optometrists for visual processing disorder, and listening therapy from audiologists for auditory processing disorder. These provide specialized exercises, activities, and therapies that help retrain the senses. Providers can also prescribe sensory diets of activities to be practiced at home to neurologically retrain the senses over time, environmental modifications, school services, and accommodations. Some schools have OTs that can provide treatment as part of their individual education programs (IEPs). Certain OTs, dietitians, and other feeding specialists can address feeding and food difficulties. QEEG brain mapping from neurofeedback providers may assist diagnostically by suggesting which SPD conditions may exist, and neurofeedback can be a helpful treatment for all SPDs. Detecting and treating coexisting conditions remains imperative as well.

SENSORY PROCESSING DISORDERS AND ADHD

Sensory deficits in children with ADHD are more common than in children without ADHD. One study showed that 64 percent of children with ADHD demonstrated a sensory processing condition, and the three most prevalent sensory processing conditions were tactile defensiveness (82 percent), poor antigravity (vestibular) difficulties (81 percent), and dyspraxia (69 percent) (Huecker & Kinnealey, 1998). Another study of children with either ADHD or SPD found that 40 percent had symptoms of both (Scherer, n.d.). Children with ADHD and significant sensory problems are more likely to exhibit more aggression and delinquency (Ghanizadeh, 2011).

In addition to their high prevalence with ADHD, SPDs can also cause ADHD-like symptoms that can easily be mistaken for ADHD. Therefore, SPDs are an important and challenging area to explore in ADHD evaluations. Children and teens with SPD may experience significant inattention, excessive motor activity, restlessness, fidgeting, and self-control problems, as well as behavioral, mood, frustration-tolerance, emotional self-regulation, self-soothing, anxiety, stress, irritability, self-esteem, and social difficulties. Younger children are particularly vulnerable to manifesting hyperactivity, behavioral problems, and irritability. The hyperactivity and behavioral problems may also be a result of their vestibular, proprioceptive and other sensory seeking conditions, a reaction to sensory over-sensitivities, and/or automatic ways of managing chronic discomfort.

Amen (2013) stated that some with ADHD can have distractibility problems, causing sensory hypersensitivities which stop them from suppressing surrounding sights, sounds, and tactile sensations. This can cause them to be highly reactive to their environment. When they take ADHD medications, the underlying neurobiological distractibility can balance and the sensory issues may improve. However, those with SPDs without true ADHD will not improve or can even worsen on ADHD medications.

Some SPDs will be difficult to differentiate from ADHD without proper sensory processing evaluations, even if sensory screening measures are used. However, SPD measures and checklists can be helpful to determine if OT evaluations are needed. Additionally, these OTs can be asked to specifically determine if the child or teen has sensory processing difficulties, ADHD, or both. However, the accuracy of this discrimination will depend on the evaluator's experience and diagnostic abilities. Clinicians may identify when the child has attentional problems, and what preceded these difficulties. Attention and learning problems that occur only during sensory episodes will be more suggestive of SPD. While sometimes difficult to identify, parents and clinicians can explore the sensory triggers to understand and manage them. Examples of these are dressing, brushing teeth or hair, playing outside, climbing stairs, or when picked up.

One way to help determine if SPD conditions truly exist is to begin OT and observe which symptoms improve. If a child has decreased symptoms immediately after treatment sessions or sensory diet exercises, this could suggest SPD. If the SPD symptoms decrease but ADHD symptoms remain, this could suggest they have both conditions. A neurodevelopmental assessment may also help to distinguish these two conditions. Sometimes an indirect, but helpful, way to differentiate between SPDs and Combined ADHD is to try several stimulant medications at sufficient doses. A lack of reduction of hyperactivity and impulsivity symptoms, or if they worsen, may suggest that the child has sensory processing deficits without true ADHD. Additionally, if there is partial improvement, this may suggest that the child has both. Diagnostic assessments conducted over time and various treatments may help clarify the conditions further. Finally, Scherer (n.d.) reported it is important to distinguish between ADHD and SPD because the treatments differ. ADHD medication and behavioral management approaches will not improve or effectively treat SPD.

SENSORY PROCESSING DISORDERS

Auditory Processing Disorder (APD)

Central Auditory Processing Disorder is a brain impairment that improperly processes incoming auditory signals. APD creates intermittent inabilities to process verbal information and difficulties understanding spoken language. It can negatively impact many areas of life, including social and academic functioning. Most children with this disability have normal hearing and their auditory difficulties will not be detected during routine hearing tests (Schminsky & Baran, 1999). APD causes difficulties with what is heard, not hearing. Students with APD can pass school hearing screenings because these only measure the detection of sounds, but not the discrimination among sounds or comprehension of speech (Bellis, 2002). Listening is a highly complex process of hearing and processing sounds. Sound consists of frequency, pitch, duration, intensity, and a location source. Individuals with APD have difficulties integrating these qualities and can expend great energy blocking out sounds that are distracting, stressful, or overwhelming (Biel & Peske, 2009). APD is comprised of three separate conditions that frequently overlap: sound discrimination, auditory memory, and language processing problems (Scherer, 2004).

Children and adults with APD struggle to understand the sounds of language, particularly when background noise is present. While most individuals instantly process and interpret what is heard, those with APD scramble sounds. "Tell me how a tiger and lion are alike" to a child with APD may sound like "Tell me how lint and tanger are like" (The Understood Team, 2014). Those with APD can recognize speech in ideal listening situations. However, because they are not always in ideal listening circumstances, they can misunderstand information because fewer words may be perceived and the words they hear may be garbled and unclear. They may guess to fill in their processing gaps and may not know they misunderstood.

Many clinicians are unaware of APD and its symptoms. The medical profession only started seriously studying APD in children in 1977, and there is still much to learn. Although some experts estimate that boys are twice as likely as girls to have APD, this is still unclear (The Understood Team, 2014). APD is believed to occur mostly in young children and older adults (Matson, 2005). It is estimated that 3 to 5 percent of school-age children have APD. Some children diagnosed with APD appear to eventually outgrow it. However, a "wait and see" approach is not recommended, and due to the brain's neuroplasticity, time is critical for evaluations and treatment (Kelly, 2004). APD can also coexist with speech and language disorders or delays, LD, ADHD, and emotional difficulties (Schminsky & Baran, 1999).

While the cause of APD is not known in most cases, APD can be impacted by a number of influences, including prenatal alcohol and cigarette exposure, malnutrition, chronic ear infections, low birth weight, premature birth, brain infections, Lyme disease, head injuries, and exposure to heavy metals such as mercury or lead. Because the auditory pathways do not mature until age 10 to 12, significant progress can be made with early intervention (Scherer, 2004). While less common, prolonged middle ear infections with fluctuating hearing loss can lead to auditory problems resulting in language and learning delays long after the middle ear disorder is treated. This suggests that children with histories of chronic colds, sinus problems, and middle ear infections should be carefully monitored for their auditory, language, and learning abilities (Matson, 2005). Children who experienced frequent middle ear infections (perhaps more than three a year, especially during the first several years) are at a higher risk for developing APD, along with speech and language problems.

Those with APD can be easily misdiagnosed with ADHD because both disorders cause attentional and other similar deficits (The Understood Team, 2014). Also, since ADHD is much more commonly known, APD symptoms are frequently misdiagnosed as ADHD. APD can mimic ADHD-like problems, such as difficulties understanding and recalling spoken information, maintaining focus while other sounds are present, organizational problems, following multistep directions, auditory attentional deficits, verbal comprehension problems, social and interpersonal difficulties, and difficulties with reading and spelling. Also, hyperactivity, impulsivity, poor frustration tolerance, behavioral and emotional symptoms can result from the persistent stresses and overwhelming difficulties that APD can cause.

These children frequently have problems developing reading, spelling, and writing skills, which obviously impact academics. The building blocks for reading are learning vowels and developing phonemic awareness and these can be particularly difficult for these children. Research suggests that auditory processing deficits can be a contributing factor for dyslexia. Children with APD may not speak clearly, and can drop the endings of syllables and words, as well as confuse similar sounds. (The Understood Team, 2014).

While APD impairs the ability to understand language, a receptive language disorder can also cause this. Unfortunately, it can be difficult to discriminate between these two. Speech therapists diagnose and treat receptive language deficits, and some may be able to differentiate between APD and receptive language disorder.

Evaluation and Treatment

There are APD screening checklists and measures that can be completed by parents and teachers that may be useful to suggest when APD evaluations should occur. All children suspected of APD should first be referred to a special pediatric audiologist for hearing and APD testing since it will not be detected with standard hearing tests. While pediatricians can provide basic hearing tests, only audiologists can provide comprehensive hearing evaluations, and some audiologists can also provide specialized APD screenings and testing. Bellis (2002) shared that even transient, fluctuating, or the mildest hearing loss should be evaluated and addressed before APD testing occurs. Once hearing testing is completed, then APD screenings and full evaluations can proceed. APD screenings by audiologists can be conducted when a child is five to seven or older. If the child is at least seven and fails the APD screenings, then a full evaluation by an audiologist would be appropriate. If a child has APD symptoms, clinicians can inquire about the prior number of chronic cold, sinus problems, and ear infections (Kelly, 2004). Three or more ear infections in the first three years should trigger careful monitoring of speech, language, and auditory processing abilities. Also, children with frequent ear infections should receive a tympanogram (ear drum test) from an audiologist (Biel & Peske, 2009).

While audiologists can evaluate and diagnose APD, not all have this special training. Some OTs may evaluate for APD as well. It can be difficult to diagnose APD in children before age seven or eight (The Understood Team,

2014). Audiologists with APD testing experience may not exist in more remote areas, and not all audiologists in public schools have this special training (Bellis, 2002). Also, not all health insurance companies cover APD testing. Full APD testing conducted by audiologists consists of extended tests that require children to identify words heard with background noise, or spoken very slowly. Some believe that an APD evaluation should include an evaluation from a speech-language pathologist to assess the child's receptive and expressive language abilities, particularly because receptive language deficits can present identically as APD (University of Virginia Speech-Language-Hearing Center, 2012).

While some have suggested that a true diagnosis of APD cannot be fully determined until age 12, younger children with APD symptoms should still receive audiologist referrals (Ciocci, 2002). Ideally, when referring for APD testing, the child should be at least seven or eight years old, should be tested in their primary language, has passed a hearing screening within the past year, has an IQ score of 85 or higher, has had testing for learning disorders, ADHD has been evaluated, has had a recent speech and language evaluation that particularly explored listening skills, and has intelligible speech. The APD testing can be less accurate if any of these are not present. One author suggested that APD evaluations should be conducted after hearing, speech-language, learning disorder, and ADHD evaluations are completed, and the APD testing should not be done concurrently (Kent, 2002). Another author would not provide APD testing until a child or teen had evaluations of their language, cognition, and academic abilities, as well as other current difficulties (Bellis, 2002). Additionally, those with APD can have large differences between verbal and performance IQs (with lower verbal IQs). Hearing loss can coexist and complicate APD, but often APD will exist without peripheral hearing loss.

APD testing is not perfect, and sometimes the results can be inconclusive or difficult to interpret in children with ADHD, language problems, lower IQs (Kutscher, 2014), or other significant neurodevelopmental conditions such as nonverbal learning disorders or autism. Because ADHD, auditory processing deficits, and receptive language difficulties can appear so similar, clinicians can struggle with this diagnostic discrimination. The auditory processing testing can last one to two hours, involves many different listening tasks requiring focus and concentration, and ADHD can interfere with this process. For many with ADHD-like presentations, an ADHD evaluation should probably come first. ADHD evaluators should share their concerns about the possible presence of APD with audiologists, and can discuss the findings to attempt to determine which conditions exist.

ADHD medication may be attempted if there continues to be uncertainty. Those with true Combined ADHD, but not APD, should improve.

Receptive language testing by speech therapists may be helpful to determine if receptive language disorder exists and not APD, and this testing should be considered during the diagnostic process, particularly if ambiguity persists. QEEG brain mapping from neurofeedback providers may assist with diagnostic discrimination challenges as well.

Treating APD consists of treatment approaches, using methods of compensating, and managing the listening environment (Bellis, 2002). Treatment and management for APD should be provided by experienced audiologists. In general, management approaches will include augmenting auditory perceptual skills, enhancing language and cognitive resources, and improving the quality of the auditory signal (Schminky & Baran, 1999). Accommodation is one of the strategies used to manage this condition at home and school. Certain strategies can be basic but helpful. Some children can benefit from background music, while others benefit from a lack of noise and music in their environments.

At school, children may need their APD to be officially addressed in an IEP, and may require classroom modifications and other special education school services (Bellis, 2002). The types of classroom management and remediation approaches for children with APD are also effective for ADHD (Matson, 2005).

There are many auditory training treatment approaches, with new ones emerging frequently. Some are basic, and others are computer-based or utilize special equipment. Home-based training programs can be helpful and complement audiologist services (Bellis, 2002). Listening therapy can improve APD for some, but its effectiveness is still debated. It is provided by audiologists, as well as some OTs. Listening therapy helps improve the brain-ear connection with specials types of headphones and units. These treatments can be expensive and are usually not covered by health insurance. While it may help, it typically does not fully cure this condition. There are different types of listening therapies, including Auditory Integration Therapy (clinic-based), Tomatis (clinic-based), Integrated Listening Systems (clinic-based), Therapeutic Listening (home-based), Samonas (home-based), and The Listening Program (home-based). Finally, Bellis (2002) stated that after receiving APD services, some (particularly young children) may no longer have symptoms, while others may continue to experience these for the rest of their lives.

Visual Processing Disorder (VPD)

This condition involves the brain's deficiency in processing and perceiving incoming visual signals. VPD can occur without any vision impairments and it is often undetected in regular eye exams by optometrists and ophthalmologists. VPD is like APD because while the eyes work (as the ears for APD), the brain connection and its ability to process incoming information is faulty. It is a perceptual vision problem that can involve eye teaming, focusing, and tracking difficulties. VPD can be a lifelong condition without treatment. It can be a primary condition, or it may coexist with ADHD. Like all sensory processing conditions, VPD exists on a continuum. Similar to APD, there is a great lack of awareness by many clinicians of VPD.

Vision is tremendously complex, and requires the greatest amount of brain space of all the senses. About 30 percent of the brain's cortex neurons are utilized for vision, while 2 percent is used for hearing. Vision has a separate processing area in the occipital lobe in the back of the brain, while the hearing, smell, and taste sites are located in the temporal lobes at the sides of the brain.

VPD can cause symptoms and difficulties similar to ADHD and/or learning disorders, and these can be misdiagnosed when VPD really exists. Similar to ADHD, children with vision-based learning problems have short attention spans, make frequent errors, are highly distractible, do not complete assignments, fidget and move excessively, and are often off-task. However, their learning and behavior problems are due to discomfort using their eyes for long periods at close range, and not from true attentional deficits (Children's Vision Information Network, n.d.). VPD can be misinterpreted as ADHD and especially learning disorders due to the reading, writing, spelling, and academic problems that it can cause. Similar to APD, VPD can cause frustration and behavioral problems. VPD can also cause dysgraphia (handwriting impairments), coordination and fine motor problems.

Studies have shown that about 20 percent of school-aged children have eye teaming or eye focusing deficits that cause struggles with remaining on tasks for long periods. Eye teaming disorders include convergence insufficiency and convergence excess, and are a result of eye muscle coordination problems. These can also mimic ADHD problems because these children have difficulty using their two eyes together with close up materials necessary for reading and writing. Thus, they have eyestrain and discomfort and unknowingly take "eye breaks" to avoid academic work or other difficult tasks (Children's Vision Information Network, n.d.).

Convergence insufficiency (CI) problems can occur when near vision is utilized for screen use and reading. The symptoms of CI can make it difficult for children and teens to sustain their visual focus and this can overlap with ADHD symptoms. It is believed to be a common condition affecting about 5 percent of individuals, and five of nine official symptoms of ADHD can overlap with CI. One study found that children diagnosed with ADHD were three times as likely to have CI, and therefore, those diagnosed with ADHD should also be evaluated for CI (Granet et al., 2005). One quick test for CI is to ask the child to hold the head up and watch the tip of a pencil as it slowly is brought to their nose. If one eye swings out instead of inward, then a developmental optometrist evaluation is warranted.

Evaluation and Treatment

If a child or teen has VPD symptoms and/or learning disorder (LD) indicators, an evaluation by a behavioral or developmental optometrist is needed. Additionally, when children or teens have been diagnosed by schools with reading, math, or written expression learning problems, they should be further evaluated outside of the school to confirm if they have a true LD, VPD, or both. Also, if a child using ADHD medication experiences focusing and academic improvements, but continues to have reading and learning difficulties, then VPD testing from a specialized optometrist should be considered. Neuropsychologists may be able to detect some visual processing deficits, but optometrists will be more comprehensive. The diagnostic discrimination between LDs and VPD is important because of the prognosis and treatment. For LDs in older children, the prognosis can be poor. Vision therapy can improve VPD, but this treatment will not be considered if a learning disorder is incorrectly believed to exist.

The lack of awareness of VPD can be a barrier for optometrist referrals. Not all optometrists are trained to evaluate and treat VPD. Developmental or behavioral optometrists are doctors of optometry who evaluate and treat VPDs, have additional years of training beyond general optometrists, and provide vision therapy. Their specialized evaluations are more than just vision screenings and eye chart exams. Optometrists differ from ophthalmologists. Ophthalmologists are medical doctors who specialize in eye diseases and surgery, but do not evaluate or treat VPDs. Many ophthalmologists do not believe vision therapy is effective. Some physicians may want to refer their patients with suspected VPD to ophthalmologists, but only developmental optometrists can identify and treat VPD.

True VPDs cannot be treated with corrective lens or surgeries. Optometric vision therapy can be the most effective treatment for VPD conditions, including eye misalignment (strabismus), convergence insufficiency, binocular coordination difficulties, crossed eyes (amblyopia), and double vision (diplopia). Vision therapy is like physical therapy for the eye-brain connection, and involves doing special eye exercises and using special lenses, instruments, and visual computer activities. Vision therapy typically consists of a weekly in-office visit combined with daily at-home eye exercises. It does not improve visual acuity, which is what prescription glasses do. The results of vision therapy will vary based on the deficits, and more complex deficiencies will require longer treatments. Hopefully, this treatment can improve reading skills and academics. Unfortunately, insurance companies typically do not pay for this, and it may be an expensive treatment. To find an optometrist that offers vision therapy, go to www.COVD.com.

Irlen syndrome (formerly known as scotopic sensitivity syndrome) is a lesser known condition that is not an optical problem, but a specific visual processing condition involving wavelengths of light. This tends to be genetic and is not currently identified by most standardized vision tests or optometrists (Johnson, 2010). The Irlen Institute states that about 50 percent of children and adults with attention, reading, and learning problems have this condition, as well as some with autism spectrum disorder. They believe that some will improve significantly with the Irlen Method, while for others it can help but they will require additional services. For those with Irlen syndrome, the method involves using different colored overlays and lens to filter out certain offending waves of light to improve reading, light sensitivity, attention, and headaches. These special Irlen Spectral Filters can make print clear, comfortable, and easy to see, and improve reading flow and fluency, comprehension, and sustained attention. Those with reading and learning deficits related to language and phonics difficulties will not benefit from this method. Also, visual problems should be addressed before using this approach (Irlen Institute, 2017). While this syndrome is not commonly screened for during visual processing evaluations, parents can discuss this with behavioral optometrists, or a certified Irlen Screener or Diagnostician could be contacted to explore this condition. For more information, research, and to find an Irlen evaluator, go to www .irlen.com.

Tactile and Gustatory Processing Disorders

These are neurological deficiencies with the tactile (touch) and/or gustatory (taste) systems that can cause eating, food, social, and hygiene difficulties. Children with tactile problems may also have difficulties with vestibular and proprioceptive senses, as well as APD and VPD. Huecker and Kinnealey (1998) found that 82 percent of children with ADHD also demonstrated tactile defensiveness, and others have concurred. Children with these sensitivities may be fussy eaters and have limited foods they will tolerate due to certain textures, smells, or colors. Some children with these conditions may eat only, or will refuse to eat, creamy and smooth foods (like pudding), chewy foods (such as meat), or crispy foods (like chips). Some may strongly respond to the appearance of foods, such as foods that wiggle (Jello) or only white foods (Beil & Peske, 2009). As a consequence of their limited diets, they may also have zinc or magnesium deficiencies and should be tested for these. Experienced OTs can provide these evaluations and treatment.

Olfactory Sensory Processing Disorder

Individuals with this condition have neurological deficiencies with the olfactory system. They may also experience eating problems and food issues. These picky eaters may have limited foods they can tolerate due to discomfort with the smells, colors, or textures of certain foods. They may have social challenges and may seem odd to others because of their need to excessively smell things and their strange responses to scents, animals, and people. They may also have a zinc deficiency and should be tested for this. Experienced OTs can provide these evaluations and treatment.

Vestibular Processing Disorder

The vestibular system involves registering movement in all directions through the inner ear, proper balance, coordination, and sensory information about spatial awareness, motion, muscle tone, and being upright. This disorder causes impairments in these abilities, and can cause excessive motor activity and other ADHD-like behaviors. This can be very difficult to differentiate from true ADHD, particularly in younger children and those with predominantly hyperactive ADHD-like presentations. Additionally, those with vestibular conditions may also have true Combined or Inattentive ADHD.

Children with hyperactivity from underaroused or overinhibited lower brain centers (specifically an underaroused vestibular system) are believed to be hyperactive from their attempts to compensate for the brain's overinhibition. Curiously, these children can respond well to stimulant medications. They experience stimulants as calming because they no longer need to compensate to increase arousal. Conversely, children with hyperaroused vestibular systems and deficient inhibition from higher brain centers typically have lower attention and worsen from stimulants (Huecker & Kinnealey, 1998).

While vestibular related disorders have been linked to attentional deficits, Heckler and Kinnealey (1998) found that many children believed to have ADHD actually had a vestibular processing condition or deficits. They suggested that numerous children who appear to have ADHD may really be struggling with vestibular sensory deficits and are unknowingly trying to compensate with hyperactivity. They also found that 14 percent of children with ADHD also demonstrated gravitational insecurity, which is a form of sensory defensiveness. Children with vestibular problems may also have tactile and proprioceptive sensory problems. They may have persistent or fluctuating attentional deficits from their distractibility or overfocused and constant attempts to screen out unpleasant and difficult stimuli (Hanft, Miller, & Lane, 2000). Recurrent ear infections have also been associated with vestibular sensory processing deficits. Research has indicated that children with

ADHD (especially Combined types) have over one-third more balance and coordination problems than children without ADHD. Children with Combined ADHD have more impairments with equilibrium, postural control, and balance performance (Ghanizadeh, 2011).

Evaluation and Treatment

Children or teens with vestibular difficulties should be referred to an experienced OT for evaluation and treatment. Vestibular sensory-seeking conditions can closely mimic ADHD. Unfortunately, vestibular conditions will be very difficult to differentiate from true ADHD, particularly in young children with hyperactivity and impulsivity. Vestibular intolerance to movement and vestibular underresponsivity can mimic inattentiveness conditions. The vestibular sensory-seeking child with increased tolerance for movement can mimic hyperactivity and impulsivity problems. Also, those with more severe vestibular or multiple sensory conditions can generate significant elevations on ADHD measures, and therefore these measures may not be useful. Consequently, all young children with high levels of hyperactivity and impulsivity should receive referrals to OTs, especially if they are not positively responding to ADHD medications.

An indirect, but sometimes helpful, way to distinguish ADHD from vestibular processing disorder is to try different stimulant medications at sufficient doses. A lack of a positive response may suggest that the child has certain vestibular processing deficits. Also, a partial improvement may suggest that the child could have both. However, underaroused vestibular systems may improve on stimulants, while children with hyperaroused vestibular systems may become worse.

One school accommodation for these conditions is the use of ergonomic classroom furniture that incorporates movement into student chairs and desks. This can be helpful for children with ADHD who have higher levels of hyperactivity and impulsivity, as well as children with sensory processing vestibular or proprioceptive difficulties. OTs may also suggest other school recommendations.

Proprioceptive Processing Disorder

The proprioceptive system helps us move effectively and safely, and involves the awareness of body movements, postures, and the positions of our bodies. Its receptors are in the muscles, joints, and skin, and these help us know our body movements and postures, even without vision. Children with these difficulties seem to be lost in space, and can be excessively slow, insecure about their movements, and clumsy. They can have various difficulties with their movements, fine and gross motor coordination, muscle strength, and posture. They may also struggle to feel confident and connected to their bodies, and may have sensory-seeking traits.

This condition may seem very similar to vestibular dysfunction, and these two may overlap. As with vestibular conditions, proprioceptive disorders can closely resemble ADHD and can be difficult to differentiate, but may also coexist with Combined or Inattentive ADHD. Proprioceptive sensory seeking conditions can easily mimic hyperactivity and impulsivity problems, and in younger children can appear as predominantly hyperactive ADHD or Combined ADHD. Proprioceptive overresponsiveness and underresponsiveness can mimic Inattentive ADHD. As with vestibular processing disorders, hyperactivity and impulsivity can result from sensory seeking, under, and/or overresponder proprioceptive conditions because these children can excessively seek stimuli and inputs to the proprioceptive system to activate or calm their imbalanced nervous systems. Proprioceptive deficits often occur with tactile sensory dysfunction, vestibular sensory problems, and fine motor skills deficits. Since this condition is similar to the vestibular disorder, please refer to that section for evaluation and treatment information.

Sensory-Based Motor Disorder (SBMD)–Dyspraxia

Also called developmental dyspraxia, developmental coordination disorder, or motor learning disability, this condition impairs the ability to make smooth and coordinated movements. SBMD is composed of two different categories, Dyspraxia/Motor Planning and Postural Disorder. Dyspraxia causes difficulties with motor coordination, planning, timing, sequencing, and organization. It can result from certain neurological conditions and other sensory dysfunction issues, including tactile-based motor problems, vision-based motor problems, vestibular-based motor problems, and proprioceptive-based motor issues ("SPD Symptoms Motor Disorder: Sensory Based Motor Disorder," 2008-10). Due to its neurological basis, those with dyspraxia can also have language, speech, learning and perception problems, as well as poor muscle strength (Nordqvist, 2009).

It is estimated that dyspraxia affects at least two percent of the general population. Six percent of all children demonstrate some signs of this, and 70 percent of those affected are male (National Center for Learning Disabilities Editorial Team, n.d.b). Those born with extremely low birth weights and prematurely are at significantly higher risk. Children with this are often delayed in their developmental milestones of crawling, walking, and speech. They may also have difficulties with dressing themselves, handling a ball, and in social skills (Gibbs, Appleton, & Appleton, 2007). Dyspraxia exists on a continuum, its effects vary from person to person, and is considered a lifelong disorder. It can also impact individuals differently at various stages of life (National Center for Learning Disabilities Editorial Team, n.d.b). It can also be considered a fine and gross motor learning disability, and causes children to be clumsy, accident-prone, and uncomfortable playing sports or engaging in physical activities.

Dyspraxia often coexists with ADHD, but may create ADHD-like symptoms by itself. Pearsall-Jones, Piek, and Levy (2010) stated that up to half of those with dyspraxia also have ADHD. Others found that up to 60 percent of children with ADHD had poor motor coordination or dyspraxia and balance deficits (Spruyt & Gozal, 2011). Those with dyspraxia can develop additional problems, including low self-esteem, behavioral problems, frustration tolerance problems, social difficulties, anxiety, and depression (National Center for Learning Disabilities Editorial Team, n.d.b), all of which can resemble ADHD. Huecker and Kinnealey (1998) reported that dypraxia can easily cause attentional problems from the challenges of planning the sequence of steps necessary for motor tasks. Nordqvist (2007) shared that children with dyspraxia often struggle to sustain focus on one thing, and this may cause inattention difficulties. These children may also fidget more than others, and this can resemble hyperactivity. Other ADHD-like symptoms include organizational difficulties and struggling to recall instructions.

Evaluation and Treatment

Evaluating ADHD in children and teens with suspected dyspraxia can be challenging, and many have diagnostic complexities. Dyspraxia can coexist with ADHD, postural disorder, learning disorders, memory deficits, and sensory processing disorders and sensitivities (National Center for Learning Disabilities Editorial Team, n.d.a). Children with dyspraxia should be evaluated by primary care physicians and/or pediatric neurologists to rule out an underlying or undetected medical or neurological conditions causing or impacting the dyspraxic symptoms, including seizures, hearing, or visual deficits. Developmental physicians may be helpful in the evaluation process, too. After medical conditions are ruled out, dyspraxia can be evaluated and treated by experienced OTs who should also evaluate any potential SPDs. Physical therapy and/or speech-language pathologist evaluations and treatment may be needed as well (Gibbs, Appleton, & Appleton, 2007). After these evaluations, a neurodevelopmental assessment can be helpful to determine if other conditions exist, such as ADHD. Obviously, treating coexisting conditions will be important. Also, children with dyspraxic symptoms should be screened for an immature symmetric tonic neck reflex (STNR), which is addressed later in this chapter.

While there is no cure for dypraxia, early diagnosis and treatment is important. Since there is an overlap between this and other conditions, diagnostic and treatment planning confusion can occur, and different professionals may label or address these difficulties differently. Due to the frustrations and difficulties resulting from this condition, it is important that parents understand dyspraxia, and offer encouragement, patience, and support. These children will need help practicing various tasks, and they should start with simple physical activities that develop coordination, which should help to build confidence. Caregivers can also encourage developing supportive and accepting friendships. Family and individual psychotherapy can address the self-esteem, anxiety, depression, behavioral and social skills difficulties that often occur with dyspraxia (National Center for Learning Disabilities Editorial Team, n.d.b).

Sensory-Based Motor Disorder (SBMD)–Postural Disorder

This condition causes problems with muscle tone and coordination, motor control, balance, and the capacity to move bodies effectively. Those with postural disorder often appear as lazy and clumsy, and lag behind their peers in sports and physical abilities. Postural disorder can result from or coexist with various other sensory issues, including oral, visual, vestibular, and proprioceptive motor dysfunction ("SPD Symptoms Motor Disorder: Sensory Based Motor Disorder," 2008-10). Additionally, postural disorder and dyspraxia often coexist, and children with this combination also tend to have visual-motor difficulties. Children with postural disorders may have higher rates of sensory underresponsivity difficulties because they may have weaker muscles and may not feel their bodies appropriately (Miller, 2007).

It is believed that children with postural problems who struggle to maintain upright postures at desks and tables can have attentional difficulties because their impaired postures lessen focusing and learning abilities. Curiously, Huecker and Kinnealey (1998) found that 81 percent of children with ADHD also demonstrated poor antigravity control, which is poor upright posture and vestibular issues. For children with these difficulties, clinicians should also consider the postural condition of immature symmetric tonic neck reflex (STRN) (see next section). Refer to the sections for dyspraxia and Immature STRN for information on the evaluation and treatment of postural disorder because these are similar and can overlap.

Immature Symmetric Tonic Neck Reflex (STNR)

This is a specific postural condition resulting from a reflex problem that begins in early childhood. An immature STNR causes coordination, sitting, and posture impairments that can create behavioral and academic difficulties. Children with immature STNRs are sometimes incorrectly diagnosed with ADHD because of their difficulties sitting in one position and hyperactive-like behaviors. Additionally, they often have poor handwriting due to their difficulty holding pencils and moving their arms while in seated positions (O'Dell & Cook, 1997).

The STNR is one of the many automatic reflexes that develop after birth, such as sucking, Babinski, or coughing. All essential movements babies make result from reflexes, and motor development progresses as children gain control over their bodies. The STNR is an automatic movement that causes the top half of the body to work in opposition to the bottom half. When the top half is straight, then the bottom body half bends, and then the opposite occurs. However, the STNR can remain immature for children who did not crawl, crawled improperly, walked early, or were in playpens, walkers, or braces for lengthy periods (O'Dell & Cook, 1997). When children do not perform enough crawling in early childhood, this reflex can remain dominant and cause involuntary movements that interfere with bodily control (Pederson, 2016).

For neurotypical children, the STNR reaches peak strength during the sixth to eighth month of life and then declines by age two or three. An abnormal STRN persists beyond age two or three. A retained STRN can chronically impact academics by hindering coordinated and rhythmic movements that interfere with the postures necessary for writing and reading. It can cause great difficulties sitting at a desk in a normal sitting position with the hips and elbows bent at the same time. When the arms are bent to hold a book or write, the legs want to straighten. As a result, the child will want to stand up when writing or will have difficulty staying seated. Additionally, older children and teens will frequently slouch to extend their legs when reading or writing. This can appear disrespectful to teachers even though this position is comfortable (O'Dell, n.d.).

Children and teens with the immature STNR can seem hyperactive because of the difficulties staying seated in a proper position, as well as repeatedly getting up and down to relieve muscular tension. They may also have poor or messy handwriting, and may write in a cramped position. Copying from a board can be very difficult. As they grow older, they can experience increasingly more academic difficulties, may try to avoid written work or seem lazy, and can lack motivation or interest in school work (O'Dell, n.d.). Pederson (2016) shared a retained STNR can cause ADHD-like difficulties, including frequent fidgeting, problems relaxing, being easily distracted, squirming, and struggling to complete academic work. Obviously, ADHD medications will not improve immature STNRs (O'Dell & Cook, 1997). Researchers found that up to 75 percent of children with learning disorders may have an immature STNR. Other researchers have also written about how immature STNRs can negatively impact learning (Freides et al., 1980).

Evaluation and Treatment

Those with immature STNRs can be referred to OTs familiar with conditions involving immature reflexes, but not all OTs will be knowledgeable about this. Children and teens with dyspraxia may appear to have some immature STNR reflex symptoms, and an experienced OT should be able to distinguish between these conditions. Brain Gym® activities offered by some OTs can utilize repatterning exercises that can promote brain integration and completion of the crawling stage so the STNR can become properly integrated (Pederson, 2016). O'Dell and Cook (1997) in their books *Stopping Hyperactivity—A New Solution* and the updated 2018 version *Stopping ADD/ADHD and Learning Disabilities,* discuss approaches and exercises to address and correct an immature STNR. Treatment involves accommodations, permitting the use of comfortable postures for them, and specific exercises that promote progression from the STNR. The exercises are five days a week for 15 minutes for children five or older, and their program lasts about 26 weeks. Also, some physical therapists may be able to provide evaluations and treatment.

REFERENCES

Amen, D. (2013). *Healing ADD* (revised edition). New York: Berkley Books.

Bellis, T. J. (2002). *When the brain can't hear.* New York: Pocket Books.

Biel, L., & Peske, N. (2009). *Raising a sensory smart child.* New York: Penguin Books.

Children's Vision Information Network. (n.d.). College of Optometrists in Vision Development. *Vision and ADD/ADHD.* Retrieved on 11/04/12 from http://www.childrensvision.com/ADD.htm

Ciocci, S. R. (2002). Auditory processing disorders: An overview. *ERIC Digest,* E634. Retrieved from https://files.eric.ed.gov/fulltext/ED474303.pdf

Freides, D., Barbati, J., van Kempen-Horowitz, L. J., Sprehn, G., Iversen, C., Silver, J. R., & Woodward, R. (1980). Blind evaluation of body reflexes and motor skills in learning disability. *Journal of Autism and Developmental Disorders, 10,* 159–171.

Gibbs, J., Appleton, J., & Appleton, R. (2007, June). Dyspraxia or developmental coordination disorder? Unravelling the enigma. *Archives of Disease in Childhood, 92*(6), 534–539. doi: 10.1136/adc.2005.088054

Ghanizadeh, A. (2011, June). Sensory processing problems in children with ADHD, a systematic review. *Psychiatry Investigations, 8*(2), 89–94. doi:10.4306/pi.2011.8.2.89

Granet, D. B., Gomi, C. F., Ventura, R., & Miller-Scholte, A. (2005, December). The relationship between convergence insufficiency and ADHD. *Strabisumus, 13*(4), 163–168.

Haft, B. E., Miller, L. J., & Lane, S. L. (2000). Toward a consensus in terminology in sensory integration theory and practice: Part 3: Observable behaviors: Sensory integration dysfunction. *Sensory Integration Special Interest Section Quarterly, 23*(3), 1–4.

Hueckler, G. H., & Kinnealey, M. (1998). Prevalence of sensory integrative disorders in children with attention deficit hyperactivity disorder: A descriptive study. *The Journal of Developmental and Learning Disorder, 2*(2), 265–292.

Irlen Institute. (2017). *FAQs.* Retrieved from https://irlen.com/faqs/

Johnson, K. (2010). *The Roadmap from learning disabilities to success.* Burnt Hills, NY.

Johnson, C. D., Benson, P. V., & Seaton, J. B. (1997). *Educational audiology handbook.* San Diego, CA: Singular.

Kelly, D. A. (2004, May 3). *Auditory processing disorders: Considerations for the speech-language pathologist.* Retrieved from http://www.speechpathology.com/articles/pf_article_detail.asp?article_id=70

Kent, M. (2002, summer). Houston educational audiologists establish guidelines for referring for an auditory processing evaluation. *Educational Audiology Review, 3*–4. Retrieved from https://association-secure.org/Customers/7/ear/ear-summer-2002.pdf

Kranowitz, C. S. (2005). *The out-of-synch child.* New York: Penguin Group.

Kranowitz, C. S. (2016). *The out-of-sync child grows up.* New York: A TarcherPerigree Book.

Kutscher, M. L. (2014). *Kids in the syndrome mix of ADHD, LD, autism spectrum, Tourettes, anxiety, and more!* (2nd ed.). London: Jessica Kingsley.

Matson, A. E. (2005). Central auditory processing: A current literature review and summary of interviews with researchers on controversial issues related to auditory processing disorders. *Independent Studies and Capstones.* Paper 149. Program in Audiology and Communication Sciences, Washington University School of Medicine. Retrieved from http://digitalcommons.wustl.edu/pacs_capstones/149

Miller, L. J. (2007). *Sensational kids.* New York: A Perigee Book.

Miller, L. J., Nielsen, D. M., & Schoen, S. A. (2012). Attention deficit hyperactivity disorder and sensory modulation disorder: A comparison of behavior and physiology. *Research in Developmental Disabilities, 33*(3), 804–818. doi:10.1016/j.ridd.2011.12.005

National Center for Learning Disabilities. (2003a). *Visual processing disorders: In detail.* Retrieved from http://www.ldonline.org/article/Visual_Processing_Disorders%3A_In_Detail

National Center for Learning Disabilities. (2003b). *Visual processing disorders by age group.* Retrieved on from http://www.ldonline.org/article/Visual_Processing_Disorders_by_Age_Group

National Center for Learning Disabilities Editorial Team. (n.d.a). *Common warning signs of dyspraxia in children in grades 9–12.* Retrieved on 11/14/12 from

http://www.ncld.org/types-learning-disabilities/dyspraxia/common-warning
-signs-of-dys...

National Center for Learning Disabilities Editorial Team. (n.d.b). *What is Dyspraxia?* Retrieved on 11/15/12 from http://www.ncld.org/types-learning-disabilities /dyspraxia/what-is-dyspraxia?tmpl=compo...

Nordqvist, C. (2009, May 29). *What is dyspraxia? How is dyspraxia treated?* Retrieved from http://www.medicalnewstoday.com/articles/151951.php

O'Dell, N. (n.d.). *The Symmetric tonic neck reflex (STNR).* Retrieved on 04/17/17 from www.ndcbrain.com/assests/stnrinformation.pdf

O'Dell, N., & Cook, P. (1997). *Stopping hyperactivity.* Garden City Park, NY: Avery.

Pederson, J. (2016). *ADD/ADHD and brain gym.* Retrieved from http://eduction .jhu.edu/PD/newhorizons/Exceptional%20Learners/ADD%20ADHD/Articles /ADD%20ADHD%20and%20Brain%20Gym/

Pearsall-Jones, J. G., Piek, J. P., & Levy, F. (2010, October). Developmental coordination disorder and cerebral palsy: Categories or a continuum? *Human Movement Science, 29*(5), 787–798. doi: 10.1016/j.humov.2010.04.006

Scherer, P. (n.d.). *Is it sensory processing disorder or ADD/ADHD?* Retrieved on 09/10/12 from http://www.additudemag.com/adhd/article/print/793.html

Scherer, P. (2004, October & November). *Is it auditory processing disorder (APD) or ADHD?* Retrieved from http://www.additudemag.com/adhd/arti cle/print/731.html

Schminsky, M. M., & Baran, J. A. (1999, fall). *Central auditory processing disorders—An overview of assessment and management practices.* Deaf-Blind Perspectives, Teaching Research Division of Western Oregon University for DB-LINK. Retrieved from http://www.tsbvi.edu/Outreach/seehear/spring00/centralauditory.htm

Signs, Symptoms and Background Information on Sensory Integration. (n.d.). Retrieved on 03/11/13 from http://www.incrediblehorizons.com/sensory-integration .htm

SPD Symptoms Motor Disorder: Sensory Based Motor Disorder. (2008-10). Retrieved on 03/08/13 from http://spdlife.org/symptoms/sensory-based-motor -disorder.html

Spruyt, K., & Gozal, D. (2011, April). Sleep disturbances in children with attention-deficit/hyperactivity disorder. *Expert Review of Neurotherapeutics, 11*(4), 565–577. doi: 10.1586/ern.11.7

The Understood Team. (2014). Reviewed by Kelly Johnson on 04/14/14. *Understanding auditory processing disorder.* Retrieved from https://www.understood.org /en/learning-attention-issues/child-learning-disabilities/auditory-processing -disorder/understanding-auditory-processing-disorder

University of Virginia Speech-Language-Hearing Center. (2012). *Auditory processing.* Retrieved from www.curry.virginia.edu/community-programs/sjc/u.va.-speech -language-hearing-center/auditory-processing

"What is SPD?" (n.d.). Retrieved on 03/10/15 from http://spdstar.org/what-is-spd/

Chapter 8

PRENATAL SUBSTANCE EXPOSURE

INTRODUCTION

Prenatal substance exposure is a significant global issue that lacks the attention it deserves. In the United States alone, about 650 infants are born each day with prenatal illicit drug exposure (excluding alcohol, nicotine, and prescribed drugs), and many develop permanent neurodevelopmental damage. One national survey reported that among pregnant women, 8.5 percent disclosed current alcohol use, 15.9 percent recently smoked tobacco, and 5.9 percent currently use illicit drugs (Pilar, 2016).

Fetuses are quite vulnerable to prenatal substances exposure. Substance metabolites can easily enter the fetal bloodstream, penetrate their blood-brain barrier, negatively impact brain development, and disrupt neuronal cell development. Additionally, some children may be genetically more vulnerable to certain drugs' impact. Some drugs can cause damaging oxygen restrictions to fetuses (Minnes, Lang, & Singer, 2011). Isolating the prenatal effects of certain substances on brain development and later neurodevelopmental and behavioral health conditions can be perplexing (Pilar, 2016). Exposure effects are complicated and impacted by the timing, route, and dose of the substance use. Determining these effects can also be difficult due to polysubstance use and documentation challenges (Thompson, Levitt, & Stanwood, 2009). Symptoms of fetal substance exposure exist on a continuum from mild to severe, vary greatly, and affect individuals in different ways.

Prenatal and postnatal factors that often coexist with maternal substance use and addiction typically exacerbate the risks of poor outcomes. Many mothers have polysubstance use, poor prenatal care, inadequate diets during pregnancy, malnutrition, and poverty, along with paternal substance use (Pilar, 2016). After birth, the exposed child may be further impacted by maternal psychopathology, poverty, poor educational services, low maternal IQ, dysfunctional lifestyles, neglect, traumas, unhealthy diets and living environments, environmental neurotoxins, and foster care placement. Children's neurodevelopmental deficits can negatively impact their parents' interactions with them, causing additional difficulties (Minnes, Lang, & Singer, 2011). Lastly, there is still a great need for research and understanding of the prenatal impact of illegal substances upon children and adults later in life.

FETAL ALCOHOL SPECTRUM DISORDERS (FASD) AND PRENATAL ALCOHOL EXPOSURE (PAE)

Prenatal exposure to alcohol is the leading and most preventable cause of birth defects, intellectual disabilities, and neurodevelopmental disorders in children in the world. It is found in all ethnic and racial groups. The damage can impact many organs, the central nervous system, overall growth and size, and facial features. The neurobehavioral impairments can impair intelligence, learning, memory, language, executive functioning, visual spatial functioning, attention, and behavior. Consequently, many affected individuals struggle with academics, social functioning, and daily living skills (O'Brien & Mattson, 2011).

FASD is not a DSM-5 diagnosis, but is an umbrella term that describes a range of effects and conditions resulting from prenatal maternal alcohol consumption. The effects can produce permanent damage and deficits that can cause mild, moderate, or severe physical, psychological, neurodevelopmental (including ADHD-like difficulties), and learning impairments ("Fetal Alcohol Spectrum Disorders," 2015). One study found that 12.2 percent of pregnant women consumed alcohol (Eme & Millard, 2012). The percentage of children diagnosed with FASD is about 3.6 percent (Khazan, 2015). Besides total quantity consumed, drinking patterns can modulate effects (Ross et al., 2015).

Prenatal exposure to alcohol, as compared to other drugs, produces the most damaging effects. Most of the adverse prenatal effects reported in the past about crack cocaine ("crack babies") were really from alcohol (Eme & Millard, 2012). Indeed, many are surprised to learn that a pregnant mother's use of alcohol is far more toxic to a developing fetus than the use of cocaine, heroin, opioid products, and tobacco (Belcher, 2008).

The challenge of identifying FASD is that only the most severe condition of Fetal Alcohol Syndrome (FAS) will have the obvious physical features, which makes it more easily identified. The majority of alcohol exposed children lack some or all of the physical features (O'Brien & Mattson, 2011). They can be subtle or absent, and the dysmorphic features may resemble traits from other conditions (Belcher, 2008). Those with FASD can possess average to above average intelligence, but may still suffer from neurobehavioral difficulties. Unfortunately, there is no clear and specific neurobehavioral profile to identify individuals affected by FASDs (O'Brien & Mattson, 2011).

FAS-related behavioral difficulties are frequently misattributed to ADHD, ODD, and/or other conditions, and can cause significant diagnostic confusion. A confirmed maternal history of alcohol use during pregnancy is essential, but this can be difficult to obtain, especially for those with unclear histories. Birth mothers may be honest if asked about alcohol use during pregnancy if they are approached in a clinical and nonjudgmental manner. The exact amount of prenatal alcohol use that will cause adverse effects on children has not been determined, and probably varies with each child. However, women who are long-term alcohol abusers have the greatest risk of having a child with full FAS (Belcher, 2008).

Because many exposed children look normal, frequently clinicians and parents do not consider FASD (Khazan, 2015), and most are undiagnosed. One study indicated that only one in seven students with FAS were identified. Impaired general intellectual ability is one of the worst effects of prenatal alcohol exposure. The mean IQ for individuals with FAS who have facial anomalies is in the low 70s, while those without facial anomalies have a mean IQ in the low 80s. Approximately 25 percent with FASD have an intellectual disability, and most of the remaining have higher IQs but below normal. For those with average to above average intelligence, most will have some cognitive or neurodevelopment impairments, such as symptoms of nonverbal learning disorder, ADHD-like conditions, and executive functioning deficits (Eme & Millard, 2012). Studies reported certain cognitive functions are more sensitive to prenatal alcohol exposure than IQ, including verbal learning and memory, working memory, verbal fluency, and arithmetic abilities (Jacobson, 2011).

There are four categories that comprise FASD:

1. Fetal Alcohol Syndrome (FAS)

This is the most severe end of the spectrum, and describes individuals with the most damage ("Fetal Alcohol Spectrum Disorders," 2015). This exposure may be confirmed or unknown. FAS is diagnosed from the presence of all three in the following areas:

a. *Three distinct facial abnormalities:* (1) Smooth philtrum (an absence of the typical vertical ridge between the nose and upper lip); (2) Thin vermillion border (very small and thin upper lips); (3) Small palpebral fissures (short horizontal openings between the upper and lower eye lids with a resultant lack of normal openings for each eye).

b. *Growth problems:* confirmed prenatal or postnatal weight, height or both at or below the 10th percentile that is documented at any time, with adjustments for sex, age, prematurity of birth, ethnicity, and race.

c. *Central nervous system abnormalities* (criteria are met if one or more of the following are present): (1) Structural abnormalities (such as head circumference at or below the 10th percentile or clinically significant brain abnormalities confirmed through imaging); (2) Neurological problems, including seizures; or (3) Functional abnormalities consisting of performance that is significantly below what is expected for age, schooling, or circumstances. This is evidenced by global intellectual or cognitive deficits below the 3rd percentile or functional deficits below the 16th percentile in three or more of following: executive functioning deficits, developmental or cognitive deficits, attention or hyperactivity problems, motor functioning delays, social skills, or other areas including memory deficits, sensory problems, and pragmatic language problems (National Center on Birth Defects and Developmental Disabilities, 2005).

2. Partial Fetal Alcohol Syndrome (pFAS)

Individuals with this condition do not meet the full FAS criteria, but have a history of prenatal alcohol exposure and some of FAS symptoms including facial abnormalities, growth problems, or central nervous system abnormalities ("Fetal Alcohol Spectrum Disorders," 2015).

3. Alcohol-Related Neurodevelopment Disorder (ARND)

Those with this condition may have neurodevelopmental difficulties with behavior, learning (particularly math), academics, intellectual deficiencies, and impairments in judgement, attention, and impulse control (Centers for Disease Control and Prevention, 2015, April 16). They do not have abnormal facial features or growth problems ("Fetal Alcohol Spectrum Disorders," 2015). Children with ADHD-like symptoms who exhibit some or full criteria for ADHD, have significant and confirmed prenatal alcohol exposure but do not meet criteria for full FAS, pFAS, or ARBD, can be diagnosed with ARND. Also, "with ADHD-like features" can be added to the diagnosis of ARND to further emphasize the ADHD qualities. This can be a helpful diagnosis when clinicians believe that a child or teen has ADHD-like symptoms or even full ADHD criteria that is FASD-related. ARND and true ADHD can appear similar but are somewhat different. An ARND diagnosis requires significant and confirmed prenatal alcohol exposure, and this may limit the use of this diagnosis. Astley (2011) stated that alcohol exposure must be confirmed because ARND does not have clear or identifiable functional or physical features (such as with FAS or pFAS).

While ARND is not an official disorder, children and adolescents with FASD and ADHD-like symptoms can be diagnosed with the DSM-5 condition "other specified neurodevelopmental disorder associated with prenatal alcohol exposure with ADHD-like symptoms." This diagnosis should not be used along with full ADHD unless other neurodevelopmental symptoms are also present (American Psychiatric Association, 2013). If a child or teen meets full ADHD criteria and had prenatal alcohol exposure, it may be challenging to determine which diagnosis to use because these are generally believed to be separate conditions. It is possible to use the "other specified . . ." diagnosis as a long term rule out along with a full ADHD diagnosis to indicate that the clinician has suspected but not confirmed that prenatal exposure is the source of the ADHD-like difficulties. If an ADHD diagnosis is used when prenatal alcohol exposure existed, clinicians should state that prenatal alcohol exposure occurred. Additionally, "neurobehavioral disorder associated with prenatal alcohol exposure" is presented in the DSM-5 under the section "Conditions for Further Study" (American Psychiatric Association, 2013).

4. **Alcohol-Related Birth Defects (ARBD)**

Individuals with this condition can have problems related to their kidneys, heart, hearing and/or bones (Centers for Disease Control and Prevention, 2015, April 16).

PRENATAL ALCOHOL EXPOSURE AND ADHD

ADHD is the most frequent presentation for individuals with FASD, and 60 to 95 percent are diagnosed with ADHD. However, there is controversy if those with FASD can have true ADHD, or whether they have an ADHD-like, but somewhat different, neurodevelopmental condition. One reason FASD is often unrecognized by professionals is because it masquerades as ADHD (Eme & Millard, 2012). Research has attempted to differentiate between true ADHD and FASD. The growing consensus is that while individuals with FASD can have ADHD-like symptoms, they do not have true ADHD as it is commonly known. Chasnoff has stated that while a high number of children with FASD meet criteria for ADHD due to the alcohol-related neurochemistry changes, it is a different form of ADHD (Khazan, 2015).

Mattson and Wozniak (2011) found similarities and differences in children with ADHD and FASD. They were similar from parental reports in problems involving attention, social functioning, communication issues, and performance on an executive function test (the Wisconsin Card Sorting Test). Differences were found on laboratory measures of attention, other executive functioning measures, mathematics and numerical processing, verbal learning, balance control, motor competence, daily living skills, and eye blink conditioning.

When symptoms of both ADHD and FASD exist and discernment is difficult, clinicians can examine IQ scores. ADHD-like symptoms accompanied by a lower IQ score (85 or below), may suggest FASD. The average IQ for those with true ADHD is higher than those with FASD and ADHD. One study of children with attention and executive functioning deficits with either ADHD or heavy prenatal alcohol exposure reported a twenty-point IQ difference (105 IQ with ADHD versus 85 IQ with FASD) (Eme & Millard, 2012).

Another distinguishing research finding is children with FASD have social problems related to significantly weaker social cognition and facial emotional-processing abilities than children with true ADHD. This core deficit appears related to misperceiving social information and misunderstanding another's emotional state. A child with FASD may upset someone, but may not perceive this because the negative facial reactions cannot be recognized (Alcoholism: Clinical & Experimental Research, 2009).

Researchers have attempted to determine if a characteristic behavioral phenotype could be used as a screening tool to distinguish between FASD and true ADHD. They found two combinations of items on the Child Behavior Checklist (CBCL) measure that significantly differentiated FASD from ADHD with high sensitivity and specificity. The first combination of CBCL items is no guilt, acts young, and cruelty (with a sensitivity of 70 percent and specificity of 80 percent). The second combination is the CBCL items of no guilt, acts young, cruelty, lying or cheating, steals from home, and steals outside of the home (with a sensitivity of 81 percent and specificity of 72 percent) (Nash et al., 2006). These items could be used during evaluations and assessments to help with the diagnostic discrimination process.

Additionally, the presentations of true ADHD versus FASD and ADHD or ADHD-like symptoms can differ. Those with both FASD and ADHD or ADHD-like symptoms are more likely to present with comorbid medical, developmental, and psychological conditions. As infants they can have difficult-to-settle or slow-to-warm temperaments, followed by early-onset ADHD, as well as difficulties with self-soothing, mood, state regulation, hyperactivity, hypersensitivity to sensory stimuli, and irritability. Children with true ADHD have significant focusing and sustaining attention difficulties, while individuals with FASD tend to have more problems with encoding (or learning new material) and shifting attention. Also, children with ADHD frequently do not have intellectual disabilities (O'Malley & Nanson, 2002).

A number of studies have demonstrated that individuals with FASD have diagnostically complex neurodevelopmental presentations that include ADHD-like symptoms and difficulties with learning, executive functioning, working memory, and language (and especially a mixed receptive-expressive language disorder with deficits in social cognition and communication and/or a mathematics learning disorder). Other comorbidities include mood, anxiety, conduct disorders, and explosive behaviors. Also, because children with

FASD often struggle with understanding cause and effect relationships, standard behavioral management techniques may be less effective (O'Malley & Nanson, 2002).

EVALUATION OF FASD

At present, there are no simple tests that can assess the broad range of FASD symptoms and signs. In the future, brain imaging and other precise biomarker diagnostic tools will exist. A known history of prenatal alcohol use during pregnancy is extremely helpful but not required for the diagnosis of FASD, but is necessary for an ARND diagnosis. Most children in foster care or adoption processes (especially international adoptions) should be assessed for FASD due to the higher likelihood of the mother's use of alcohol ("Fetal Alcohol Spectrum Disorders," 2015). The ARND diagnosis requires significant and confirmed prenatal alcohol exposure by maternal self-report, the reports of others who observed consumption during the pregnancy, and/or documentation from medical or other records (Interagency Coordinating Committee on Fetal Alcohol Spectrum Disorders, 2011). Maternal self-reports are practical, but can be problematic due to lack of honesty and recall accuracy. Surveys may also promote more accuracy than in-person interviews (Behnke & Smith, 2013).

FASD is chronically underdiagnosed, and differential diagnosing can be difficult. Up to 94 percent of children and teens with FASD have one or more coexisting psychological conditions. FASD should be conceptualized as a continuum of disorders that always affects cognition but may not have physical signs. Due to their complex presentations, individuals should ideally receive a specialized FASD assessment from an experienced multidisciplinary team. Developmental or experienced pediatricians can explore medical issues. Neuropsychologists can assess the cognitive and neurobehavioral challenges. Speech therapists can address speech and language issues, and OTs can address motor and sensory processing concerns. Psychiatrists should be consulted for medication options. School psychologists, education specialists, and school social workers can help with school needs and challenges (Elias, 2013).

TREATMENT OF FASD

The most effective treatment approach is to create an individualized and comprehensive plan that is specific to the child's conditions and needs. Numerous studies indicate that early intervention is best, and generally children diagnosed before age six seem to do better (Belcher, 2008). The education of family members is critical because it can lead to a paradigm shift in the understanding and attitude of others toward the child. Without the diagnosis, those with FASD are often viewed as difficult, confusing, selfish, criminal, or sociopathic. However, with an accurate diagnosis and perspective, they can be seen as someone with neurological impairments and brain-functioning difficulties who needs assistance and treatment to manage their challenges (Tao et al., 2013). Also, those with FASD can present years younger developmentally, and this can help explain their immaturity and social problems. Teachers and parents should consider lowering their expectations and focusing more on their developmental level than comparing them to peers. Neurodevelopmental testing can assist with this enhanced understanding as well (Nauert, 2014).

Children and adolescents with FASD may require a number of services, including specialized educational interventions and services through IEPs, school advocacy and educational therapist assistance, developmental services, parent education and training, behavioral management and modification training, social skills training, occupational therapy, speech therapy, psychiatric medications from psychiatrists, developmental pediatricians providing primary medical care, specialized medical treatments, and referrals for community support services. Experienced psychotherapists who provide family therapy and individual therapy (possibly using expressive or play therapy) can be impactful as well ("Fetal Alcohol Spectrum Disorders," 2015).

Psychiatric medication management can be challenging since there are no specific medications for FASDs. If there are FASD with ADHD-like symptoms, the first-line treatment is stimulant medication, and more than one is often needed. Children who experience severe disruptive or explosive behaviors may need mood stabilizers (Belcher, 2008). However, medications for ADHD can produce mixed results for children with FASD. They seem to have a differential response to dextroamphetamine (Dexedrine) and methylphenidate (Ritalin, Concerta), and these can be less effective for them (Elias, 2013). Generally, individuals with neurochemical or structural central nervous system changes are often overly sensitive to the effects and side effects of psychiatric medications. However, their response to stimulants may improve with as they grow older. A negative response in a child under five may change to a positive response when six or seven. Individuals with FASD can also have unpredictable medication responses, and stimulants can possibly increase aggression or impulsivity (O'Malley & Nanson, 2002). Finally, neurofeedback can be a promising treatment for FASD to potentially produce permanent long-term brain changes and improvements.

PRENATAL MATERNAL USE OF NICOTINE

In the United States, nearly one in six pregnant women reported recently smoking cigarettes. Among its many hazards, smoking can cause impaired oxygen exchange in the placenta (Pilar, 2016). Cigarette smoke contains over 7,000 chemicals, and many are toxic. Nicotine and its metabolite cotinine easily pass through the placenta, with concentrations far greater in fetuses than mothers. Even maternal exposure to secondhand smoke can cause chronic neurodevelopment difficulties (Ross et al., 2015). Thompson, Levitt, and Stanwood (2009) reported that there is clear evidence that active and passive smoke exposure can increase risks of preterm birth, sudden infant death syndrome (SIDS), and lower birth weight. All of these are high risk factors for later behavioral conditions as well.

After alcohol, in utero nicotine exposure is the second greatest prenatal risk for ADHD. Many studies have found a significant association between prenatal environmental tobacco smoke exposure and ADHD or ADHD-like behaviors, and this includes controlling for numerous confounding variables (Behnke & Smith, 2013; Braun et al., 2006; Ross, et al., 2015). Various studies have also demonstrated nicotine exposure is associated with externalizing behaviors, deficient language development, poor reading skills in later childhood, lesser arithmetic and spelling abilities, and higher rates of delinquency, substance use, and criminal behavior in adolescents and adults (Behnke & Smith, 2013), as well as learning disabilities (Thompson, Levitt, & Stanwood, 2009). Researchers detected a two- to fourfold increased risk for ADHD in children associated with prenatal environmental tobacco smoke exposure (Braun et al., 2006). Also, nicotine exposure increases the risk of neurodevelopment conditions and future substance abuse (Pliszka, 2015). The children of women who smoked tobacco had lower verbal and auditory functioning intelligence scores, lower working memory scores, and greater impulsivity and oppositionality (Pilar, 2106). Tobacco exposure has also been implicated in anxiety and depression in young children through late adolescence (Minnes, Lang, & Singer, 2011).

PRENATAL MATERNAL USE OF ILLICT DRUGS AND ABUSE OF OPIOID PRESCRIPTIONS

Unfortunately, there is a lack of substantial research on the effects of prenatal illicit drug use and prescription medication abuse. What is known is that the type of drug, the frequency of use, and when used during the fetal development are meaningful. Individuals who abuse substances often use more than one, and so polysubstance abuse (including alcohol and nicotine use) should be considered when exploring prenatal drug impact. Some drugs can cause short-term effects on a newborn and infant (such as drug withdrawal and neurobehavioral symptoms), as well as long-term effects.

Identification of prenatal maternal drug use is obviously important. The two basic methods are maternal self-reports and infant biological specimens. Newborn drug testing is common in hospitals but not in outpatient settings. As with alcohol and nicotine, verbal maternal self-reports are practical, but can be problematic due to lack of honesty and recall accuracy. Surveys may promote more accuracy (Behnke & Smith, 2013). The reports of relatives and friends who observed maternal use during pregnancy, and/or documentation from medical or other records can help (Interagency Coordinating Committee on Fetal Alcohol Spectrum Disorders, 2011). One of the clearest sources of information will be a newborn's positive test for drugs at the hospital. However, alcohol exposure will not typically be present in this infant testing.

Marijuana

Cannabis is the most frequently used illicit substance during pregnancies, and can cause mild withdrawal symptoms in newborns (Pilar, 2016). Marijuana can remain in the body for up to 30 days, which increases fetal exposure. Smoking marijuana creates up to five times the amount of carbon monoxide as cigarettes, and this may impact fetal oxygenation (Behnke & Smith, 2013). Nearly 5 percent of pregnant women reported smoking marijuana during the first trimester, with decreased use during later trimesters. Some studies found stunted growth outcomes and decreased birth weight, while others found little to none of these effects (Ross et al., 2015).

Other cannabis exposure research found an association with low birth weight, negative neurodevelopmental outcomes, and increased rates of psychological conditions. By age six, exposed children exhibited executive functioning deficits, including increased inattention, hyperactivity, and impulsivity symptoms, that remained into early adulthood. School-age children with exposure demonstrated disorganized speech and visual problem-solving impairments (Pilar, 2016). Another study found inattention and impulsivity problems at age 10 were associated with this exposure (Behnke & Smith, 2013). Other research found that pregnant women who smoked one or more joints a day during the first trimester were found to have children with reading and spelling deficits. Prenatal exposure was also associated with deficits in attention, memory, impulsivity, planning, and problem solving through age 16. Children age 10 with this exposure during the first and third trimesters had more depression symptoms. Prenatal exposure among 16- to 21-year-olds at least doubled their chances of both tobacco and cannabis use

(Minnes, Lang, & Singer, 2011). Lastly, as cannabis becomes increasingly legalized across the United States, this prenatal exposure is expected to become more prevalent.

Cocaine

In-utero cocaine exposure has varying research results regarding its physical effects, including severe and global physical malformations, while other studies found no physical impact. However, dosage, timing, and exposure may have caused variances. Some research reported growth restrictions that continued until age 10. There is consistent evidence that cocaine exposure causes decreased executive functioning, poor cognitive performance in language skills, and behavioral difficulties. Research found this exposure is associated with language development impairments, but adoption or foster care offers some protection from language delays. One study found first trimester cocaine exposure was associated with more anxious, depressed, and withdrawn behaviors. Other research indicated children age nine with higher exposures had delinquent and aggressive behaviors. Also, children age 12 with higher exposures had executive functioning deficits (Ross et al., 2015).

Cocaine can easily cross the placenta and blood-brain barrier, and create significant toxic fetal effects. The developing brain areas regulating executive functioning, attention, and memory are especially vulnerable to cocaine (Behnke & Smith, 2013). Recreational prenatal cocaine use was found to cause a subtle but dominant developmental phenotype that resembles ADHD. Detailed research has shown this exposure can cause chronic negative effects on the attention and cognitive systems. Also, some children with this exposure were found to have increased risks for special needs programs (Thompson, Levitt, & Stanwood, 2009). Research found exposed children ages four to seven performed below standard norms on selective and sustained attention tests, while another study found exposed children had greater inattention on measures. Exposed children age six had higher rates of ADHD and ODD. One study reported cocaine-exposed boys had greater likelihoods of aggression, disregard for safety, and substance use, while another found exposed girls had significantly more delinquent behaviors. However, several studies did not find that exposure predicted behavioral problems (Minnes, Lang, & Singer, 2011).

Research has indicated that cocaine exposure does not predict problems with IQ or overall development in children. However, several studies indicated that exposure was associated with subtle language delays and alterations in attention, working memory, and visual-motor ability. One study found exposed children had a 79 percent increased odds of having an

Individual Education Program (IEP), while another found 2.8 times the risk of learning disabilities. Conversely, other studies have not found cocaine exposure to cause significant academic difficulties (Behnke & Smith, 2013).

Opioids

Opioids includes heroin and prescription medications. Opioid usage rates during pregnancy are difficult to obtain, and vary greatly from one to 21 percent. Although more people abuse prescription pain medications, most of the research involves mothers using heroin or opioid agonist medications (Minnes, Lang, & Singer, 2011). Children with opiate in-utero exposure often have low birthweight and smaller head circumference (Ross et al., 2015). Heroin exposure does not seem to cause congenital malformations, although opioid exposure causes a worse impact than cocaine exposure on infant autonomic and central nervous systems (Minnes, Lang, & Singer, 2011). Newborns with opioid exposure can cause significant withdrawal problems and often requires hospitalization and medication after birth (Behnke & Smith, 2013).

Prenatal opioid exposure has often been associated with childhood behavioral problems. One study found that exposed 10-year-olds were more likely to have ADHD or other disruptive behavior diagnoses (Minnes, Lang, & Singer, 2011). Pre- and elementary school-age children demonstrated cognitive and motor impairments, inattention, hyperactivity, and increased rates of ADHD with heroin exposure (Ross et al., 2015). Exposure has also been associated with perceptual and memory problems in older children. However, longitudinal studies have not shown consistent deficiencies in executive functioning and cognition (Behnke & Smith, 2013). The prevalence of cognitive impairments from methadone exposure has been questioned (Ross et al., 2015). Some studies of prenatal methadone and buprenorphine use reported normal results, while others found lower cognitive functioning scores (Pilar, 2016).

Methamphetamine and Amphetamine

These psychostimulants can be ingested, smoked, or snorted. These may be used illegally, or methamphetamine may be used appropriately through prescriptions by mothers with ADHD. The frequency of its use and abuse has risen steadily, and exceeds cocaine use in many United States regions (Thompson, Levitt, & Stanwood, 2009). Just over 1 percent of the population in North and Central America use amphetamine-type stimulants, and 5 percent of pregnant women in high use areas within the United States self-reported methamphetamine use (Ross et al., 2015).

Although methamphetamine and amphetamine use during pregnancy has become more widespread, there is little research on long-term consequences. Yet this exposure has been associated with low birth weight, decreased academics, increased stress, and lower scores on measures of attention, visual motor integration, verbal and long-term spatial memory (Thompson, Levitt, & Stanwood, 2009). One study of unspecified prenatal amphetamine use suggested a potential link with peer problems and externalizing behaviors. Another study found teens had higher rates of repeating grades and significantly lower mathematics test scores (Behnke & Smith, 2013).

Research found methamphetamine-exposed children had subtle, but significant, decreases in volume or size in specific brain regions, and these correlated with reduced sustained attention and delayed verbal memory. Other research found exposed children at age five demonstrated behavioral problems, as well as increased parental stress and psychological symptoms. Finally, children who experienced continuous prenatal amphetamine exposure had negative physical, emotional, cognitive, and social effects, with higher rates of ADHD, aggression, and learning problems attributed to memory, attention, and motivation deficiencies (Ross et al., 2015).

REFERENCES

Alcoholism: Clinical & Experimental Research. (2009, July 20). *Children with fetal alcohol spectrum disorders (FASD) mave more severe behavioral problems than children with attention deficit hyperactivity disorder (ADHD), study finds. ScienceDaily.* Retrieved from www.sciencedaily.com/releases/2009/07 /090716164335.htm

American Psychiatric Association. (2013). *Diagnostic and statistical manual of mental disorders* (5th ed.). Washington, DC: Author.

Astley, S. (2011, November 1). *What prenatal alcohol exposure is necessary for an ARND diagnosis? Experience from the Washington state fetal alcohol syndrome diagnostic and prevention network clinic.* Retrieved from http://www.niaaa.nih.gov/sites/default /files/ICCFASD_ARNDProgram_D_508.pdf

Belcher, H. (2008, August). *Fetal alcohol syndrome: An undiluted danger.* Retrieved from https://www.kennedykrieger.org/sites/kki2.com/files/8-08.pdf

Behnke, M., & Smith, V. C. (2013, March). Prenatal substance abuse: Short- and long-term effects on the exposed fetus. *Pediatrics, 131*(3), e1009–e1024. doi: 10.1542/peds.2012-3931

Braun, J. M., Kahn, R. S., Froehlich, T., Auinger, P., & Lanphear, B. P. (2006, December). Exposures to environmental toxicants and attention deficit hyperactivity disorder in U.S. children. *Environmental Health Perspectives, 114*(12), 1904–1909. Retrieved from http://www.ncbi.nlm.nih.gov/pmc/articles /PMC1764142/

Centers for Disease Control and Prevention. (2015, April 16). *Facts about FASDs.* Retrieved from www.cdc.gov/ncbddd/fasd/facts.html

Elias, E. (2013, June). *Improving awareness and treatment of children with fetal alcohol spectrum disorders and co-occurring psychiatric disorders.* The Disability Service Center JBS International Inc. Retrieved from http://www.jbsintertional.com/sites /default/files/FASDpaperfinal_INT.pdf

Eme, R., & Millard, E. (2012, January). Fetal Alcohol Spectrum Disorders: A literature review with screening recommendations. *The School Psychologist.* Retrieved from http://www.apadivisions.org/division-16/publications/newsletters/school -psychologist/2010/01/fetal-alcohol-disorders.aspx

Fetal Alcohol Spectrum Disorders. (2015, November 21). Retrieved from https: //www.healthychildren.org/English/health-issues/conditions/chronic/Pages/Fetal -Alcohol-Spectrum-Disorders.aspx

Interagency Coordinating Committee on Fetal Alcohol Spectrum Disorders (2011, October 31 to November 2). *Consensus statement on recognizing alcohol-related neurodevelopment disorder (ARND) in primary health care of children.* Rockville, MD. Retrieved from http://www.niaaa.nih.gov/sites/default/files/ARNDConference Consensus StatementBooklet_Complete.pdf

Jacobson, J. L. (2011, October 31). *Differential diagnosis of ARND: Other toxic exposures.* Retrieved from http://www.niaaa.nih.gov/sites/default/files/ ICFASD_ARNDProgram_D_508.pdf

Khazan, O. (2015, January 15). When ADHD isn't what it seems. *The Atlantic.* Retrieved from http://theatlantic.com/health/archive/2015/01/when-adhd-isn't -what-it-seems/384537/

Mattson, S., & Wozniak, J. R. (2011, October 31). *Specificity of the neurobehavioral profile of ARND: Comparisons with ADHD.* Retrieved from http://www.niaaa.nih.gov /sites/default/files/ICCFASD_ARNDProgram_D_508.pdf

Minnes, S., Lang, A., & Singer, L. (2011, July). Prenatal tobacco, marijuana, stimulant, and opiate exposure: Outcomes and practice implications. *Addiction Science & Clinical Practice, 6*(1), 57–70.

Nash, K., Rovet, J., Greenbaum, R., Fantus, E., Nulman, I., & Koren, G. (2006). Identifying the behavioural phenotype in fetal alcohol spectrum disorder: Sensitivity, specificity, and screening potential. *Archive of Women's Mental Health, 9*(4), 181–186. Retrieved from http://link.springer.com/article/10.1007/s00737 -006-0130-3#page-2

National Center on Birth Defects and Developmental Disabilities, Centers for Disease Control and Prevention, Department of Health and Human Services. (2005, May). *Fetal alcohol syndrome: Guidelines for referral and diagnosis,* 3rd Printing. Retrieved from www.cdc.gov/ncbddd/fasd/documents/FAS_guidelines...

Nauert, R. (2014). *Less ADHD than meets the eye among kids with fetal alcohol syndrome.* Retrieved from http://psychcentral.com/news/2014/04/25/less-than-meets-the -eye-among-kids-with-fetal-alcohol-syndrome/68966.html

O'Brien, J., & Mattson, S. N. (2011, February). *Neurobehavioural profiles of individuals with fetal alcohol spectrum disorders.* Encyclopedia on Early Childhood Development. Retrieved from ww.child-encyclopedia.com/fetal-alcohol-spectrum -disorders-fasd/according-experts/neurobehavioural-profiles-individuals-fetal

O'Malley, K. D., & Nanson, J. (2002). Clinical implications of a link between fetal alcohol spectrum disorder and attention-deficit hyperactivity disorder. *The Canadian Journal of Psychiatry, 47*(4), 349–354.

Pilar, M. (2016). *Brain development effects: Prenatal exposure to drugs and alcohol.* Retrieved from https://pro.psychcentral.com/brain-development-effects-prenatal-exposure-to-drugs-and-alcohol/0012502.html

Pliszka, S. (2015). Comorbid psychiatric disorders in children with ADHD. In R. Barkley (Ed.), *Attention deficit hyperactivity disorder: A handbook for diagnosis and treatment* (4th ed., pp 140–168). New York: Guilford Press.

Ross, E. J., Graham, D. L., Money, K. M., & Stanwood, G. D. (2015, January). Developmental consequences of fetal exposure to drugs: What we know and what we still must learn. *Neuropsychopharmacology, 40*(1), 61–67. doi: 10.1038/npp.2014.147

Tao, L., Temple, V., Casson, & Kirkpatrick. (2013). *Health watch table—fetal alcohol spectrum disorder (FASD).* Retrieved from http://vkc.mc.vanderbilt.edu/etoolkit/physical-health/health-watch-tables-2/fetal-alcohol-spectrum-disorder/

Thompson, B. L., Levitt, P., & Stanwood, G. D. (2009, April). Prenatal exposure to drugs: Effects on brain development and implications for policy and education. *Nature Reviews Neuroscience, 10*(4), 303–312. doi: 10.1038/nrn2598

Chapter 9

PSYCHOLOGICAL CONDITIONS

Note: For all of the conditions in this chapter, experienced clinical psychologists and psychotherapists who work with children and adolescents with ADHD and any of the following disorders could provide evaluations and the psychotherapy treatment.

ANXIETY DISORDERS

Anxiety is one of the most common psychological conditions in children and adolescents. It is easily misdiagnosed as ADHD, and is the most common cause of ADHD-like symptoms (Silver, 2006). Anxiety can be transient from brief stressors, or chronic from long-term stressors or an anxiety disorder. It can impair concentration and cause inattention and sleep difficulties due to worry, rumination, and excessive preoccupations. Anxiety can also cause fidgeting, persistent movement, and restlessness which mimics hyperactivity. About 20 to 25 percent of people with true ADHD also have anxiety disorders (Spruyt & Gozal, 2011). Those with Inattentive ADHD can have higher rates, and anxiety can worsen true ADHD. ADHD itself often generates anxiety, stress, and worry due to the difficulties it can cause.

Anxiety disorders generally persist longer than about one month, are pervasive, debilitating, and difficult to manage without treatment. Anxious children and teens can act irrationally or quickly to discharge nervousness. Because anxiety conditions can be genetic in nature, family history is important (Silver, 2009, Spring).

Inappropriate content and interactions on social media, as well as excessive use, may be associated with anxiety and depressive disorders. Inadequacy feelings, negative self-comparisons to others who seem more interesting, difficulties with emotional regulation, and worries about being left out or having poor connections with peers may result from unhealthy social media use, and can cause or increase anxiety and depression (Hoge, Bickham, & Cantor, 2017). Further, the pace and content of the constant stimuli from social media and video game use, particularly with excessive and persistent use, can cause chronic stress and anxiety. With excessive use, continual states of arousal and hypervigilance can create ongoing stress and increased cortisol release which may impact sleep and prefrontal cortex functioning over time. Screen time (and particularly video games) should not be used before homework, and not before or after studying for tests because it can impair executive functioning abilities and decrease new learning (M. Wehrenberg, personal communication, December 07, 2018).

Evaluation and Treatment

Children and teens may not be able to articulate the content and details of their thoughts and feelings, so clinicians should proceed slowly to explore their anxiety-provoking stressors and triggers. To discern if anxiety is secondary or coexists with ADHD, clinicians can explore when each set of symptoms started and the specific content of the thoughts. When the majority of the thoughts are ADHD-related (like worry about forgetting homework and "getting in trouble") and the anxiety began after the ADHD symptoms manifested, then this can suggest that the anxiety is secondary. Parent and self-report anxiety measures can be used. Known or undetected traumatic and abusive experiences should be explored for children or teens with anxiety as well.

If a child or teen has ADHD-like symptoms that disappear when the anxiety subsides, this could suggest an anxiety condition. However, if the ADHD symptoms persist while anxiety symptoms fluctuate, then true ADHD and an anxiety condition may both exist (Lougy, DeRuvo, & Rosenthal, 2007). Furthermore, if ADHD symptoms improve with ADHD medication treatment but the anxiety does not, then both conditions may exist. Some with ADHD who have secondary anxiety will experience anxiety improvements after effective ADHD medications. For those with intermittent responses to stimulant medication, there may be an underlying but undiagnosed anxiety, depression, or other condition. Additionally, ADHD symptoms may worsen when anxiety or other symptoms escalate.

Coexisting anxiety may also improve after parents receive education about ADHD and accept the disability. Improvement may also be seen if school plans and accommodations are provided for ADHD. However, if the anxiety persists, an experienced psychotherapist should address it, along with family therapy or parental involvement to facilitate better understanding and management of the difficulties. Family or other issues that are upsetting or destabilizing should also be addressed. Psychiatric medication may be helpful to treat the anxiety, particularly with more severe conditions.

Excessive and concerning social media use may require greater supervision and management, or specialized psychotherapy. Lastly, neurofeedback and Walsh's Advanced Nutrient Therapy may improve anxiety.

Social Anxiety Disorder (SAD)

Individuals with this condition have an irrational fear of embarrassing or humiliating themselves, and being watched, judged or evaluated by others. The anxiety and discomfort can be extreme and interfere with daily functioning. SAD is common, with up to 13 percent of the general population experiencing symptoms at some point. The difference between normal shyness and SAD is the severity and persistence of the symptoms. Those with SAD know that their fear is out of proportion, but are unable to control it. The anxiety can occur in a certain situation (specific SAD) or in all situations (generalized SAD). Common triggers include interacting with strangers, making eye contact, and initiating conversations (Cuncic, 2014). SAD and ADHD can also coexist. Those with ADHD may experience social anxiety from increased social and academic problems, rejection, and lower self-esteem.

A newer form of SAD called social media anxiety disorder can occur when individuals use social media excessively and experience increased anxiety when not using it. The condition is persistent and can cause users to become obsessively focused on social media activity. Symptoms include excessive social media use and account checking, withdrawal from others, difficulties reducing or stopping use, loss of interest except for social media, neglect of important life activities, heightened anxiety when unable to check accounts, depression, interpersonal conflicts due to use (Fader, 2018), fear of missing out (FOMO) on more interesting experiences, nondigital interpersonal skill deficits, and negative self-comparisons (M. Wehrenberg, personal communication, December 07, 2018).

Evaluation and Treatment

Social anxiety measures can be utilized. The prior information provided for evaluation and treatment of anxiety conditions can be applicable for this condition.

Obsessive Compulsive Disorder (OCD)

OCD is a common and often chronic condition with a neurobiological basis. The obsessions cause children and adults to experience recurrent, intrusive, and uncontrollable disturbing or uncomfortable thoughts, mental images, and urges. Compulsions frequently, but not always, occur; they are behaviors, rituals, or urges that are repeated over and over after obsessions in attempts to neutralize or erase them. These symptoms are time-consuming and interfere with relationships, school and work (National Institute of Mental Health [NIMH], 2016). The more common categories of obsessions are fears of harm, unwanted sexual thoughts, contamination, loss of control, perfectionism, and religious thoughts. The more common types of compulsions are cleaning and washing, repeating, checking, counting, and ordering (International OCD Foundation, 2016). OCD is believed to affect about 1 percent of children in the United States.

While everyone worries or may have odd routines at times, those with OCD have extreme difficulty controlling their thoughts and behaviors, even when they know these are excessive. Individuals with OCD often spend at least one hour each day on their obsessions and compulsions, and symptoms can fluctuate over time. They do not enjoy the compulsions, but they can provide temporary relief. They may attempt to avoid situations that trigger obsessions, and some may use substances to medicate themselves. Children and teens can hide their symptoms due to embarrassment. Yet many may not realize that their OCD behavior is not normal, but parents and teachers often recognize their symptoms. Clinicians may not recognize that the symptoms are significant, and may incorrectly minimize them as part of a child's quirkiness or behavioral problem (Obsessive-Compulsive Disorder, 2012).

Most with OCD are diagnosed by age 19. A family history is associated with OCD and individuals with a first-degree relative with this are at a greater risk. Also, those who have experienced abuse or traumas are at a greater risk. In certain cases, full OCD or symptoms can manifest up to six months after a streptococcal infection, or strep throat (called Pediatric Autoimmune Neuropsychiatric Disorders Associated with Streptococcal Infections or PANDAS) (NIMH, 2016).

Since OCD and ADHD can coexist, it can be challenging to diagnose both conditions. When discussing OCD, children and teens may be secretive or feel shameful. Rates of coexisting OCD and ADHD vary between 6 to 16 percent (Geller & Brown, 2009). There are a number of commonalities between OCD and ADHD. Both can cause procrastination and problems with planning. Hoarding and disorganization can occur, but those with OCD may hoard due to the discomfort of discarding items while those with ADHD hoard from disorganization. Both can suffer from distracting thoughts and over-focusing. However, OCD focusing and attention problems often result from distractions with obsessions and compulsions, while ADHD causes more random thoughts that can distract focusing. Also, ADHD-related overfocusing often occurs from immersion in activities they love (like video games). Both can cause difficulties with controlling impulses. OCD can create rigid routines that must be followed while ADHD can cause sudden urges which are acted upon without thinking. Additionally, those with OCD can be mistaken for having hyperactivity due to their compulsively driven behaviors (Brasic, 2012).

Some with OCD can suffer from extreme perfectionism that compels them to do classwork or homework perfectly, or they will erase and start over (Silver, 2009, fall). These children and teens can have classwork that is not finished due to their extreme slowness and meticulousness, and homework can take agonizing hours because of their rigidly high standards. Finally, Amen (2013) has discussed an ADHD subtype called Overfocused ADD that is a combination of both ADHD and OCD-like symptoms that includes excessive worrying, obsessional thinking, compulsive behaviors, trouble shifting attention, and argumentative tendencies.

Evaluation and Treatment

OCD measures should be used because those with this condition may not mention all symptoms, and can feel uncomfortable during interviews, particularly with obsessions that involve sexual or aggressive themes. Clinicians can explore the symptoms to determine if these may be related to other issues, such as family problems or undetected traumas. While ADHD and OCD can coexist, OCD can cause ADHD-like symptoms. If ADHD symptoms exist mostly or solely when OCD symptoms occur and are absent when no OCD problems occur, this could suggest that true ADHD does not exist. However, if the ADHD symptoms exist when OCD symptoms are fewer or not present, then ADHD and OCD may coexist.

OCD can coexist with a number of other conditions, and so this will make the diagnostic detective work more complicated. These include anxiety disorders, depression, disruptive behavior disorders, learning disorders, tic disorders, and trichotillomania (compulsive hair pulling) ("Obsessive-Compulsive Disorder," 2012).

OCD specific psychotherapy and psychiatric medications are the most effective treatments for OCD. Generally, OCD therapy is recommended before medication. One of the most effective therapy treatments for OCD is exposure response prevention. This is a cognitive behavior therapy focusing on gradual exposure to the thoughts and experiences of the obsessions while choosing not to perform the compulsions. Parents should ask if psychotherapists provide this. Any therapy for children and teens should include sessions with the parent/s to help better understand and manage the conditions. Other problems or family issues that are upsetting or destabilizing should be addressed as well. Relationship-focused, play therapy, or other therapies not specifically focused on the OCD will probably be less or ineffective.

Psychiatric medication may be helpful or even necessary to treat OCD. Therapy and medication together may be the most effective approach, particularly for more severe OCD. Selective serotonin reuptake inhibitor (SSRI) medications are typically the most effective. However, stimulant medications can exacerbate OCD symptoms in those without true ADHD and OCD, and this can help discriminate between OCD and ADHD. For those with both, unless the OCD is mild, often the OCD is treated first (Silver, 2009, Fall). Neurofeedback and Walsh's Advanced Nutrient Therapy may be helpful treatments as well.

Children Ages Three to Six with School and/or Nap Transitions

Children ages three to six could potentially have behavioral difficulties, irritability, and ADHD-like presentations if they are struggling with transitioning into or from half to full days of preschool, kindergarten, first grade, or daycare. Children may struggle with the structure and new routines of these settings, as well as separations from parents. Additionally, these younger children may be taking shorter or less frequent naps to none at all, and this may further impact their adjustment. The transition process may take months. If school transitions and nap problems are causing the difficulties and true ADHD and persistent separation anxiety are not present, then these problems should most likely be transitory and occur only during these changes. As the child ages and adjusts to these settings, the ADHD-like problems should remit, unless they have enduring separation anxiety. However, if true ADHD exists, then these transitions may be more difficult for the child and problems could persist. Lastly, ADHD and separation anxiety could coexist.

Depressive Disorders

Silver (2006) reported that depression is the second most common cause of ADHD-like symptoms after anxiety. Depressive symptoms can resemble ADHD, including focusing and memory difficulties, decreased motivation, academic underachievement, sleep impairment, mood problems, irritability, agitation, and restlessness. Depression can also coexist with and worsen true ADHD. About 20-30 percent of people with true ADHD also have depressive disorders. Those with Inattentive ADHD can have more depression and general unhappiness (Barkley, 2015, March 19a). Children with ADHD, particularly older children and adolescents, are at risk for developing depressive conditions due to their ADHD-related difficulties. Amen (2013) has discussed Limbic ADD, which is a combination of ADHD and depression symptoms. The issues with inappropriate and excessive social media use discussed previously with anxiety also apply to depressive conditions. Studies indicate that spending more time on social media can increase unhappiness and loneliness. There are concerns that the increased rates of depression in adolescents may be related to the pervasive increase in excessive screen and social media use.

Evaluation and Treatment

While some depression symptoms may occur briefly, depressive conditions symptoms should persist for at least two weeks and exhibit a change from prior functioning. When children or teens present with depression and possible ADHD-like indicators, clinicians should explore when the symptoms for each were first noticed. It is also important to investigate the specific content of the depressive thoughts and moods to determine if the depression is related to the possible ADHD (such as sadness about poor academics or social problems). Depression that is secondary to ADHD typically generates symptoms that are briefer or more transient, and are often connected to specific triggers and events associated with ADHD-related problems. In contrast, depressive disorders are frequently more chronic, have more symptoms and greater severity, and last weeks to months.

Depression and mood problems can impair concentration and cause hyperactivity. If ADHD symptoms exist mostly or solely during depressive phases, and ADHD symptoms are absent when mood problems improve or mood is normal, then this could suggest that true ADHD does not exist. If the ADHD symptoms exist when depressive symptoms are decreased or not present, then ADHD and a depressive condition may coexist. Also, children or adolescents with intermittent responses to stimulant medication may have an underlying mood condition (Lougy, DeRuvo, & Rosenthal, 2007).

When distinguishing between ADHD and depressive conditions, it can be helpful to determine triggers, stressors, and depression sources. Generally, if the depression has existed for longer periods, began earlier in the child's life, is pervasive and debilitating, and if the child has struggled with managing their sadness and depressive symptoms, then these factors can be suggestive of a separate mood disorder. Depression problems can be genetic in nature, so a family history can suggest that a true mood condition with or without true ADHD exists. Clinicians can use depression measures to further explore the symptoms and to elicit potentially more honest information. Additionally, those with depression can experience more sleep quality and quantity difficulties, including partial sleep deprivation, and these can also worsen ADHD. Individuals can also have an agitated depression which is a mixture of anxiety and depression that can resemble ADHD.

For children and adolescents with ADHD and depression, the depression symptoms and low self-esteem may decrease with effective ADHD-focused therapy, school accommodations, and medication, particularly when the depression is secondary. However, if the depression persists after effective ADHD treatment, an experienced psychotherapist should be consulted. Therapy should include the family to better understand, support, and manage the condition. Family or other problems that are upsetting or destabilizing should also be addressed. Psychiatric medication may be helpful to treat the depression, particularly if therapy is less effective.

With significant depression and true ADHD, medication treatment should first target the more serious condition. Since suicide is a significant risk with depression, this topic should always be explored in diagnostic interviews. Those with ADHD and depression have higher risks for suicide than with either condition alone. When children or adolescents present with suicidal risks, safety plans should be created and documented. Most parents should participate in therapy sessions when these risks exist, and they will be essential participants in the safety plans and risk management efforts. Higher levels of care beyond outpatient therapy may be necessary, such as intensive outpatient programs, partial hospitalization programs, and psychiatric inpatient hospitalizations. Lastly, neurofeedback and Walsh's Advanced Nutrient Therapy can improve depression.

Bipolar Disorder

This chronic mood disorder causes dysregulation of mood, behavior, activity, and sleep, along with significant interpersonal and other impairments. It is a brain-functioning condition that causes intense and persistent rages, prolonged temper tantrums, mood problems, lesser need for sleep, higher levels of irritability, and significant frustration tolerance problems. A meta-analysis of bipolar conditions found a prevalence of 1.8 percent in children. Bipolar disorder often emerges during childhood and adolescence, and its presentation differs from adult bipolar. Symptoms in children can fluctuate in intensity and their durations are often shorter than adult episodes. Also, pediatric versions may have more rapid cycling with accelerated phases of manic and depression symptoms (Faedda et al., 2016).

Pavuluri et al. (2006) discussed how pediatric bipolar differs from adult onset bipolar condition. The child and adolescent versions tend to exhibit significant episodic mood fluctuations, mixed mood states of depression and mania symptoms, high rates of comorbidity with other psychological conditions, and rapid cycling. Children with this can have rapidly fluctuating moods consisting of sadness, irritability, elation, and excitability that often result from environmental triggers. Also, this condition is chronic and refractory, with some symptoms occurring after treatment (West et al., 2011).

The symptoms for pediatric bipolar disorder can be difficult or inadequate to evaluate using adult criteria. The mania symptoms of flight of ideas, increase in goal directed activities causing painful consequences, and grandiosity can be hard to determine in children (Faedda et al., 2016). Proper identification and treatment are critical because this serious condition can cause school failure, aggression, high suicide rates, and high-risk behaviors including substance abuse and sexual promiscuity. Sadly, it can have high rates of recurrence, even though initial recovery can occur (Henry et al., 2008).

ADHD and childhood mania can be confused because they share several common features, including impulsivity, hyperactivity, distractibility, irritability, defiance, and behavioral problems. This can cause screening and detection difficulties because clinicians and psychological measures may be unable to differentiate mania (particularly lower level mania) from true ADHD symptoms. Pediatric bipolar conditions can cause false positives for ADHD (Henry et al., 2008). Many children and adolescents with bipolar-like presentations will not qualify for full DSM-5 bipolar I or bipolar II disorders, and may acquire other diagnoses. Milder bipolar disorder and severe ADHD can appear similar in some individuals. When they coexist, the onset of bipolar disorder may be earlier than bipolar disorder without ADHD.

ADHD, ODD, conduct disorder, learning disorders, and substance abuse are common coexisting conditions with bipolar disorder. ADHD is the most common, and 66 to 75 percent of prepubescents with bipolar will also meet criteria for ADHD. Coexisting conditions can complicate the diagnostic process, and it is more common to see a child or teen with bipolar with other superimposed conditions. Also, because other disorders will be more familiar to clinicians, they are often recognized and addressed first, including ADHD. Due to diagnostic challenges, clinicians may need to extend the diagnostic window for bipolar disorder and evaluate repeatedly over time (Youngstrom et al., 2005).

Significant sleep disturbance is much more common in bipolar disorder than ADHD. One researcher found it was 6.5 times more prevalent in children with bipolar than ADHD. Another study found that children with bipolar had substantially reduced total sleep and markedly increased nocturnal activity when compared to children with ADHD and controls, and these could be indicators to differentiate pediatric bipolar from ADHD. Research found that actigraphy (a wrist watch-like device) was helpful in measuring activity levels to differentiate the two (Faedda et al., 2016).

Children and teens with ADHD, but not bipolar, typically have less depression and mood problems, sleep longer once they fall asleep, show guilt and remorse after they break things or make mean statements during frustration episodes, and have shorter tantrums. Children with ADHD also tend to calm down faster when frustrated, usually within five to 30 minutes.

The controversial condition disruptive mood dysregulation disorder (DMDD) was created to distinguish children ages six to 17 with persistent and extreme irritability and recurrent severe temper outbursts (that may include aggression) from more traditional bipolar symptoms (Faedda et al., 2016). However, some clinicians believe DMDD symptoms are really a type of pediatric bipolar condition that does not meet DSM-5 criteria, and further research is necessary to determine its validity. Those supporting DMDD believe it is separate from adult bipolar because children with extreme irritability do not grow up to develop bipolar disorder and are more likely to have unipolar depression or anxiety disorders. While pediatric bipolar disorder occurs more commonly in girls, DMDD is more common in boys. Additionally, DMDD can resemble ODD, and DMDD may reflect the top 15 percent of ODD (Iliades, 2014).

To qualify for the DMDD, three or more severe tantrums should occur each week, and are excessive for the child's age and the situation. There is also an angry or irritable mood that occurs between the tantrums that persists without breaks. Also, there can be no mania or hypomania episodes, and the symptoms must have existed for at least a year. The symptoms must have been observed before age 10, but the condition cannot be diagnosed before age six (Iliades, 2014).

Finally, Amen (2013) has discussed two types of combinations of ADHD and bipolar-like symptoms. The first is Temporal Lobe ADD and includes irritability, temper without provocation, aggression, dark thoughts that can be suicidal or homicidal, mild paranoia, periods of confusion and panic or fear, as well as memory, learning and/or auditory processing difficulties. The second subtype is Ring of Fire ADD that includes cyclic changes of mood, rigid thinking, mean and demanding behaviors, excessive and rapid speech, grandiosity, irritability, and racing thoughts (Amen, 2013).

Evaluation and Treatment

Bipolar disorder is one of the most heritable psychological conditions. While some researchers have cautioned not to overinterpret family histories of bipolar disorder (Youngstrom et al., 2005), it can be helpful to explore this.

As with other disorders, clinicians should explore if the bipolar-like symptoms are the sole result of stressors. If negative parent-child relationships exist, it is important to determine if these began before or after the bipolar-like symptoms began. Additionally, true bipolar conditions will persist over time. For younger children, monitoring, time, and re-evaluations will often be needed to determine if the condition will persist or not.

Research indicates that parent-report measures can be the most accurate in assessing childhood bipolar disorder. Parent reports, and particularly mothers, have higher diagnostic accuracy than either teacher or child self-reports. Some of the most common and effective child bipolar measures are the Child Mania Rating Scale–Parent Version, the Parent Young Mania Rating Scale, and the Parent–General Behavior Inventory (West et al., 2011). Additionally, while the BASC and CBCL broadband measures do not have bipolar scales, they can help identify pediatric bipolar when the externalizing scales are highly elevated (Youngstrom et al., 2005).

At this time, there are two main ways of trying to determine if a child or teen has bipolar, true ADHD, or both. The first method involves conducting a thorough evaluation and/or psychological testing that includes a clinical interview, bipolar and other psychological measures, and exploring other potential conditions. For clinicians who lack experience diagnosing bipolar disorder, it may be necessary to obtain a testing from an experienced clinical psychologist.

The second method is to try several stimulant and/or bipolar medications at sufficient doses and monitor the response. In theory, if the child or teen has true Combined ADHD without bipolar, their hyperactivity and impulsivity will improve on stimulants, but the bipolar symptoms will not improve or will worsen. For those with bipolar conditions without true ADHD, stimulants or antidepressants will often make them worse. However, bipolar medications should improve the bipolar symptoms, and may improve the ADHD-like symptoms that have resulted from the bipolar condition. If bipolar and ADHD both exist, ADHD or bipolar medications should improve the respective condition, and overall partial progress can result. While this is not the most reliable or safest way to differentiate the two, some families attempt this. This approach will be safest with an experienced psychiatrist and careful monitoring. Generally, if bipolar disorder is suspected, it is best to treat this first with medication, and then re-assess and treat the ADHD.

Another approach to determine if a person has true ADHD and/or bipolar disorder is to use special blood and urine tests to determine which specific biochemical imbalances exist. Bipolar disorder alters certain neurochemical functioning in certain ways, and in addition to various psychiatric medications, specific nutrients can help to balance these issues. Please refer to the Walsh Biochemical Imbalances section presented in Chapter 3 for more information. QEEGs from neurofeedback providers may also provide some diagnostic information.

The most effective treatment for bipolar disorder is psychiatric medication. Family therapy treatment with experienced therapists can be helpful for caregivers to better understand, manage, and live with this difficult condition. Behavioral management approaches may need to be modified with more focus on rewards and less on negative consequences. Support groups may be helpful, but few seem to exist. Individual therapy may not be effective until the child is stabilized on medication, and results will probably depend upon the child or teen's openness to help, acceptance of the problems, and motivation for change. Fluctuating safety issues involving threats and aggression towards others and/or themselves may occur. Intensive outpatient programs or psychiatric hospitalizations may be necessary at times if they are not on effective medications, deteriorate in functioning, or become unstable. West et al. (2011) stated that clinicians who work with bipolar conditions often know that positive responses to treatment can be poor. Walsh's Advanced Nutrient Therapy can be a helpful treatment. Finally, neurofeedback may improve some brain-functioning issues, and could reduce medication usage, but a full remission may be unlikely.

Intermittent Explosive Disorder (IED)

Children age six to adults with this condition have significant anger issues that result in aggressive impulsive acts, including verbal aggression, physical violence toward people or animals, or damage to property. The anger episodes are greatly out of proportion, brief, and not preplanned. These angry or impulsive outbursts occur at least twice a week for three months, or at least three severe episodes involving property damage or assaults involving injury within one year. Aggressive behavior would not be considered part of IED when it occurs in children or teens who use aggression for a reason or have something to gain. While aggressive behavior occurs in other conditions, IED should be considered if the episodes are beyond what is expected from these other conditions. While it can coexist with ADHD, it should be distinguished from frustration tolerance difficulties within ADHD and bipolar disorder, as well as temper tantrums in younger children, head injuries, substance use, and psychotic conditions (Grohol, 2016).

IED is believed to have a lifetime incidence from 5 to 7 percent. It can be a destructive condition, frequently seen in the young and mostly males. In the worst cases, dozens of serious aggression episodes can occur over time that can necessitate medical treatment or cause significant property damage. One study found that first degree relatives of those with IED had significantly greater risk of developing the condition. A number of studies have found that it seems associated with abnormally low levels of serotonin, a neurotransmitter that assists in regulating aggression. Another study found that people with IED demonstrated similar performances to those with prefrontal cortex damage (Harvard Medical School, 2011). Legal difficulties are not uncommon with more severe cases from the crimes of violent behaviors.

Evaluation and Treatment

It will be important to explore other conditions to determine if IED-like behaviors are better explained by them. Also, because poor frustration tolerance, aggressive physical or verbal outbursts are typical in those with Combined ADHD, ODD, conduct disorder, and bipolar disorder, care should be used when diagnosing IED along with these. Only when the outbursts are chronic, severe, and beyond what is expected for these other disorders should IED be diagnosed in addition to them. For treatment, cognitive behavioral therapy that utilizes coping skills and relaxation training along with cognitive restructuring has shown some promise. Although research has been limited, there are medications that reduce aggression and prevent rages. These include mood stabilizers (lithium and anticonvulsants), selective serotonin reuptake inhibitors (SSRIs) antidepressants, and antipsychotic medications (Harvard Medical School, 2011). Neurofeedback and Walsh's Advanced Nutrient Therapy may also help.

Oppositional Defiant Disorder (ODD)

ODD is a pattern of anger, irritability, argumentativeness, and defiance lasting for a minimum of six months, with four or more of the symptoms on this checklist. These behaviors are beyond what is considered normal for the child's peers, occur with at least one person that is not a sibling, and cause significant difficulties. For children below age five, the behaviors occur on most days for at least six months. For children ages five and older, they occur at least once a week for six months or longer (Mayo Clinic Staff, 2015).

About 60 percent of those with Combined ADHD have ODD. All children and adolescents with Combined ADHD should be screened for ODD because of this high coexistence. Children and teens with ADHD and ODD have greater difficulties with emotional control, aggression, and have more conflictual and negative relationships with family members (Barkley, 2015, March 19a). Parents are often overwhelmed and highly frustrated by this combination. The ODD component seems to magnify and accelerate the ADHD challenges, and over time highly negative familial relationships and discord can occur. Parents commonly demonstrate chronic bitterness, resentment, frequent yelling, avoidance of their children, passive compliance with children's demands, and even desperate episodes of ineffective corporeal punishment and physical abuse. Verbal and physical escalations and altercations can be become increasingly frequent without treatment.

ODD can evolve from untreated ADHD because these individuals can have more difficulties completing tasks and chores they dislike, as well as poor frustration tolerance. It is easier to refuse, complain, or argue with parents when they are asked to do things they do not want to do. When parents and teachers make requests, they can become easily stressed, overwhelmed, and frustrated, causing noncompliance and oppositionality. Children and teens with ODD often lie, blame others, swear and deny that they didn't do things they actually did, and exhibit anger. A negative and reinforcing cycle can form because the more difficult they become, the more adults resent them and stop asking them to do things.

Evaluation and Treatment

When evaluating this condition, clinicians should be careful to rule out other potential causes of ODD. In many cases, ODD can be considered a secondary condition. If ADHD is not the cause, ODD can result from abuse, highly conflictual divorce or parental separations situations, domestic violence, dysfunctional family environments, or other traumatic experiences. Clinicians should explore if the child has ongoing or unresolved traumas or upsetting situations not related to ADHD. Because families with children and teens with ODD typically have dysfunctional relationships, clinicians should explore if the ODD (and ADHD) seemed to exist first before the negative relational difficulties, or if family problems and/or negative parental interactions occurred first. Of course, both scenarios may exist.

For those with ODD and ADHD, ADHD treatment is critical. Fortunately, effective ADHD medication at sufficient doses often improves ODD. Family therapy focused on treating ADHD and ODD can help parents specifically understand, accept, and manage ODD behaviors, as well as improve parent-child relationships. This therapy should teach behavioral management approaches, including helping parents learn to not emotionally react to negative behaviors and attitudes, maintain clear and realistic expectations for daily behaviors, and consistently apply consequences for desired and unwanted behaviors. Family issues or other problems that are upsetting or destabilizing should also be addressed. Individual therapy may be necessary to address coexisting conditions, significant difficulties, and/or trauma, and will probably be more effective after ADHD medication and family therapy occur. Resistance may initially occur, and rewards for therapy participation can be utilized. Parents may require their own individual therapy to help them accept the conditions, reduce bitterness, work on their own triggers, improve relations, and address other personal or family issues.

Treatment for substance use may also be needed because teens with ODD tend to have more of these problems. Finally, neurofeedback and Walsh's Advanced Nutrient Therapy may also be helpful treatments.

Rebuilding positive parent-child relationships will be important. One potent way to accomplish this is through the use of together time. Barkley and Benton (1998) discuss this at length. During together time, parents spend at least 20 minutes with the child or teen daily doing an activity the child likes, and making positive observational comments. The goal is to not teach or correct, but to connect, spend enjoyable time together, and reverse the negative relational dynamics.

Conduct Disorder (CD)

This is a serious behavioral condition where the rights of others and societal norms are violated and disrespected. It is associated with more impulsive and reckless behavior, defiance, substance use, aggression, serious school behavioral difficulties, delinquent and criminal behaviors. A diagnosis of CD is given when the pattern of difficult behavior exists for over a year, and is much more extreme than is socially acceptable. CD has been associated with significant family problems and conflicts, child abuse, poverty, genetic defects, parental substance abuse, and poverty. CD behavior can also be an early sign of bipolar disorder and depression, so these conditions should be monitored and considered (Rogge & A.D.A.M. Editorial Team, 2015). It often coexists with and causes tremendous relational problems between youth and parents. Higher levels of bitterness, anger, disengagement, aggression, dysfunctional family dynamics, and parenting problems are not uncommon in these families.

One study found 14 percent of children with ADHD had CD, while other studies reported higher rates. Those with ADHD and CD have more foster care placements, significantly more learning disorders than ADHD alone, and their parents have higher rates of psychological conditions and divorce. Finally, CD is the strongest predictor of higher rates of future substance use (Pliszka, 2015).

Evaluation and Treatment

ADHD can coexist with conduct disorder, so any child or teen with CD symptoms should be evaluated for ADHD. Due to the similarities of ODD and CD, please refer to the evaluation and treatment section for ODD. However, CD is usually more difficult to treat than ODD and has a worse prognosis. Fortunately, if a child or teen has ADHD and CD, medication for ADHD can improve some CD symptoms. Similar to ODD, successful treatment will also involve identifying and treating coexisting conditions (including ADHD, learning disorders, depression, and substance use), dysfunctional family issues, chronic relational problems, trauma and/or abuse. Addressing police involvement and legal issues resulting from vandalism, theft, aggression, and substance use may also be necessary.

Effective treatment for CD should occur early and heavily involve the parents. Research has indicated that children and teens with CD are more likely to have ongoing difficulties if their families do not receive comprehensive and early treatment. Without this, individuals with CD may be unable to effectively adapt to the demands of later life and can continue to have a downward spiral of interpersonal, substance abuse, employment, criminal, and aggression problems. Due to these challenges, treatment should not be expected to be brief (American Academy of Child and Adolescent Psychiatry, 2015). Unfortunately, treatment attendance and compliance may be problematic. Again, similar to ODD, family psychotherapy will be a critical part of helping families change, and should include teaching effective parenting and behavioral management skills, addressing family problems, and improving the highly negative parent-child relationships. After family therapy and ADHD medication use, individual therapy (if they will participate) may be needed to teach emotional management skills and work on other conditions and problems. Parents may require their own individual psychotherapy to address their resentments, frustrations, and relational challenges. Finally, neurofeedback and Walsh's Advanced Nutrient Therapy may be helpful treatments.

Substance Abuse

Because the brain experiences dramatic changes during adolescence, substance use can have serious impact on brain development. Additionally, teens who repeatedly abuse substances have much greater risks of developing serious substance abuse conditions later in life. Older children and adolescents with ADHD have higher rates of substance experimentation and abuse, including nicotine, alcohol, marijuana, illegal, and over-the-counter drugs. Those with ADHD have higher substance use rates due to their higher levels of thrill-seeking, risk taking, impulsivity, poor planning and anticipation of negative consequences, and self-medicating behaviors. The direct and after-effects of substance use can cause ADHD-like symptoms, including problems with focusing and concentration, disorganization, behavior, academics, motivation, mood changes, irritability, delinquent behaviors, and lack of compliance with chores or daily expectations. Also, substance use can cause additional behavioral and lifestyle changes, including secretive behaviors, a change in friends, theft, cessation of previously enjoyed activities, a lack of parental compliance, and new interests in drug-related themes and music.

Evaluation and Treatment

While many teens experiment to some degree with risky behaviors, adolescents with ADHD use nicotine, alcohol, and drugs at earlier ages than their peers and have higher rates of substance abuse. To help distinguish between true ADHD and substance use, clinicians can explore when the ADHD symptoms began and when the substance use first occurred. When ADHD symptoms existed prior to use, this can suggest true ADHD. It may be helpful for clinicians to explore substance use with adolescents alone and then together with their parents in a neutral manner to obtain the most accurate information due to teens' tendency to be less honest about their use. Clinicians should explore the first use, last use, and typical frequency of use over the last 12 or more months for all substances used. Attempting to understand the reasons for their use is helpful as well.

Substance use can be addressed in a number of ways. First, education about substances and about adolescent substance use will be important. Increased parental monitoring and supervision should occur, and the trust of the teen will need to be rebuilt over time. Peer groups and boredom may play substantial roles in the use, and will need to be addressed. Other related factors and issues should be explored and addressed, and professional assistance should be considered. Parents should create clear expectations with standard groundings for any future alcohol and/or drug use. Additionally, random drug screening can be conducted periodically by parents to monitor usage. Drug kits are sold online and at pharmacies and are inexpensive, but more costly and sensitive kits that can test for a greater range of substances (including nicotine) may be more useful. Random testing can help adolescents with peer pressure because they can tell peers, "I can't use. My parents test me and I'll get in big trouble."

Adolescent drug and alcohol counselors can be utilized when substance experimentation first occurs for less intensive services, and may be the safest approach. Teens with repeated substance use should receive treatment from adolescent substance use intensive outpatient programs (IOPs) or more intensive services from counselors. These providers typically also work with families to provide treatment, as well as education on substance use, guidance for parents when more serious usage occurs, and can address other use issues. For repeated nicotine use, adolescents can start with treatment or referrals from primary care physicians. Older children and adolescents who take effective ADHD medications tend to have less substance use, so medication should be considered if not currently utilized. If medication is used, providers should explore if it is taken consistently and if the medication and dosage are effective. Neurofeedback and Walsh's Advanced Nutrient Therapy may be helpful, but will probably not be the primary treatments, particularly with more severe abuse.

Gaming Disorder

Also called video game disorder or addiction, this is a pattern of recurrent, excessive, and persistent video game use (online or offline) that causes significant impairments in personal, family, relational, or educational functioning. It may be episodic or continuous, but persists for at least 12 months. However, for severe symptoms, the duration may be shorter. It can affect children and adults. This is in the International Classification of Diseases (ICD-11) and in the DSM-5 as a condition to be further researched (Lopez, 2018). In the United States, over 90 percent of children and adolescents spend significant amounts of time playing video games. Reported prevalence rates of gaming disorder vary, ranging from 1 to 9 percent (Gentile et al., 2017). Excessive video game use seems more detrimental than other forms of screen use (M. Wehrenberg, personal communication, December 07, 2018). Some studies have suggested that the most addictive video games are fantasy role-playing games, particularly for children who are unpopular or shy (Dewar, 2009–2013).

The amount of daily entertainment screen media use in children and teens is alarming. While some studies indicate lesser daily usage, one large 2015 study by Common Sense Media reported that American adolescents spend about nine hours a day on screen media, and tweens ages eight to 12 use about six hours per day. One interesting large study examined the occurrence of future ADHD symptoms with higher digital media use and found that adolescents with heavy use were twice as likely as infrequent users to develop new ADHD symptoms (Ra et al., 2018).

Conversely, research has shown that ADHD is the most significant predictor for developing video game and internet addiction in children and adolescents. Those with ADHD may have a predisposed vulnerability to the intense stimulation and experience of video games. "Getting to the next level" can be a highly addictive and immediate reward for players, and the quickly changing images and sounds require less attentional and working memory abilities. Pathological gaming and ADHD seem to share a bidirectional relationship, where ADHD makes video games highly appealing, while the gaming itself seems to worsens ADHD symptoms. Excessive gaming also reduces other activities, interests, exercise, and social experiences which promote healthy brain functioning over time (Weiss et al., 2011). Additionally, the other issues concerning screen time previously discussed in the anxiety section also apply to this condition.

Evaluation and Treatment

This diagnosis should not be based on excessive video game playing alone, and should include significant impairments in life areas (Gentile et al., 2017). Gaming disorder can mimic ADHD because it can cause difficulties with lower grades, behaviors, falling asleep and shorter sleep duration, executive functioning, social functioning, and other ADHD-like symptoms. These usually occur immediately after video game use, particularly after longer periods of play. Because it can cause ADHD-like presentations and also coexist with true ADHD, discriminating between these is important.

The American Academy of Pediatrics recommends that the total amount of screen time per day be limited to up to two hours. Additionally, no screen devices should be located in bedrooms, and no screen time, particularly video game use, within 60 minutes before sleep. Because gaming disorder often presents with other conditions, clinicians should screen for and treat these, including ADHD, anxiety, depression (Gentile et al., 2017), and social phobia. After studying for tests, screen use and video gaming should not be used because these can negatively impact executive functioning and learning (M. Wehrenberg, personal communication, December 07, 2018).

Because children and teens with ADHD are at higher risks of developing video game addiction, parents should protect them by limiting and monitoring their use. Rules and limits for screen time and video games are some of the most important things parents can do. Children and teens can earn daily screen time and video game use after they perform their chores, homework, and other expected behaviors each day. Families should routinely use kitchen or phone timers to manage video game and screen use, and can use timer limits within devices.

Warner (2007) presented additional approaches parents can utilize to reduce and manage the risk of gaming disorder. Screen devices should be located and used in community areas of the home. Parents should check and follow age-based ratings and content descriptions of video games before children acquire them. Parents can use clear expectations with negative consequences for not complying with these, as well as parental approval of all new games. Discussions should be regularly held with children and adolescents regarding internet safety, particularly if they use multiplayer online role-playing games. Caregivers should talk to the parents of their children's friends about the video games they play, what they are permitted to play, their children's limits on content, and the amount of time they are permitted to play. Caregivers should also play games with their children so they can learn more about them.

Medication treatments for ADHD can help with gaming difficulties. One study found that eight weeks of methylphenidate reduced their game usage and addiction test scores (Weiss et al., 2011). Psychotherapy can involve learning to manage cravings for gaming and enforcing limits on usage and the types of games played. Victoria Dunckley's book *Reset Your Child's Brain* presents a four-week plan to reverse the effects of excessive screen time (M. Wehrenberg, personal communication, December 07, 2018). Neurofeedback and Walsh's Advanced Nutrient Therapy may be helpful to various degrees.

REFERENCES

Amen, D. (2013). *Healing ADD* (revised edition). New York: Berkley Books.

American Academy of Child and Adolescent Psychiatry. (2015). *Conduct disorder.* Retrieved from http:www.aacap.org/AACAP/Families_and_Youth/Facts_for _Families/FFF-Guide/Conduct-Disorder-033.aspx

Barkley, R. (2015, March 19a). *ADHD: Nature, course, outcomes, and comorbidity.* Retrieved from www.continuingedcourses.net/active/courses/course003.php

Barkley, R., & Benton, C. (1998). *Your defiant child.* New York: Guilford Press.

Brasic, J.R. (2012, July 9). *Pediatric obsessive-compulsive disorder differential diagnoses. medscape reference.* Retrieved from www.ocdandfamilies.org/2012 /07/16/ocd-and-adhd-why-the-overlap-with-poll/

Checklist of OCD symptoms. (2005). Tourettes Syndrome Foundation of Canada. Retrieved from www.tourette.ca/learn-diagnoses.php and www.gapacademy.ca /files/checklist_ocd.pdf

Cuncic, A. (2014, May 16). *Overview of social anxiety disorder.* Retrieved from http://socialanxietydisorder.about.com/od/overviewofsad/a/overview.htm

Dewar, G. (2009-2013). *Video game addiction: An evidence-based guide.* Retrieved from http://www.parentingsscience.com/video-game-addiction.html

Faedda, G., Ohashi, K., Hernandez, M., McGreenery, C., Grant, M., Baroni, A., Polcari, A., & Teicher, M. (2016). Actigraph measures discriminate pediatric bipolar disorder from attention-deficit/hyperactivity disorder and typically developing controls. *Journal of Child Psychology and Psychiatric, 57*(6), 706–716.

Fader, S. (2018). *Social media obsession and anxiety.* Retrieved from http://adaa.org /social-media-obsession

Geller, D. A., & Brown, T. E. (2009). ADHD with Obsessive-Compulsive Disorder. In T. E. Brown (Ed.), *ADHD comorbidities: Handbook for ADHD complications in children and adults* (pp. 177–188). Arlington, VA: American Psychiatric.

Gentile, D. A., Bailey, K., Bavelier, D., Brockmyer, J. F., Cash, H., Coyne, S., & Young, F. (2017, November). Internet gaming disorder in children and adolescents. *Pediatrics, 140*(Suppl 2), S81–S85. doi: 10.1542/peds.2016-1758H

Grohol, J. (2016). *Intermittent explosive disorder.* Retrieved from https://psychcentral .com/lib/intermittent-explosive-disorder/

Harvard Medical School. (2011, April). *Treating intermittent explosive disorder.* Retrieved from http://www.health.harvard.edu/newsletter_article/treating-inter mittent-explosive-disorder

Henry, D. B., Pavuluri, M. N., Youngstrom, E., & Birmaher, B. (2008). Accuracy of brief and full forms of the Child Mania Rating Scale. *Journal of Clinical Psychology, 64*(4), 368–381.

Hoge, E., Bickham, D., & Cantor, J. (2017, November). Digital media, anxiety, and depression in children. *Pediatrics, 140*(Suppl 2), S76–S80. doi: 10.1542/peds .2016-1758G

Iliades, C. (2014, October 25). *Disruptive mood dysregulation disorder current concepts and controversies.* Retrieved from http://www.psychiatryadvisor.com/childadolescent -psychiatry/disruptive-mood-dysregulation-disorder-current-concepts-and- controversies/article/379374/

International OCD Foundation. (2016). *What is OCD?* Retrieved from https//iocdf .org/about-ocd/#obsessions

Lopez, G. (2018, December 6). *Video game addiction is real, rare, and poorly understood.* Retrieved from https://www.vox.com/science-andhealth/2018/12/6/18050680 /video-game-addiction...

Lougy, R. A., DeRuvo, S. L., & Rosenthal, D. (2007). *Teaching young children with ADHD.* Thousand Oak, CA: Corwin Press.

Matheis, L. (2016, March 14). *Identifying signs of anxiety in children.* Retrieved on from https://www.anxiety.org/causes-and-symptoms-of-anxiety-in-children

Mayo Clinic Staff. (2015, February, 06). *Oppositional defiant disorder (ODD)—Symptoms.* Retrieved from https://www.mayoclinic.org/diseases-conditions/oppositional -defiant-disorder/basics/symptoms/con-20024559

Mayo Clinic Staff. (2017, August, 16). *Depression (major depressive disorder)—Symptoms & causes.* Retrieved from https://www.mayoclinic.org/diseases-conditions /depression/symptoms-causes/syc-20356007

National Institute of Mental Health [NIMH]. (2016, January). *Obsessive-compulsive disorder.* Retrieved from https:www.nimh.nih.gov/health/topics/obsessive -compulsive-disorder-ocd/index.shtml

Obsessive-Compulsive Disorder. (2012). Reviewed May 5, 2012 by Ben Joseph and Elana Pearl. Retrieved from http://kidshealth.org/en/parents/ocd.html?view =ptr&WT.ac=p-ptr

PANDAS Network. (2017). *What is PANDAS?* Retrieved from https://www.pandas network.org/understanding-pandaspans/what-is-pandas/

Papolos, D., & Papolos, J. (2006). *The bipolar child* (3rd ed.). New York: Broadway Books.

Pavuluri, M. N., Henry, D. B., Devineni, B, Carbray, J.A., & Birmaher, B. (2006). Child mania rating scale: Development, reliability, and validity. *Journal of the American Academy of Child & Adolescent Psychiatry, 45*(5), 550–560.

Pliszka, S. (2015). Comorbid psychiatric disorders in children with ADHD. In R. Barkley (Ed.), *Attention deficit hyperactivity disorder: A handbook for diagnosis and treatment* (4th ed., pp 140–168). New York: Guilford Press.

Ra, C. K., Cho, J., Stone, M. D., De La Cerda, J., Goldenson, N., Moroney, E., & Leventhal, A. (2018, July). Association of digital media use with subsequent symptoms of attention-deficit/hyperactivity disorder among adolescents. *Journal of the American Medical Association, 320*(3), 255–263. doi: 10.1001/jama.2018.8931

Rogge, T., & A.D.A.M. Editorial Team. (2015, March 04). *Conduct disorder: Medlineplus medical encyclopedia.* Retrieved from https://medlineplus.gov/ency /article/000919.htm

Silver, L. (2006). *The Misunderstood child: Understanding and coping with your child's learning disabilities* (4th ed.). New York: Three Rivers Press.

Silver, L. (2009, Spring). *Is it anxiety or ADHD?* Retrieved from www.addditudemag .com/adhd/article/print/5231.html

Silver, L. (2009, Fall). *Is it OCD or ADD/ADHD?* Retrieved from www.additude mag.com/adhd/article/print/6113.html

Spruyt, K., & Gozal, D. (2011, April). Sleep disturbances in children with attention-deficit/hyperactivity disorder. *Expert Review of Neurotherapeutics, 11*(4), 565–577. doi: 10.1586/ern.11.7

Warner, D. E. (2007, December). Video games: When does play become pathology? *Current Psychiatry, 6*(12), 27–38.

Weiss, M. D., Baer, S., Allan, B. A., Saran, K., & Schibuk, H. (2011, December). The screens culture: Impact on ADHD. *Attention Deficit Hyperactive Disorders, 3*(4), 327–334. doi: 10.1007/s12402-011-0065-z

West, A. E., Celio, C. I., Henry, D. B., & Pavuluri, M. N. (2011, January). Child mania rating scale-parent version: A valid measure of symptom change due to pharma-cotherapy. *Journal of Affective Disorders, 128*(1-2), 112–119.

Youngstrom, E. A., Findling, R. L., Youngstrom, J. K., & Calabrese, J. R. (2005). Toward an evidence-based assessment of pediatric bipolar disorder. *Journal of Clinical Child and Adolescent Psychology, 34*(3), 433–448.

Chapter 10

PSYCHOLOGICAL TRAUMA
AND DISSOCIATION

Note: Throughout this and the next chapter, psychological and emotional trauma will be referred to as "trauma." There is overlap throughout this and the next chapter because some children who have experienced trauma and abuse may have also experienced neglect and pathogenic care, while many children who have experienced neglect and pathogenic care will have also encountered multiple traumas.

UNDERSTANDING TRAUMA

Sadly, trauma and abuse in children and adolescents is common. One in four children and adolescents experience at least one significant traumatic event inside or outside their home before age 18 (Costello et al., 2002). One in 10 children experience sexual abuse before age 18. While most who experience severe or life-threatening events will manifest posttraumatic symptoms soon after the exposure, only about 30 percent will manifest symptoms beyond the first month (American Academy of Child and Adolescent Psychiatry, 2010). Children can suffer from traumatic stress and reactions long after the event has ceased. Younger children may lose previously acquired skills (such as language or toileting abilities), while adolescents may exhibit atypical aggression, self-destructive, or reckless behavior (Siegfried et al., 2016).

There are different types of trauma, including community violence, complex trauma, domestic violence, early childhood trauma, medical trauma, traumatic grief, physical abuse, sexual abuse, refugee trauma, disasters, terrorism and violence (The National Child Traumatic Stress Network, n.d.), and neglect. Additionally, there are single episodes of trauma, repetitive trauma, complex trauma that is recurrent and chronic, developmental trauma from ongoing adverse childhood experiences including abuse or neglect within close relationships, intergenerational and historical trauma that affects familial generations and cultural groups, and vicarious trauma where professionals become impacted by the patient's trauma ("Types of Trauma," n.d.).

Studies have shown maltreated children can demonstrate a great range of difficulties, including withdrawal, aggression, oppositional behavior, substance use, self-injury, compulsive behaviors, mood difficulties, anxiety, eating disorders, academic and learning impairments, and diminished self-esteem. Their behavioral problems may result from feeling overwhelmed or unconscious attempts to dispel negative emotional states. Forty percent of traumatized children have an anxiety, disruptive behavior, or mood disorder. Another type of trauma, exposure to domestic violence, was found to increase the risk and severity of internalizing and externalizing problems, academic, relational, vocational, and legal problems from childhood to adulthood (D'Andrea et al., 2012). Research reported that physically abused children tend to exhibit more externalizing problems, while sexual abuse can produce more posttraumatic stress disorder (PTSD) and internalizing symptoms, and sexual behavior problems in children. Peer rejection can be particularly devastating for trauma exposed children and teens because it places them at significant risk for academic underachievement, ongoing social problems, and behavioral difficulties (Briscoe-Smith & Hinshaw, 2006).

While more difficult to detect, psychological maltreatment or emotional abuse is a common type of child abuse that is more damaging than many realize. It differs from dysfunctional parenting because it is a severe, chronic, and escalating pattern of emotionally abusive and neglectful parenting. It often coexists with other types of abuse and neglect, and its occurrence with and without other forms of abuse and neglect is more common than recognized. Although psychological abuse is the most common form of maltreatment, official reports to child welfare agencies are rare. Youth with histories of psychological maltreatment have demonstrated elevated rates of hyperactivity, inattention, aggression, noncompliance, depression, anxiety, PTSD, and suicidality. Other research reported that when there is psychological maltreatment with sexual or physical abuse, there were greater difficulties than abuse alone (Spinazzola et al., 2015).

TRAUMA AND ADHD

Because trauma and abuse are so prevalent in children and adolescents, it is important to understand how they can cause ADHD-like symptoms, as well as coexist with true ADHD. ADHD symptoms occur in 25 to 45 percent of severely maltreated children (Putnam, 1997). Maltreated and traumatized children may experience symptoms which can closely mimic ADHD, including behavioral problems, hypervigilance, poor frustration tolerance, risk-taking behaviors, and self-regulation difficulties. They may experience inattention due to internal preoccupation with intrusive memories, dissociation, anxiety, and avoidance of trauma-related material. The PTSD symptoms of avoidance and reexperiencing can cause hyperactivity, restlessness, disorganization, and agitated play. The PTSD hyperarousal symptoms can cause poor concentration, hypervigilant motor activity, sleeping difficulties, angry outbursts, irritability, and ODD traits (American Academy of Child and Adolescent Psychiatry, 2010).

Additional trauma-related symptoms resembling ADHD are difficulties with learning, concentration, listening, anger control, overwhelming stress, and depression. Children with intrusive trauma-related thoughts and memories may be agitated or confused which can resemble impulsivity (Siegfried et al., 2016). Also, repeated childhood maltreatment can increase risks for developing chronic difficulties with impulse control, emotional regulation, attention, cognition, dissociation, and interpersonal relationships. Research has clearly demonstrated maltreated children have problems maintaining attention and integration of their cognitive functions, either as generalized or episodic impairments (D'Andrea et al., 2012). Researchers using neuropsychological tests found maltreated children demonstrated worse executive functioning, attention, and concentration abilities than nonmaltreated children (D'Andrea et al., 2012). Studies have also shown that children exposed to almost any form of maltreatment can experience increased aggressive, delinquent, and antisocial behaviors (Kendall-Tackett & Giacomoni, 2003).

In addition to trauma causing ADHD-like presentations, a number of studies indicate that youth with ADHD are more likely to develop traumatic stress than those without ADHD. Some researchers have proposed that children with ADHD should be considered a high-risk group for developing traumatic stress (Siegfried et al., 2016). Other studies have documented that ADHD diagnoses were more frequent in interpersonal trauma victims (D'Andrea et al., 2012). Ford et al. (2000) reported significantly high rates of sexual and physical abuse among children who had ADHD, ODD, and particularly both conditions. Researchers found that 45 to 73 percent of children with ODD were exposed to physical maltreatment, and 18 to 31 percent were sexually maltreated. Additionally, 25 percent of children with ADHD experienced physical abuse and 11 percent experienced sexual abuse. Sadly, 91 percent of children with ADHD and ODD were found to have a history of abuse. This study suggests that children with ADHD and ODD are at greater risk for having abuse experiences and warrant trauma evaluations. Additionally, research has demonstrated that trauma can worsen true ADHD, and ADHD can complicate the effects of trauma. Youth with both trauma and ADHD have demonstrated increased lifetime rates of almost all psychological disorders and more severe outcomes (Siegfried et al., 2016).

ADHD AND ABUSIVE CAREGIVERS

For decades, research has indicated that children and teens with ADHD and PTSD have high comorbidity rates. One group of researchers hypothesized that children with ADHD are at higher risk for trauma due to their persistent behavioral problems, including difficult, defiant, and dangerous behaviors. Also, their abusive parents and caregivers may have their own difficulties, including ADHD, substance abuse, impulse control difficulties, impatience, and poor frustration tolerance (Cuffe, McCullough, & Pumariega, 1994).

Other studies have shown that parents of children with ADHD experience more stress and dysfunctional interactional styles with their children. Additionally, these parents report more feelings of incompetence, self-blame, depression, and isolation. Mothers of children with hyperactivity are separated or divorced more often than mothers of children without ADHD. One group of researchers presented the possibility that caregivers of children with difficult temperaments and ADHD may experience higher levels of parental stress and distress which can lead to abusive parenting. This toxic parenting can then increase aggressive tendencies and behavioral problems in those with ADHD, with a negative cycle forming (Briscoe-Smith & Hinshaw, 2006). Also, children who have poor relationships with caregivers are less compliant with them, and this can further contribute to the negative spiral. Consequently, while not the child or adolescent's fault, those with ADHD, ODD, and behavioral problems can elicit excessive negative and abusive reactions from parents.

Since ADHD is highly genetically transmitted, many parents of children with ADHD will also have this. These parents can become easily overwhelmed and frustrated with their challenging children, contributing to abusive behavior and excessive discipline. Becker-Blease and Freyd (2008) found that 77 percent of abused children had a parent with ADHD. Parents who are abusive with their children may also have their own childhood histories of abuse and neglect, and may unknowingly participate in the intergenerational cycle of family violence. Some parents may believe that abusive corporal punishment is normal or necessary, and their discipline approaches should be explored during evaluations.

THE NEUROBIOLOGICAL EFFECTS OF TRAUMA

The neurobiological effects of trauma can cause brain changes that create ADHD-like symptoms. Traumatic events, particularly those that occur early in the child's life and over time, can cause significant brain functioning alterations. Abuse, neglect, and deprivation that occur before age two can cause severe neurological damage that may create ADHD-like presentations. Infants and very young children need certain levels of human touch, interaction, and brain stimulation for proper brain development, and physiological damage can result when this is lacking (Ladnier & Massanari 2000). Some researchers have proposed that child neglect and abuse may create developmental deficits and difficulties which could cause hormonal changes and an inability to learn self-regulation (Follan et al., 2011). Additionally, when children experience significant and chronic fearful experiences early in life, their ability to tolerate and regulate stress, arousal, and emotions can be affected. They can lose the ability to distinguish between safety and threat. They also become impaired in their abilities to interact with others, and may falsely perceive threats in social situations where none exist (National Scientific Council on the Developing Child, 2010). These traumatic experiences can then cause impairments in their ability to trust and connect with others, causing serious relationship difficulties with their caregivers, teachers, and peers.

The overwhelming stresses of trauma can disrupt normal developmental processes and cause chronic and abnormal changes through system overactivity (Dahmen et al., 2012). Children who experience trauma and maltreatment can have damaged neurobiological "alarm systems" that alert them to danger. They may become stuck in imbalanced brain states of constant alert mode waiting for danger. As a result, they can overreact to normal situations, have difficulty trusting others, be impulsive, and struggle with self-regulation and calming down. Over time, an extended state of stress and hyperarousal that produces stress hormones and neurochemicals can damage the brain (Perry et al., 1995).

Trauma can cause hypothalamic-pituitary-adrenal axis disturbances to produce abnormal cortisol concentrations that can cause harmful long-lasting effects, including brain dysfunction in the prefrontal regulatory system and hippocampus. Additionally, continuing stress can change the prefrontal connectivity in attention networks to create ADHD-like behavior (Dahmen et al., 2012). Chronic trauma can impair the development and functioning of the prefrontal cortex (National Scientific Council on the Developing Child, 2010). Enduring and higher doses of cortisol and adrenaline in children who experience abuse and neglect can actually shrink parts of the brain responsible for learning and memory (Rutledge, 2014). One study even showed children with PTSD, compared to those without PTSD, had decreased volumes of certain portions of the brain (D'Andrea et al., 2012).

The monoamine systems (which involve the neurotransmitters dopamine, serotonin, and noradrenaline) are important parts of the brain's stress-response neural networks. Chronic hypervigilance from trauma can cause sympathetic nervous system hyperarousal that results in inattention, hyperactivity, and impulsivity. When a person is threatened and the monoamine system stress response is activated in a chronic and repetitive way, the involved neural networks will become damaged and change. The brain will shift to act as if it is under constant threat, and ADHD-like and other behavioral symptoms can result (Perry, 2009).

Developmental trauma can cause a number of medical and neurodevelopmental conditions (B. D. Perry, personal communication, April 14, 2014). Trauma, neglect, maltreatment, prenatal exposure to alcohol and drugs, and impaired early bonding all adversely influence the child's developing brain and disrupt the normal developmental process. These interfere with normal patterns of experience-guided neurodevelopment by creating abnormal patterns of neural and neurohormonal activity. The neurobiological organization of higher parts of the brain depend upon the input from the lower parts. Developmental trauma will cause sequential damage from the lower to the higher parts of the brain. If the incoming neural activity in these monoamine systems is normal, then the higher brain areas will organize in healthier ways. However, if the patterns are extreme or dysregulated, then the higher areas will have abnormal brain pattern organization causing developmental problems and conditions, including ADHD-like difficulties (Perry, 2009).

THE EVALUATION OF TRAUMA

All children and teens should be screened for trauma and neglect during ADHD evaluations. However, this can be challenging because traumatized children and adolescents can have confusing or diagnostically complex presentations, especially when their trauma history is not known or appreciated. Therefore, it is critical that clinicians ask about a range of possible traumatic experiences. If this is not done, some traumas may not be disclosed. If any are identified, they should be further explored, including when they occurred and their duration. Clinicians should practice neutrality and objectivity while discussing trauma topics, and not make assumptions or conclusions about a child or teen's functioning, diagnoses, or situation until the evaluation process is completed. When inquiring about trauma, clinicians should phrase questions in direct, concrete, and clear terms, such as "Has anyone ever hit you?," "Was a bruise or mark left on your body?," "Has anyone ever touched your private parts, talked about private parts, or showed you their private parts in a way that made you scared or uncomfortable?" and "Have you ever seen anyone hit any of your family members?" Questions that are vague ("Have you ever experienced a trauma?" or "Have you been abused") and not age appropriate can produce inaccurate and inadequate information (Assessment of Complex Trauma, n.d.).

Clinicians should also be aware of confidentiality issues and not make blanket promises to families that "nothing bad will happen" regarding the consequences of disclosure. Clinicians should know their state mandatory child abuse and neglect reporting laws and inform families of these obligations at the very start of clinical services.

To screen for trauma items, clinicians should specifically ask families if the child or teen has experienced or witnessed the topics listed in the checklist "Identify the Types of Potential Psychological Trauma." Clinicians can first specifically ask parents and children together about the various traumas. Families can be reluctant, embarrassed, or unwilling to disclose family secrets and sources of shame. Clinicians should use a matter-of-fact tone during the questioning and review of trauma items to help normalize the process. Parents may be more open about these topics if their children are not in the room. Conversely, it can also be helpful to speak with children and adolescents without the parents present.

Some children or parents may not be comfortable enough to discuss traumatic experiences, so more time may be needed until greater trust is established. Some children and teens may be embarrassed, ashamed, or afraid to disclosure traumatic experiences, particularly at initial sessions with clinicians. Avoidance may present as denial of traumas. Parental denial of a child's trauma may occur when the parent is truly unaware of it, if they are ashamed or fear repercussions (such as additional domestic violence, or the authorities contacted), or if they are the perpetrator. Children and adolescents should be referred for specialized forensic evaluations if clinicians suspect abuse that is not confirmed with disclosure or other evidence (American Academy of Child and Adolescent Psychiatry, 2010).

While trauma is difficult to discuss, it should not be assumed what will or will not be shared during clinical interviews. Some may share openly, while others refuse to speak. In evaluating trauma, a challenge is to obtain information to make accurate understandings and facilitate appropriate care and treatment, while creating a safe environment and not "pushing" excessively for answers. Because each person's reactions to trauma is individualistic, providers should not assume that certain traumas are more impactful than others. Additionally, parents may have their own strong reactions during this trauma evaluation process and/or their own traumatic pasts.

The impact of trauma is partially determined by a person's experience of the event, and it may not be predictable. This impact is highly individualized and depends on a variety of factors, including the severity and frequency of the trauma, the caregivers' reactions, the level of support for child, the meaning or context of the trauma (to the child, family and within the culture or community), the personal history of child (prior or current psychological or medical conditions and stressors), coping abilities, and prior exposure to other traumas or neglect (Emotional and Psychological Trauma, 2005). Risk and protective factors, resilience and adaptive capacities, and temperament can influence whether a child will have longer-term and more severe trauma responses (Siegfried et al., 2016). Also, complex trauma often has more impact than single events, and the relationship to the abuser will be affected with interpersonal traumas.

Children and teens should be interviewed alone when they live in families who have suspected domestic violence, abusive behaviors, parental mental illness, severe family stressors, or highly dysfunctional environments. When exploring ADHD with these families, clinicians should try to explore which came first, the unhealthy environment or ADHD symptoms, and unfortunately this may not be clear.

When children and adolescents report sexual abuse, clinicians should refer families to their local or county child advocacy center (CAC). These CACs are designed to forensically evaluate sexual abuse in children and adolescents, and their findings are often used in the subsequent legal proceedings. CACs address the legal issues related to the abuse, and often provide sexual abuse treatment and supportive case workers.

If trauma symptoms are new, appear suddenly, or are a change from prior functioning, this may indicate a more recent traumatic experience. While a full trauma assessment or evaluation is not typically part of an ADHD evaluation, it may be needed. Also, when possible, multiple sources of information are helpful (Assessment of Complex Trauma, n.d.).

Children's neglect and traumatic experiences may be difficult to determine unless there are accurate witnesses or others who are aware of the child's experiences, such as non-offending reliable family members. Most children will be unable to recall traumas if these occurred before about age three, yet the effects of preverbal and early traumas can persist and cause long-term damage. Also, children in foster care or orphanages notoriously lack adequately documented early childhood history. When traumatic experiences are not clear or confirmed, these may need to be conceptualized as long-term "suspected" or "rule out" conditions.

In the absence of a child specifically reporting trauma, abuse, or other compelling evidence, a trauma or full PTSD diagnosis should not be made. Children and adolescents can present with trauma-like symptoms without disclosures. Clinicians should be suspicious, but not assume that trauma happened, and should directly ask children and parents whether abuse or trauma exposure has occurred. If the child or caregiver cannot confirm that trauma exposure, then trauma or abuse should not be assumed (American Academy of Child and Adolescent Psychiatry, 2010).

The use of trauma measures can be quite helpful in identifying symptoms and related difficulties. It is amazing sometimes how honest children and teens will be about their traumas symptoms when completing written measures, while denying or minimizing these during face-to-face interviews. Additionally, clinicians can use DSM criteria for PTSD to explore further the trauma symptoms. Finally, children may display abuse-related or traumatic themes in their play or art, and play or art-based evaluations can help in assessing trauma in some cases.

DISTINGUISHING BETWEEN TRAUMA AND TRUE ADHD

To discern if known maltreatment or traumatic events are causing or compounding ADHD-like symptoms, clinicians should try to explore when the traumas began (if known), and when the ADHD-like symptoms first emerged. If the ADHD-like symptoms began before the trauma, this may suggest that both exist. However, as stated previously, children and teens with true ADHD experience trauma and abuse more frequently. Recent and current traumas can easily cause ADHD-like and behavioral symptoms. Therefore, delaying the ADHD evaluation process in these cases may be more prudent, and treating the trauma might be more important. Also, individuals can have delayed reactions to traumas, so trauma reactions or ADHD-like symptoms may not appear immediately. A diagnosis of ADHD should not be given after recent or current traumatic situations unless there is clear evidence the ADHD symptoms began before the trauma.

When distinguishing between ADHD and trauma, clinicians should use their psychological detective skills to investigate how much the child or teen thinks about the traumas now, what symptoms exist, and how their trauma affects them currently. Clinicians should also explore the themes and content of their negative moods, repetitive negative thoughts, anxiety, depression, and trauma symptoms. What do they specifically fear, do they think of the traumas and how often, do they have trauma-related trust problems, and do they have chronic anger or self-blame? If possible, clinicians can examine the settings where ADHD-like symptoms occur to determine if there is a connection to trauma triggers. The clinician can also explore if focusing and behavioral problems occur across multiple settings, or if they appear to be related to being overwhelmed and preoccupied by trauma-related memories, feelings, or negative beliefs. Also, in theory, if a child or teen has persisting ADHD-like difficulties that are purely trauma related, then the maltreatment or trauma effects would be expected to be more severe and chronic (and may also result from early pathogenic care).

There are three main ways of trying to determine if a child with trauma, maltreatment, neglect, dissociation, or attachment disorders also has true ADHD. The first method is to use trauma-focused evaluations or psychological assessments. Evaluations should utilize a thorough clinical interview and parent, teacher, and child self-report measures, including trauma, ADHD, dissociation, attachment disorder, and broadband measures. For clinicians who lack trauma diagnostic experience, it may be necessary to obtain psychological or neurodevelopmental testing from an experienced clinical psychologist who has adequate knowledge of trauma, dissociation, and attachment disorders to distinguish ADHD from these conditions. Projective psychological tests may also be helpful. However, if a child refuses to disclose or discuss their traumatic experiences, testing may only be able to suspect, but not confirm, trauma.

Some research has suggested caution in interpreting ADHD measures of traumatized children. One group of researchers gave the Connors' ADHD Parent Rating Scale-48 (CPRS-48) to parents of sexually abused and nonsexually abused children aged eight to 14, and found that the abused children had significantly higher scores on all of the ADHD scales than the nonabused children. Further, they compared the CPRS-48 parent ratings of traumatized children who had full PTSD to the ratings of nontraumatized children, and did not include participants who had ADHD or other disorders. Their findings indicated that children with PTSD had significantly higher total ADHD scores (Saight et al., 2015).

The second method is to try several stimulant medications at sufficient doses to treat ADHD-Combined-like conditions. In theory, if children or adolescents have true Combined ADHD, their hyperactivity and impulsivity will improve with the right medication and dose, but trauma, dissociation, and attachment disorder symptoms will not. While this is not the best way to diagnose ADHD, this can be attempted if diagnostic confusion persists. This approach will not help distinguish trauma from Inattentive ADHD, and those without true ADHD may experience increased hyperactivity, impulsivity, and other difficulties while on stimulants.

The third method is to provide specialized psychotherapy focused on traumas, dissociation, and/or attachment disorders. The more extensive the trauma, maltreatment, attachment, and dissociative problems, the longer therapy can take. If children or adolescents have true ADHD and trauma (and attachment and/or dissociative problems), focused trauma therapy should provide improvements in the trauma-related difficulties, while the ADHD symptoms may reduce but will probably remain. However, if the child only has trauma and not true ADHD, then the ADHD-like symptoms should decrease and eliminate eventually with trauma treatment. The difficulty with this approach is that it will take time and some families may feel desperate for results sooner.

Clinicians should discuss the pros and cons of these diagnostic approaches with the family. With all these approaches, trauma and ADHD rating scales can be utilized to track progress. Additionally, long-term monitoring, regular re-evaluations, treatments for other identified conditions, and obtaining a more comprehensive neurodevelopmental assessment can be helpful, particularly for those with diagnostic complexity. The CDASS checklist "Risk Factors Associated with ADHD" in Chapter 13 may also help to identify causes of true ADHD to improve diagnostic accuracy. Finally, as mentioned previously, QEEG testing from neurofeedback providers and special blood and urine tests utilized with the Walsh biochemical imbalances approach can help discriminate trauma from true ADHD and other conditions.

TRAUMA TREATMENT

Trauma treatment should be provided by experienced or supervised psychotherapists. There are a number of evidence-based psychotherapies, including Trauma-Focused Cognitive Behavioral Therapy and Integrative Treatment of Complex Trauma for Children and Adolescents. Trauma-focused play and expressive therapies can be productive as well. Psychiatric medications may be helpful in reducing symptoms for those with more severe symptoms, but will not treat the trauma itself. Trauma processing generally should not occur until the child or teen is more stable and able to tolerate the challenges of discussing trauma in therapy. They should not have more severe difficulties, such as suicidal risks, nonlethal self-harming behaviors, substance use, severe depression, anxiety, and PTSD symptoms. They may first require more intensive services through higher levels of care. If other destabilizing conditions exist with the trauma, these may require treatment first. Also, therapists should provide education about the effects of trauma with families, and teach the effective use of emotional management and coping skills before the actual trauma work begins.

For those with trauma and ADHD, there are no standard recommendations about which to treat first, or simultaneously. Providers must determine the order of their treatment focus, and should discuss this with the family (Siegfried et al., 2016). However, if more severe ADHD exists, it may be necessary to first address it. The ADHD symptoms may prevent the child from focusing adequately, staying on task during sessions, or participating effectively in therapy (especially for younger children), and medication may improve this. The trauma may intensify true ADHD symptoms, and trauma therapy may initially increase anxiety resulting from discussing distressing topics. Some children with ADHD can also struggle with completing trauma narratives and other therapy tasks due to their inattention and hyperactivity. Psychotherapists will require more patience because children with ADHD may need more redirection, time for activities and breaks.

Perry's Neurosequential trauma treatment model incorporates a neurodevelopmental perspective that can be helpful for more impaired children or teens who were highly traumatized or neglected beginning at younger ages. Lower neural networks must be intact and well-regulated to efficiently influence the higher functions of speech, language, and socioemotional communication. Therefore, if these children are overanxious, dysregulated, and impulsive, they may have difficulties benefiting from higher-level neurodevelopmental treatments, like talk therapy. Lower-level treatments and repetitive motor activities, such as yoga, balancing exercises, massage, movement, music, and somatosensory interventions would be more effective. These approaches could offer repetitive and patterned neural impact to the brainstem and monoamine neural networks that could be more regulating and organizing, thereby reducing impulsivity, anxiety, and other symptoms related to their dysregulated systems (Perry, 2009). Treatment services should begin at more basic levels and then progress to talk therapy as the treatment advances and the brain catches up (B. D. Perry, personal communication, April 14, 2014). Lastly, neurofeedback and Walsh's Advanced Nutrient Therapy can help.

UNDERSTANDING DISSOCIATION

Dissociation is an automatic self-protection process that occurs in some children and adults who have experienced severe and recurrent traumas. Dissociative disorders are a disruption and/or discontinuity in the normal integration of consciousness, memory, identity, perception, emotion, motor control, body awareness, and behavior (American Psychological Association, 2013). Symptoms of dissociation have been correlated with traumatic histories of significant sexual abuse and/or physical abuse, natural disasters, and war traumas. These symptoms in children have also been associated with neglectful, rejecting, and inconsistent parents (International Society for the Study of Dissociation, 2004), as well as parents who are unpredictable, frightening, or are highly contradictory communicators (International Society for the Study of Trauma and Dissociation, 2014). Any discussions about the effects of traumatic experiences, significant neglect, and attachment disorders should include dissociation. Unfortunately, many clinicians lack awareness of dissociation, so it is commonly undiagnosed.

Dissociation can be considered adaptive with chronic and severe childhood trauma because it reduces the overwhelming distress. However, if the dissociation continues to occur over time and particularly when the trauma has ended, it can be maladaptive. Various studies indicate that from 2 to 10 percent of the population experiences dissociation. In the hours or weeks following severe trauma, about 73 percent will experience dissociation. However, for most people these experiences will subside within a few weeks after the trauma ends (International Society for the Study of Trauma and Dissociation, 2014).

Dissociation can be chronic, transient, gradual, or sudden, and symptoms vary and exist on a continuum. Because it is an automatic defense process, people typically do not know they dissociate. For individuals who are aware, they often display confusion, embarrassment, and a desire to hide the symptoms. Putnam (1997) reported that the loss of time and blackout experiences that are not from neurological problems or substance use are the hallmarks of dissociation.

Many children and teens with chronic dissociation are diagnostically complex, and often present with a range of difficulties and diagnoses obtained from various providers. While it is uncommon for young children to demonstrate adult-like dissociation, traumatized young children may exhibit a range of dissociative symptoms such as trance-like states, perplexing forgetfulness, emotional and behavioral fluctuations, hearing voices, and seemingly real imaginary playmates (Silberg & Dallam, 2009).

Sometimes the dissociative experiences of children make it difficult to differentiate between pathological dissociation and normal imaginative play. Dissociative imaginative play is often accompanied by intense posttraumatic symptoms (night terrors, fearfulness, intrusive traumatic memories or thoughts). Pathological imaginary friends may be at war with each other, splitting between "good" and "evil" or raging against pretend playmates. The child may also report hearing or may act out internal voices, and these may be related to abusive caretakers. Some children may talk loudly to themselves in different voices or exhibit unpredictable and out of context tantrums. Others may have trance-like states where they rigidly and compulsively reenact traumatic events. School-age children may project differentiated identities onto stuffed animals or toys. With more severe conditions, the frequency of dissociative identity disorder-like symptoms increase with age, and teens can have more adult-like presentations (Silberg & Dallam, 2009).

Dissociation can appear as inattention and impulsivity in traumatized children and thereby closely mimic ADHD symptoms. One researcher found that children with dissociation met criteria for ADHD, but nonmaltreated children with ADHD did not meet criteria for dissociative disorders

(D'Andrea et al., 2012). Children and teens with dissociation can also have significant behavioral and other symptoms, and frequently have two or three psychological diagnoses, including ADHD. They have greater affective and anxiety symptoms, suicidal risks, and academic problems. Older children and teens are typically more symptomatic, with two-thirds having conduct problems and half exhibiting sexual behavior problems (Putnam, 1997).

EVALUATION AND TREATMENT FOR DISSOCIATION

As previously stated, children and adolescents with dissociation are often complex, frequently have multiple coexisting conditions, and require experienced or supervised clinicians. Readers can refer to the prior section on trauma for information on the diagnostic process to help distinguish between ADHD, trauma, and dissociation. To help with this discrimination, clinicians should use dissociation checklists and also consider symptoms that are specific to dissociation but not ADHD, including blackouts, significant loss of memories, PTSD symptoms, freezing, persistent and vivid imaginary playmates, distinct personality states, depersonalization, and derealization.

Dissociative disorders should be considered before diagnosing ADHD, even though both can coexist (Silberg & Dallam, 2009). Children and adolescents with dissociation should be evaluated for other frequently coexisting conditions, including ADHD, conduct disorder, bipolar disorder, psychotic conditions, seizure disorder, borderline personality disorder in older teens (Putnam, 1997), PTSD, attachment disorders, eating disorders, OCD, affective disorders, substance abuse, and developmental disorders (International Society for the Study of Dissociation, 2004).

The treatment of dissociation is typically incorporated into trauma psychotherapy, and may require more experienced psychotherapists. Education about and management of dissociative experiences will be important, particularly for more serious conditions. Treatment should utilize a comprehensive approach that addresses their traumas, coexisting conditions, relational and academic challenges. Psychiatric medications do not directly treat dissociation, but may be helpful to address comorbid disorders. Lastly, an excellent resource for information on dissociation is the International Society for the Study of Trauma and Dissociation website (ISST-D; www-.isst-d.org).

REFERENCES

American Academy of Child and Adolescent Psychiatry. (2010, April). Practice parameter for the assessment and treatment of children and adolescents with posttraumatic stress disorder. *Journal of the American Academy of Child and Adolescent Psychiatry, 49*(4), 414–430.

Becker-Please, K., A., & Freyd, J. J. (2008). A Preliminary study of ADHD symptoms and correlates: Do abused children differ from nonabused children? *Journal of Aggression, Maltreatment, and Trauma, 17*(1) #51, 133–140.

Briscoe-Smith, A. M., & Hinshaw, S. P. (2006, November). Linkages between child abuse and attention-deficit/hyperactivity disorder in girls: Behavioral and social correlates. *Child Abuse & Neglect, 30*(11), 1239–1255.

Costello, E. J., Erkani, A., Fairbank, J. A., & Angold, A. (2002, April). The prevalence of potentially traumatic events in childhood and adolescence. *Journal of Traumatic Stress, 15*(2), 99–112.

Cuffe, S. P., McCullough, E. L., & Pumariega, A. J. (1994, September). Comorbidity of attention deficit hyperactivity disorder and post-traumatic stress disorder. *Journal of Child and Family Studies, 3*(3), 327–336.

Dahmen, B., Putz, V., Herpertz-Dahlmann, B., & Konrad, K. (2012, September). Early pathogenic care and the development of ADHD-like symptoms. *Journal of Neural Transmission, 119*(9), 1023–1036. doi: 10.1007/s00702-012-0809-8

D'Andrea, W., Ford, J., Stolbach, B., & Spinazzola, J. (2012). Understanding interper- sonal trauma in children: Why we need a developmentally appropriate trauma diagnosis. *American Journal of Orthopsychiatry, 82*(2), 187–200.

Department of Health and Human Services, State of Victoria (2012a, June). *Child development and trauma specialist practice resource: 9 to 12 years.* Retrieved from http://www.dhs.vic.gov.au/__data/assets/pdf_file/0007/586186/child-development -trauma-9-12years-2012.pdf

Department of Health and Human Services, State of Victoria (2012b, June). *Child development and trauma specialist practice resource: 12 to 18 years.* Retrieved from http://www.dhs.vic.gov.au/__data/assets/pdf_file/0004/586192/child-development -trauma-12-18years-2012.pdf

Emotional and psychological trauma: Causes and effects, symptoms, and treatment. (2005). Retrieved from www.traumasources.org/emotional_trauma_overview.htm

Follan, M., Anderson, S., Huline-Dickens, S., Lidstone, E., Young, D., Brown, G., & Minnis, H. (2011). Discrimination between attention deficit hyperactivity disorder and reactive attachment disorder in school age children. *Research in Developmental Disabilities, 32*(2), 520–526. doi: 10.1016/j.ridd.2010.12.031

Ford, J. D., Racusin, R., Ellis, C. G., Daviss, W. B., Reiser, J., Fleischer, A., & Thomas, J. (2000). Child maltreatment, other trauma exposure, and posttraumatic symptomatology among children with oppositional defiant and attention deficit hyperactivity disorders. *Child Maltreatment, 5*(3), 205–217.

International Society for the Study of Dissociation. (2004). Guidelines for the evaluation and treatment of dissociative symptoms in children and adolescents. *Journal of Trauma & Dissociation, 5*(3), 119–150.

International Society for the Study of Trauma and Dissociation. (2014, October 14). *Dissociation FAQ's.* Retrieved from www.isst-d.org/default.asp?contentID=76.

Kendall-Tackett, K., & Giacomoni, S. M. (Eds.). (2003). *Treating the lifetime health effects of childhood victimization.* Kingston, NJ: Civic Research Institute.

Ladnier, R. D., & Massanari, A. E. (2000). Treating ADHD as attachment deficit hyperactivity disorder. In T. Levy (Ed.), *Handbook of attachment interventions* (pp. 27–65). San Diego, CA: Academic Press.

The National Child Traumatic Stress Network. (n.d.). *Trauma types.* Retrieved on 04/12/19 from https://www.nctsn.org/what-is-child-trauma/trauma-types

National Scientific Council on the Developing Child. (2010). *Persistent fear and anxiety can affect young children's learning and development: Working Paper No. 9.* Retrieved from http://developingchild.harvard.edu/resources/persistent-fear-and-anxiety-can-affect-young-childrens-learning-and-development/

Perry, B. (2009). Examining child maltreatment through a neurodevelopmental lens: Clinical applications of the neurosequential model of therapeutics. *Journal of Loss and Trauma, 14*(4), 240–255. doi: 10.1080/15325020903004350

Perry, B. D., Pollard, R. A., Blakely, T. L., Baker, W. I., & Vigilante, D. (1995). Childhood trauma, the neurobiology of adaptation, and use-dependent development of the brain: How 'states' become 'traits.' *Infant Mental Health Journal, 16*(4), 271–291.

Putnam, F. (1997). *Dissociation in children and adolescents.* New York: Guilford Press.

Rutledge, N. (2014, May/June). Neuroscience and social work—Toward a brain-based practice. *Social Work Today, 14*(3), 20–27.

Saigh, P., Yaskik, A., Halamandaris, P., Bremner, J. D., & Oberfield, R. (2015). The parent ratings of traumatized children with or without PTSD. *Psychological Trauma: Theory, Research, Practice, and Policy, 7*(1), 85–92.

Siegfried, C. B., Blackshear, K., & National Child Traumatic Stress Network, with assistance from the National Resource Center on ADHD: A Program of Children and Adults with Attention-Deficit/Hyperactivity Disorder (CHADD). (2016). *Is it ADHD or child traumatic stress? A guide for clinicians.* Los Angeles & Durham, NC: National Center for Child Traumatic Stress. Retried from https://www.nctsn.org/sites/default/files/resources/is_it_adhd_or_child_traumatic_stress.pdf

Silberg, J. L., & Dallam, S. (2009). Dissociation in children and adolescents: At the crossroads. In P. F. Dell & J. O'Neill (Eds.), *Dissociation and the dissociative disorders: DSM-V and beyond* (pp 67–81). New York: Routlege Press.

Spinazzola, J., Hodgdon, H., Liang, L., Ford, J. D., Layne, C. M., Pynoos, R., & Kisiel, C. (2015, July/August). Unseen wounds. *Monitor on Psychology, 46*(7), 69–73.

Symptoms and Behaviors Associated with Exposure to Trauma. (2015, July 12). Retrieved from http://www.nctsn.org/trauma-types/early-childhood-trauma/Symptoms-and-Behaviors-Associated-with-Exposure-to-Trauma

Types of trauma (n.d.). Retrieved on 04/10/19 from http://yourexperiencesmatter.com/learning/trauma-stress/types-of-trauma/

Chapter 11

NEGLECT, ATTACHMENT DISORDERS, AND EARLY PATHOGENIC CARE

NEGLECT

Neglect during childhood, and particularly the early years, can cause a cascade of psychological, physical, relational, and neurobiological impairments and difficulties. Those who experience significant neglect may have inadequate or inconsistent food intake and/or malnutrition that cause developmental and growth concerns. Neglect can cause impaired concentration and memory, and academic difficulties due to poor school attendance. Chronic neglect can be particularly psychologically damaging due to heightened stress, lower levels of emotional regulation, and poor understanding of emotions. Neglected children often experience a lack of self-worth, a higher number of trauma exposures, and increased risk for developing anxiety, depression, PTSD (Hildyard & Wolfe, 2002), behavioral problems, and dissociative conditions. Adolescents who experience neglect are at higher risk for experiencing substance abuse, delinquent and criminal behavior, legal involvement, academic underachievement, and pregnancies.

Significant neglect can also lead to serious relational difficulties. Persistent long-term misattunement between a parent or caregiver and a child can cause devastating chronic attachment problems. Misattunement occurs when primary caregivers do not adequately match, reflect, or engage an infant or young child's emotional state, or do not sufficiently respond to the child's attempts for expression. This attunement process is important in developing relationships and emotional management. Generally, the younger the child when this is experienced, the more damage will result.

UNDERSTANDING ATTACHMENT DISORDERS

Attachment disorders are relatively new in the clinical literature, first appearing in the DSM in 1980, and research is still lacking (Follan et al., 2011). One study found the prevalence of attachment disorders to be 1.4 percent in a general population of a mostly deprived urban population (Minnis et al., 2013). At its essence, attachment is the interconnectedness between humans. Attachment theory states that all children have positive or negative attachments. Attachments that are positive are protective, while attachments that are negative create higher risks for poorer long-term social and psychological outcomes. Successful attachment results from two factors: first, each person must be able to read the other person' s verbal and nonverbal cues, and second, each person must be able to respond appropriately to these cues. When the caregiver and/or child cannot consistently participate in this required give and take dynamic, then healthy attachment will not occur (Chasnoff, 2015).

When caregivers are abusive or neglectful, infants and young children will not have their needs met and the child can react negatively to the caregiver. When parents do not receive positive feedback and reinforcement from the child, they may become frustrated, respond in more unhealthy ways, and disengage to varying degrees. Thus, a negative interactional spiral can form, with stress and frustration further reinforcing unhealthy parent-child relations which disrupt attunement and ultimately attachment (Chasnoff, 2015).

Children can experience a range of insecure attachment difficulties from maltreatment experiences, misattunement, and toxic parenting styles which are highly inconsistent, unresponsive, unpredictable, and/or abusive. However, formal attachment disorders occur when the normal attachment process is seriously derailed. To qualify for an attachment disorder, a child or adolescent must have experienced pathogenic caregiving during the first five years of life. Pathogenic care involves severe and persistent neglect and/or abuse that ignores a child's essential needs. This may result from a lack of sufficient care, a loss of caregivers, or frequent changes in caregivers. This damaging care may also occur in foster care or institutional placements (Dahmen et al., 2012). A history of neglect is believed to be more impactful than abuse in the development of attachment disorders (Minnis, Rabe-Hesketh, & Wolkind, 2002).

In more severe and chronic pathogenic caregiving, young children can experience failure to thrive and bodily damage due to malnutrition, physical harm, and lack of medical and dental care. Additionally, Chasnoff (2015) reported that some infants and young children with certain neurodevelopmental, medical, or fetal substance exposure conditions may not properly interpret and respond to the caregiver's nurturing cues. Therefore, an attachment disorder could result from the child's inability to adequately participate in the attachment process, even if the parents are healthy.

Reactive Attachment Disorder and Disinhibited Social Engagement Disorder

There are two main attachment disorders. The first is reactive attachment disorder (RAD), where children are inhibited, withdrawn, avoidant, and minimally connect with others. The second type is disinhibited social engagement disorder (DSED), and occurs when children or teens are excessively friendly with others or strangers, and do not seek comfort appropriately from their caregivers. Children who are adopted or in foster care are more likely to be diagnosed with these conditions than children raised by biological parents (Pritchett et al., 2013). While RAD and DSED are considered separate conditions, a mixed profile of both has been found to be common (Follan et al., 2011). Additionally, they should only be diagnosed if extreme insufficient care is known (American Psychiatric Association, 2013). Research has found that attachment disorder behaviors appear to be strongly genetically influenced (particularly in boys), suggesting that some may be more predisposed when neglect or significant toxic parenting occur (Minnis et al., 2007).

Children diagnosed with RAD often experience neglect conditions during their first months, and features are evident between nine months and five years. While some believe it is unclear whether RAD exists in children older than five (American Psychiatric Association, 2013), others have stated that it can persist through childhood (Lehmann et al., 2018). An abnormal pattern of relationships with caregivers developing before age five is a key feature. RAD nearly always occurs as a result of chronic, grossly inadequate child care. Children with RAD demonstrate fearfulness, hypervigilance, a lack of response to caregiver's attempts at comforting, social problems with peers, aggression towards self and others, withdrawal reactions, and misery. Young children with RAD can show strong contradictory or ambivalent responses when parting or reuniting with caregivers. It is more severe than insecure attachment, and the relational problems occur with others and not just primary caregivers (World Health Organization, 1992). These children can also demonstrate emotional regulation difficulties, such as sudden crying outbursts, persistent irritability, and lack of expected positive affect (Boris & Zeanah, 2005). They may not initiate interactions or show interest in caregivers, and can lack social reciprocity (Zeanah et al., 2016). RAD appears associated with maltreated children in foster care who are more unemotional and lack empathy and remorse. Fortunately, RAD can decrease in supportive foster placements (Lehmann et al., 2018).

DSED is a pattern of abnormal social functioning that often persists after neglect ends (World Health Organization, 1992). Children with DSED fail to genuinely connect with caregivers and are willing to seek comfort from almost anyone else (Boris & Zeanah, 2005). As with RAD, those with DSED typically experience neglect during the first months of life, yet unlike RAD, neglect that occurs after age two does not seem to cause DSED. By age four, clinging tends to be replaced by indiscriminately friendly and attention-seeking behaviors. As the condition develops into middle childhood, signs include physical and verbal overfamiliarity and false or shallow emotions, especially with adults (American Psychiatric Association, 2013). While they may have developed attachments, attention-seeking behavior persists and emotional and/or behavioral problems can continue. They often have social problems and difficulties forming close peer relationships, particularly in adolescence (World Health Organization, 1992). DSED can persist for some into early adulthood (Lehmann et al., 2018).

Challenges with Defining and Diagnosing Attachment Disorders

Attachment disorders are one of the most poorly understood and least researched psychological disorders (Thrall et al., 2009), and their conceptualizations can be difficult. An attachment disorder can be separate and distinct from the attachment insecurity discussed by Ainsworth, Bowlby, and others in earlier attachment literature. Formal attachment disorders generally involve relationships and settings rather than specific relational patterns between a child and primary caregiver. Curiously, children can have secure attachments with attachment disorders. One interesting study found that while children with RAD had greater risks for insecure attachments, 30 percent were found to have both a secure attachment and an attachment disorder (Minnis et al., 2009). This research suggests that insecure attachment and formal attachment disorders are not the same thing (Pritchett et al., 2013).

Some authors believe there are other disturbed attachment relationships that could be considered disorders, including those that are extremely fearful, self-endangering, vigilant, role-reversed with caregivers, and excessively compliant. In studies of children who are adopted from institutions, most seem to form attachments to their adoptive parents, but the quality of the attachments are poor and frequently insecure, atypical, and/or disorganized. Some clinicians define attachment disorders in broader terms that differ from the RAD or DSED versions. They use the term to describe children or adults with neglect and trauma who have many interpersonal and psychological symptoms. However, diagnostic precision can be lost when expanded symptoms are included instead of using the recognized DSM diagnoses (Boris & Zeanah, 2005).

Diagnosing attachment disorders can be difficult for several reasons. First, there is a lack of standardized evaluation methods and measures. Second, it can be challenging to distinguish between attachment disorders and other coexisting conditions. Children with attachment difficulties typically exhibit diagnostic complexity, with multiple symptoms that can meet criteria for other disorders. By adolescent years, it is unlikely that a clear attachment disorder diagnosis can be made without one or more coexisting conditions (Thrall et al., 2009). Third, the issue of whether attachment disorders can be reliably diagnosed in older children and adults has not been fully determined (Boris & Zeanah, 2005). However, emerging research suggests that older children and adolescents can have RAD and DSED and extensive comorbidities (Zeanah et al., 2016). Lastly, accurate diagnoses are dependent on knowing if pathogenic care occurred, but this may be unknown and can make a full diagnosis difficult.

ATTACHMENT DISORDERS AND ADHD

Studies indicate there is a high degree of comorbidity between attachment disorders and ADHD. They share the common symptoms of inattention, excessive activity levels, and social disinhibition. There also seems to be an association between the severity of ADHD and the degree of maltreatment in children with early neglect and maltreatment (Follan et al., 2011). One study found that indiscriminate social interactions in maltreated children that is common with DSED appears to persist over time, and has been associated with hyperactivity and inattention (Minnis, Rabe-Hesketh, & Wolkind, 2002).

Despite their comorbidities, attachment disorders can also mimic ADHD symptoms, and diagnostic confusion can result, particularly if history is lacking. Children who start their lives with impaired attachments are at a substantial risk of having later developmental difficulties that include behavioral problems, lack of emotional regulation, low self-esteem, and problems with social and peer relations (Pritchett et al., 2013). Yet the excessive friendliness seems to occur for different reasons. In ADHD, this seems to be due to impulsivity, while in DSED, it appears to be the child's unconscious attempt to control an unpredictable situation or to win the approval of an adult. Further, it is important to discriminate between the two because the treatments are different (Follan et al., 2011). Many with attachment disorders also have ODD, which is also common with ADHD.

Through the use of an attachment disorder measure, the Relationship Problems Questionnaire (RPQ), and a standard child behavioral health screener (the Strengths and Difficulties Questionnaire), researchers were able to discriminate attachment disorder behaviors from hyperactivity, conduct, anxiety, and depression problems (Minnis et al., 2007). Another study found that researchers could discriminate between ADHD and attachment disorders using certain attachment disorder evaluation tools (the CAPA-RAD semi-structured parental interview, a waiting room observation, and the RPQ). They found that eight core items from the CAPA-RAD had especially good reliability (Follan et al., 2011). These include children who avoid eye contact (unrelated to initial shyness when meeting new people), had frozen watchfulness (act frozen and as if invisible), were hypervigilant (jumpy and watchful despite lack of actual threats), and exhibited unpredictable reunion responses with their primary caregivers (difficult to know if they will be friendly or not after separations) (Minnis et al., 2013).

CHILDREN AND ADOLESCENTS IN FOSTER CARE

Most children and adolescents in foster care have experienced some form of serious neglect, maltreatment, and/or abuse. Additionally, research has found that children and teens had higher rates of psychological conditions before, during, and later in life after they were in foster care. The prevalence of ADHD in children in foster care is up to twice as high as the general population (Dahmen et al., 2012). One study found that the most common diagnoses for children and teens in foster care (in order of prevalence) were conduct disorder or ODD, major depression, ADHD, and PTSD (McMillen et al., 2005). Yet another study found that 25 percent of children ages two and 17 in the United States who were in foster care were diagnosed with ADHD, and about 50 percent of these children had other psychological conditions (American Academy of Pediatrics, 2015).

Evaluating and treating those in foster care can be confusing and challenging for providers due to their complicated presentations and difficulties that may include complex trauma, neglect, inherited conditions, multiple co-existing conditions, attachment disorders, early relational inadequacies, and prenatal exposure to substances. Children and teens in foster care often require more extensive diagnostic and longer-term treatment services by experienced or supervised clinicians. Sadly, however, because of state financial limitations for services and a lack of quality foster care caseworkers and treatment providers, many in foster care receive inadequate care. For successful recovery and success later in life, those in foster care require stable and long-term placements with committed and loving caregivers, as well as effective treatments.

EARLY PATHOGENIC CARE WITH ADHD
OR ADHD-LIKE FEATURES

There is evidence that early and severe neglect and pathogenic care is a risk factor for the development of ADHD or ADHD-like symptoms later in a child's life (Tarver, Daley, & Sayal, 2014). It is believed that separation from primary caretakers in early childhood is one the greatest stressors. Adverse events can negatively impact brain development which may contribute to the development of ADHD, ADHD-like conditions, and behavioral dysregulation difficulties. At the neuroanatomical level, early separations from primary caregivers, impoverished social environments, and stress can cause decreased hippocampal neurogenesis, reduced synaptic density, dendritic loss, and reduced prefrontal cortex activity that may suppress synaptic reorganization within porto-limbic circuits with reduced anatomical connectivity and the reduction of consequent gray matter (Kasparek, Theiner, & Filova, 2015).

Interestingly, there appears to be significant overlap between children with true ADHD and those who experience early pathogenic care. Researchers listed 16 studies of children with pathogenic care and ADHD-like symptoms. They had measurable neurobiological and brain deficiencies, as indicated by EEG findings, neuroimaging, neuropsychological testing, and brain anatomy measures. The studies also demonstrated that children with pathogenic care along with ADHD-like symptoms and children who have ADHD without pathogenic care had similarities in brain abnormalities. These abnormalities negatively impact neural networks essential for attention and executive functions. However, the children with early pathogenic care had more severe subcortical abnormalities in the limbic system which could cause interference from emotional states on prefrontal executive functioning. Ultimately, the research indicated that children with true ADHD and those with pathogenic care and ADHD-like symptoms had similar and yet different neurobiological abnormalities (Dahmen et al., 2012).

Epigenetics, the study of the interaction between genes and the environment, is believed to contribute to the expression of ADHD in children with pathogenic care. Yet, not all children with pathogenic care develop ADHD or ADHD-like symptoms. Hopefully, future research will help to identify which children are most vulnerable so that early therapeutic services can remodel the neurobiological network when they are more easily reversed (Dahmen et al., 2012).

These studies suggest that early pathogenic care is associated with its own version of ADHD, even though full ADHD criteria may not be met. This condition could be called "early pathogenic care with ADHD-like features" if partial ADHD criteria are met, and "early pathogenetic care with ADHD" if full criteria are met. To qualify for these conditions, ADHD symptoms would occur in those who experienced pathogenic care during the first five years of life. The earlier, more severe, and chronic the pathogenic care, the higher the risk. Those with pathogenic care with ADHD or ADHD-like presentations may be diagnostically complex, and could experience other neurodevelopmental, trauma, dissociation, attachment, relational, and fetal substance exposure difficulties. When fetal substance exposure and pathogenic care have both occurred, it may be difficult to determine which of these have caused the ADHD or ADHD-like difficulties. Future research should help to better understand these challenges. Due to certain brain functioning similarities between early pathogenic care and true ADHD, medication for ADHD may be helpful, but its effectiveness and responsiveness may vary. Neurofeedback and Walsh's Advanced Nutrient Therapy may be helpful treatments.

EVALUATION AND TREATMENT FOR
NEGLECT AND ATTACHMENT DISORDERS

Children and teens who experience neglect are often exposed to trauma, so there will be some overlap with this section and the prior chapter on trauma.

Attachment disorders can cause unclear and confusing symptoms for many reasons. Since attachment disorders arise from toxic caregiving involving neglect and/or abuse, the evaluation and treatment of trauma should be a component of working with attachment disorders. Children's neglect and traumatic experiences can be difficult to determine unless there are accurate witnesses or children can disclose this. If neglect, abuse, and pathogenic care have not been clear or confirmed, attachment disorders may need to be long-term "suspected" or "rule out" conditions. Also, developmental delays and neurodevelopmental conditions commonly coexist with attachment difficulties, and can cause the dilemma of which came first. Repeated evaluations over time to improve diagnostic accuracy may be needed. Yet another diagnostic challenge involves neglected children who may also have prenatal fetal substance exposure, which can cause neurodevelopmental, ADHD, or ADHD-like difficulties. Children with attachment disorders often have ODD as well.

Although difficult, it is essential that children with attachment disorders have a stable and long-term home with a primary caregiver to form a secure attachment. This relationship is important for the evaluation and treatment. Observations of the child and caregiver interactions should provide clinical data, including separations, reunions, and how the child interacts with the main caregiver as compared to an unfamiliar adult. A child should demonstrate clear preferences for the attachment figure for support and comfort if there is a healthy attachment. A separation is expected to be mildly stressful for younger children (Boris & Zeanah, 2005). Observations of the child and caregiver in the waiting room, office, and with assigned tasks designed to explore their relationship can be useful.

In addition to trauma and dissociation measures, the use of attachment disorder checklists and screening measures can be of value. For those with high scores, clinicians can use specialized observations and the reactive attachment disorder and disinhibited social engagement disorder assessment (RADA), which helps to provide a more detailed interview assessment (Lehmann et al., 2018). As discussed earlier, research suggests that another diagnostic method to distinguish between true ADHD and attachment disorders is to use the RPQ Parent measure and certain previously presented items from the CAPA - RAD. Clinicians should also consider whether infants and young children have neurodevelopmental, medical, or fetal substance exposure conditions that may have impaired them from responding to the caregiver's nurturing cues in appropriate ways (Chasnoff, 2015).

If the child is new to a caregiver (six months or less), the information from this new caregiver about the child's social functioning and behavioral issues may be less helpful. Children and teens with attachment difficulties may "honeymoon" with new caregivers initially, and their true relational problems may not manifest for months. Therefore, a diagnosis of an attachment disorder should probably be delayed at least six months after a child receives a placement with a new caregiver.

Children and adolescents with neglect and trauma can have relational deficits that exist on a continuum. For those with significant neglect, some clinicians may be tempted to assume that attachment difficulties exist. However, this may or may not be true, and individual evaluations should determine their challenges. While children and teens with ADHD typically have social problems, those with attachment disorders are usually more severe. Clinicians can use clinical interviews, projective tests, and social anxiety measures to explore the child's issues with trust and close relationships.

As mentioned previously, a lengthier method for distinguishing ADHD from attachment disorders is to provide specialized attachment disorder and trauma-focused psychotherapy, and then monitor if ADHD symptoms persist. Therapy may be a blend of family and individual sessions, and more extensive difficulties will require greater time and efforts. In attachment-focused therapy, a main goal is to help the child or adolescent increase their attachment to long-term caregivers, and this cannot be achieved without the caregivers' involvement in therapy and a stable long-term placement. Treatment should incorporate education about their conditions and coaching caregivers to provide specialized parenting and behavioral management approaches. Identifying and treating other coexisting conditions, including traumas and dissociation, is important as well. Progress will depend on the other coexisting conditions, the caregiver's capacity to utilize these skills and persist with treatment, and the child's receptivity to the healing process. Some of the larger challenges can include helping the child trust and verbalize more with others, increasing positive interactions, and managing the complex relational and behavioral problems.

There are some evidence-based attachment disorder therapies, such as Parent-Child Interaction Therapy and Child-Parent Psychotherapy, and Dyadic Developmental Psychotherapy is promising. Medication will not treat attachment disorders, but can be helpful to address the child's other conditions. Lastly and once again, neurofeedback and Walsh's Advanced Nutrient Therapy may improve some brain-functioning issues in children and adolescents with neglect and attachment disorders.

REFERENCES

American Academy of Pediatrics. (2015, October 23). *Children in foster care three times more likely to have ADHD diagnosis.* Retrieved from www.sciencedaily.com/re leas-es/2015/10/151023083721.htm

American Psychiatric Association. (2013). *Diagnostic and statistical manual of mental disorders* (5th ed.). Washington, DC: Author.

Boris, N. W., & Zeanah, C. H. (2005, November). Practice parameter for the assessment and treatment of children and adolescents with reactive attachment disorder of infancy and early childhood. *Journal of American Academy of Child and Adolescent Psychiatry, 44*(11), 1206–1219. https://doi.org/10.1097/01.chi.0000177056.41655.ce

Chasnoff, I. J. (2015, March 20). *Prenatal drug exposure and disruption of attachment.* Retrieved from https://www.psychologytoday.com/blog/aristotles-child/201503/prenatal-drug-exposure-an...

Dahmen, B., Putz, V., Herpertz-Dahlmann, B., & Konrad, K. (2012, September). Early pathogenic care and the development of ADHD-like symptoms. *Journal of Neural Transmission, 119*(9), 1023–1036. https://doi.org/10.1007/s00702-012-0809-8

Follan, M., Anderson, S., Huline-Dickens, S., Lidstone, E., Young, D., Brown, G., & Minnis, H. (2011, January). Discrimination between attention deficit hyperactivity disorder and reactive attachment disorder in school age children. *Research in Developmental Disabilities, 32*(2), 520–526. https://doi.org/10.1016/j.ridd.2010.12.031

Hildyard, K. L., & Wolfe, D. A. (2002). Child neglect: Developmental issues and outcomes. *Child Abuse and Neglect, 26*(6–7), 679–695. doi:10.1016/S0145-2134(02)00341-1

Kasparek, T., Theiner, P., & Filova, A. (2015). Neurobiology of ADHD from childhood to adulthood: Findings of imaging methods. *Journal of Attention Disorders, 19*(11), 931–943. https://doi.org/10.1177%2F1087054713505322

Lehmann, S., Monette, S., Egger, H., Breivik, K., Young, D., Davidson, C., & Minnis, H. (2018, September). Development and examination of the reactive attachment disorder and disinhibited social engagement disorder assessment interview. *Assessment,* 1–17. doi: 10.1177/1073191118797422

McMillan, C. J., Zima, B. T., Scott, L. D., Auslander, W. F., Munson, M. R., Ollie, M. T., & Spitznagel, E. L. (2005, January). Prevalence of psychiatric disorders among older youths in the foster care system. *Journal of the American Academy of Child and Adolescent Psychiatry, 44*(1), 88–95. https://doi.org/10.1097/01.chi.0000145806.24274.d2

Minnis, H., Green, J., O'Connor, T. G., Liew, A., Glaser, D., Taylor, E... & Sadiq, F. A. (2009). An exploratory study of the association between reactive attachment disorder and attachment narratives in early school-age children. *Journal of Child Psychology and Psychiatry, 50*(8), 931–942. https://doi.org/10.1111/j.1469-7610.2009.02075.x

Minnis, H., Macmillan, S., Pritchett, R., Young, D., Wallace, B., Butcher, & Gillberg, C. (2013, May). Prevalence of reactive attachment disorder in a deprived population. *The British Journal of Psychiatry, 202*(5), 342–346. doi: 10.1192/bjp.bp.112.114074.

Minnis, H., Rabe-Hesketh, S., & Wolkind, S. (2002). Development of a brief, clinically relevant, scale for measuring attachment disorders. *International Journal of Methods in Psychiatric Research, 11*(2), 90–98. https://doi.org/10.1002/mpr.127

Minnis, H., Reekie, J., Young, D., O'Connor, T., Ronald, A., Gray, A., & Plomin, R. (2007, June). Genetic, environmental and gender influence on attachment disorder behaviors. *The British Journal of Psychiatry, 190,* 490–495. https://doi.org/10.1192/bjp.bp.105.019745

Pritchett, R., Pritchett, J., Marshall, E., Davidson, C., & Minnis, H. (2013). Reactive attachment disorder in the general population: A hidden essence disorder. *The Scientific World Journal, 13,* Article ID 818157, 6 pages. http://dx.doi.org/10.1155/2013/818157

Tarver, J., Daley, D., & Sayal, K. (2014, November). Attention-deficit hyperactivity disorder (ADHD): An updated review of the essential facts. *Child: Care, Health, and Development, 40*(6), 762–774. doi: 10.1111/cch.12139

Thrall, E. E., Hall, C. W., Golden, J. A., & Sheaffer, B. L. (2009, Spring). Screening measures for children and adolescents with reactive attachment disorder. *Behavioral Development Bulletin, 15*(1), 4–10. http://psycnet.apa.org/doi/10.1037/h0100508

Vervoot, E., De Schipper, J., Bosmans, G., & Verschueren, K. (2013). Screeing symptoms of reactive attachment disorder: Evidence for measurement invariance and convergent validity. *International Journal of Methods of Psychiatric Research, 22,* 256–265. doi: 10.1002/mpr.1395

World Health Organization. (1992). *International statistical classification of diseases and related health problems, Tenth Revision (ICD-10).* Geneva: World Health Organization.

Zeanah, C. H., Chesher, T., Boris, N. W., & the American Academy of Child and Adolescent Psychiatry. (2016, November). Practice parameter for the assessment and treatment of children and adolescents with reactive attachment disorder and disinhibited social engagement disorder. *Journal of American Academy of Child and Adolescent Psychiatry, 55*(11), 990–1003. https://doi.org/10.1016/j.jaac.2016.08.004

Part III

THE COMPREHENSIVE DIAGNOSTIC ADHD SCREENING SYSTEM (CDASS) CHECKLISTS FOR CHILDREN AND ADOLESCENTS

Chapter 12

INSTRUCTIONS FOR USING THE COMPREHENSIVE DIAGNOSTIC ADHD SCREENING SYSTEM (CDASS) CHECKLISTS AND SUMMARY FINDINGS FORM

The Comprehensive Diagnostic ADHD Screening System (CDASS) is intended to assist clinicians in the ADHD evaluation process for children and adolescents. The CDASS screening checklists are presented in Part III for the types of ADHD, the indicators of ADHD, risk factors associated with ADHD, common coexisting conditions, and most of the conditions described in Part II. The CDASS is designed to:

1. Help increase the accuracy of diagnosing true ADHD
2. Help identify medical, sleep, psychological, trauma, neglect, neurodevelopmental, sensory process, and fetal substance conditions that may coexist with true ADHD
3. Help identify conditions that may exist when true ADHD does not

Purchasers of this book are given nonassignable permission to reproduce the CDASS checklists and Summary Findings form for use with their own clients and patients. The license is limited to the individual purchaser, and does not grant the right to reproduce these materials for other purposes.

Please refer to the sample checklist below while reading the instructions on how to use the CDASS.

213

Sample CDASS Checklist

CDASS Checklist for **XYZ Condition**

YES __**X**__   NO_____   Unknown or Unclear_____

KEY:
Y = Yes; O = Often; S = Sometimes; R = Rarely; ? = Unknown; N = No; P = In Past Only

Item	Indicator	Y	O	S	R	?	N	P
1	Symptom 1		X					
2	Symptom 2			X				
3	Symptom 3		X					
4	Symptom 4				X			
	Calculate column totals here	0	2	1	1	0	0	0

Record when symptoms began: *Most started at beginning of second grade (age 7.5)*

HOW TO USE THE CDASS CHECKLISTS

The checklists are tools intended to screen children and adolescents ages four to 17. Parents or primary caregivers will be the main providers of information for most of these, but children and adolescents should also be involved with checklist questions when appropriate. Generally, the older the child, the more important that child's participation will be. However, even young children can share information about themselves that parents may not know, such as sleep or vision difficulties, depression, anxiety, or abuse.

Clinicians should first explain to families how the CDASS will be used. They should be told that completing these checklists will require active participation and a number of sessions. The recommended process for the greatest accuracy involves the clinician reading the checklist items, and families verbally providing ratings for each item. While some parents may complete these checklists on their own with no difficulties, others may struggle with responding to various items or entire checklists, and will require clinician assistance. Users can put a date in the margin at the end of each session until all checklists are completed. Clinicians should instruct families to be honest with responses. They should not deny or minimize answers to avoid embarrassment or please the evaluator. If families will not wait for the CDASS checklists or the diagnostic process to be completed and expect answers about ADHD or treatment immediately, clinicians should address these expectations.

Evaluators should try to determine who should complete the checklists (and other measures) by the end of the clinical interview phase. The caregiver who knows the child well and spends the most time with that child should complete the checklists. However, asking both parents to complete the CDASS, if possible or appropriate, can be helpful. If both parents verbally respond to checklist items, they may have different answers, and the two responses for each item can be recorded in different colored pens. Responses from children and adolescents can receive their own pen color as well.

To be the most objective, evaluators should maintain clinical neutrality while reading the checklist items and recording responses with families. While clinicians can clarify questions about items, they should not make unnecessary comments or nonverbal responses that may influence respondents' answers. Additionally, evaluators should consider and discuss with families any cultural issues and factors which may impact their responses to checklist items.

To utilize the CDASS checklist properly, users should be diligent to review all items, and should be cautious if they choose to not complete certain items or entire conditions. Clinicians can miss disorders when checklists are skipped if it is falsely assumed that a potential condition did not exist when in fact, it did. As users gain more experience with the CDASS, greater speed and accuracy should be achieved. Additionally, with time, clinicians' understanding of a large number of disorders should improve.

The basic timeframe for rating the presence and frequencies for the checklist items is the past 90 days. Some symptoms may not neatly fit in this timeframe, and may have fluctuated over the prior months or years. Users should do their best to determine if symptoms are recent, fluctuate, or only occurred in the past. Some difficulties may be subtle or vague, and it can be unclear when the symptoms began or last occurred. If children, adolescents, or parents are uncertain whether an item or items occurred in the past 90 days, users can note this in the margins. Users may also need to return to unclear items or entire checklists to increase response precision.

For positive answers to the checklist items, users should be specific by marking the "O" column if the symptom occurs *Often* or frequently, "S" if it occurs *Sometimes,* or "R" if it occurs *Rarely.* As much as possible, clinicians should ask families to qualify affirmative responses with O, S, or R. *Yes* should be used only when O, S, and R cannot be utilized. "P" indicates that the item occurred only in the *Past,* does not exist presently, and should not be used if it still occurs. When past items are reported, their occurrence could be important, and users may wish to explore their previous severity, frequency, duration, and last occurrence. If the answer is *Unknown* or *Unclear,* the question mark "?" column should be marked. If the item does not occur, then "N" for *No* should be checked. Items should not be left blank.

After all the items have been marked in the columns, the user should calculate the totals at the bottom of the checklist. For example, if there were 3

"O" or *Often* responses, the number 3 would be written in the "O" column at the bottom of the checklist (see the sample checklist).

Asterisks next to items indicate that the item is important and often occurs frequently. While these items are not critical for determining the condition, they should be considered. Clinicians can put stars next to items that parents may say occur "Very Often," and can also write any comments in the margins.

When the symptoms were first noticed should be written on the lines below the checklists ("Record when symptoms began"). If some checklist items began or occurred at different times, users should do their best to use an approximate time frame for the beginning of the majority or most significant symptoms. They could also indicate when certain symptoms item numbers started by indicating their item numbers (for example, "Items 1, 3, 4 and 11 started in the middle of third grade, at age 8.5"). Please see the sample checklist presented earlier for example.

There are no specific numerical scoring guidelines or standardized norms for the CDASS checklists to determine whether the child or teen actually has the suspected condition. Rather, if there are a number of *Often* and *Sometimes* responses for a condition, then it can be considered as "suspected," and the child or adolescent should be referred to the appropriate qualified providers for further evaluation. Generally, the more items marked as *Often* and *Sometimes,* the greater the risk the condition may exist. Obviously, *Often* responses should have greater significance than *Sometimes.*

Discretion should be utilized when determining if a possible condition is considered to exist or not, and when additional evaluations are suggested. Depending on the disorder, even a few *Often* responses may or may not be suggestive that it is present. The significance of mostly *Sometimes* responses should be determined on a case-by-case basis. If a number of *Sometimes* are made along with *Often* responses, this can be more suggestive that the condition may exist. If there are a number of *Sometimes* responses and it is unclear if the child should receive a new referral, the evaluator can review the responses again with the parent. The clinician can also discuss the pros and cons of obtaining specialist referrals for suspected conditions. The advantages include the possibility of accurately identifying and treating the potential condition, while the disadvantages include expense, time spent, and the condition may not exist. If uncertainty persists, a cautious approach could be to make the referral to a specialist for a more qualified opinion. It may be safer to overidentify suspected disorders and spend the time and effort to evaluate these properly, rather than risk the possibility of not addressing them.

After the checklist has been completed for a condition, the user should mark the blank lines after *YES, NO, Unknown or Unclear* at the top of each checklist. The user must indicate with an "X" or check mark if they believe it may exist or not. They should indicate *YES* if there are a number of *Often* and *Sometimes* checklist items. This will indicate that the condition may exist and should be further evaluated. Users should indicate *NO* when the condition is not believed to be present because there are no indicators or minimal ones. They should check *Unknown or Unclear* when parents may not be able to answer the items and/or there are only minimal positive responses. *Unknown or Unclear* would indicate that the disorder may exist and should be considered for further evaluation to see if it is present.

When the CDASS checklists are completed, users should record all the conditions identified as *YES* and *Unknown or Unclear* on the "CDASS Summary Findings" form at the end of this chapter. These will now require further exploration and evaluation to determine if they are present or not. At this point, either further evaluations within the expertise of the clinician should occur, or referrals to other providers should be obtained. These specialists are suggested in the "Evaluation and Treatment" sections for the disorders in Part II. If parents use the checklists alone, the identified *YES* and *Unknown or Unclear* conditions should be shared with the appropriate providers.

Clinicians can record their own notes or statements from reporting parents in the item's margins. Adding clarifying statements may be particularly helpful when the user is trying to determine whether a condition should be more fully considered. When the checklists indicate a number of concerning items, clinicians need to further explore these, including their frequency, intensity level, and duration. For example, when using the checklist for auditory processing disorder, a child may receive a number of "O" and "S" responses. However, an experienced clinician may be able to discuss these further with the parents to determine that the auditory processing-like symptoms really seem more related to inattention and not true auditory processing deficits.

The CDASS checklists are intended to be screeners for possible conditions during the evaluation process. Diagnoses should not be determined only by this or any other single measure. The final diagnosis of any disorder should be based on multiple sources of information, including clinical interviews, observations and examinations, measures and instruments, and the expertise of properly trained and licensed professionals. For parents, these screening tools are not intended to replace working with qualified clinicians, and the checklist results should be shared with all clinicians to support the diagnostic process.

INSTRUCTIONS FOR THE CDASS SUMMARY FINDINGS FORM

After all the checklists and entries have been reviewed and completed, the user should complete the single page "CDASS Summary Findings" form at the end of this chapter. This should assist the user to integrate and organize the findings of the CDASS checklists.

Item Number One on the "CDASS Summary Findings" form asks the user to list only the suspected types of ADHD that may be present. This information will come from this checklist within Chapter 13. If there are suspected types of ADHD, and true ADHD has not been fully diagnosed, then "Rule Out" for the ADHD type should be listed. Fully diagnosed ADHD conditions should be listed in item five and not here.

Item Number Two asks the user to indicate *Yes, No,* or *Unknown or Unclear* if there were a concerning or significant number of *Yes, Often,* and *Sometimes* responses from the "ADHD Indicators" Checklist in Chapter 13. The more items indicated, the greater the possibility that true ADHD exists.

Item Number Three asks the user to list the risk factors associated with ADHD from this checklist in Chapter 13. The more risk items listed here, the greater the chance that true ADHD exists. However, clinicians should explore if these indicators are related to or better explained by other conditions besides ADHD.

Item Number Four asks the user to list all the identified suspected and possible CDASS conditions that may require further evaluations. All *YES* or *Unknown or Unclear* determinations for the CDASS conditions from the Chapter 14 checklists should be listed here as Rule Outs, unless they have been accurately diagnosed previously. This should help the user know which suspected disorders have been detected, and which referrals are now needed. In this section users can also write *Yes* and *Unknown or Unclear* after the condition to help indicate which are *Yes* conditions and may be of greater concern. CDASS users may have generated a long list of possible disorders listed within this item four that will require decisions regarding which referrals will be made. Each of these should be explored to determine if they are causing ADHD-like symptoms when true ADHD does not exist, or do they coexist with true ADHD.

Item Number Five asks the users to list all the conditions and diagnoses that they or others have fully determined and diagnosed at the completion of the CDASS, including ADHD. Clinicians should not list ADHD in this section if they are not ready to do so. To be accurate in diagnosing ADHD, it is important that the disorders listed in this section and in Item Number Four are determined to not be exclusively causing ADHD-like symptoms and are not creating a misdiagnosis of ADHD. Of course, these conditions may coexist with true ADHD and can worsen its presentation. Once the form is completed, evaluators can give parents and other providers copies of this form.

SUMMARY OF CDASS INSTRUCTIONS

1. ***Complete Chapters 13 and 14 checklists.*** Over the past 90 days, indicate an "O" if the checklist item has occurred *Often* or frequently, "S" if it has occurred *Sometimes,* "R" if it has occurred *Rarely* to very occasionally, Question Mark "?" if it is *Unknown or Unclear,* and "No" if it does not occur. Some items may be only "Yes" or "No." Clinicians should encourage respondents to qualify affirmative responses with O, S, or R. Indicate "P" if the item has occurred only in the past but not recently. Below checklists write when the majority or most significant symptoms began.

2. ***Indicate Yes, No, or Unknown or Unclear for each condition above completed checklists.*** After the checklist has been completed for the condition, check *Yes, No,* and *Unknown or Unclear* in section above checklist items. Check *YES* if there are a number of checklist items that are *Often* and/or *Sometimes.* This will indicate that it may exist and should be further evaluated to see if it exists. Check *NO* when the condition is not believed to be present because there are no to minimal checked symptoms. Check *Unknown or Unclear* when it is unclear if it exists because the parent may not know the answer and/or there are minimal responses for the condition. This will indicate that the condition may exist and should be considered for further evaluation to see if it is present.

3. ***Complete the "CDASS Summary Findings" form.*** This is presented at the end of this chapter and should be completed after all the Chapter 13 and 14 checklists are completed. Sections one to three should be completed based on these checklists from Chapter 13. All *YES* and *Unknown or Unclear* determinations for the CDASS conditions from checklists within Chapter 14 should be listed in section four and considered for further evaluations. These conditions may or may not be causing ADHD-like presentations, and may coexist with true ADHD. Section five is for conditions that have been fully determined and diagnosed from all providers.

The Comprehensive Diagnostic ADHD Screening System (CDASS) Summary Findings Form

Date: _____

Child's Name and Birthdate:_____

Parent/s or Caregiver/s Providing Information:_____

Person Completing this Form:_____

1. List the **Type of Suspected ADHD** indicated from checklists in Chapter 13 (print "See Below" if clinician has fully determined and diagnosed an ADHD type; Print "Unclear" or "None" if applicable):

_____

2. Indicate results from **ADHD Indicators** Checklist (Chapter 13). Was there a concerning or significant number of *Yes, Often,* and/or *Sometimes* responses from this checklist to suggest the presence of true ADHD?

       YES_____   NO_____   Unknown or Unclear_____

3. List "YES" Items from the **Risk Factors Associated with ADHD** Checklist (Chapter 13):

_____   _____
_____   _____
_____   _____

4. List **Suspected Possible and Rule Out Conditions That May be Causing ADHD-Like Symptoms and/or May Coexist with True ADHD that Require Additional Evaluations** (List the *YES* and *Unknown/Unclear* results for the CDASS conditions from the Chapter 14 checklists; Print "Rule Out" in front of these):

_____   _____
_____   _____
_____   _____
_____   _____

5. List **Currently Determined and Fully Diagnosed Conditions from All Providers** (If applicable, indicate type of ADHD, and all other diagnosed conditions):

_____   _____
_____   _____
_____   _____

Chapter 13

CDASS CHECKLISTS FOR TYPES OF ADHD, ADHD INDICATORS, RISK FACTORS ASSOCIATED WITH ADHD, AND COMMON COEXISTING CONDITIONS

Types of ADHD

CDASS Checklist for **Inattention Difficulties**

YES_____   NO_____   Unknown or Unclear_____

KEY:
Y = Yes; O = Often; S = Sometimes; R = Rarely; ? = Unknown; N = No; P = In Past Only

Item	Indicator	Y	O	S	R	?	N	P
1	Does not give close attention to details or makes hasty/thoughtless mistakes							
2	Has difficulty maintaining focus/ attention to activities/play							
3	Seems to not listen when spoken to							
4	Has problems following instructions, does not finish scholastic work/ chores from inattention							
5	Has problems with organization							
6	Dislikes/avoids tasks requiring focus (including homework)							
7	Loses items							

KEY:

Y = Yes; O = Often; S = Sometimes; R = Rarely; ? = Unknown; N = No; P = In Past Only

Item	Indicator	Y	O	S	R	?	N	P
8	Is easily distracted by things occurring around them							
9	Is forgetful with everyday activities (Mayo Clinic Staff, 2017, August 16a)							
	Calculate column totals here							

Record when symptoms began:_____

Predominantly Inattentive ADHD Presentation

To qualify, the child or adolescent will have six or more (five or more for ages 17 and above) symptoms on this checklist. Some symptoms should occur prior to age 12, have persisted for at least six months, are present in two or more settings (school, day care, social settings, home), affect their functioning, and are not the result of another condition (Centers for Disease Control and Prevention, 2017, August).

CDASS Checklist for **Hyperactivity and Impulsivity Difficulties**

YES_____   NO_____   Unknown or Unclear_____

KEY:

Y = Yes; O = Often; S = Sometimes; R = Rarely; ? = Unknown; N = No; P = In Past Only

Item	Indicator	Y	O	S	R	?	N	P
1	Taps or fidgets hands/feet or move excessively in seat							
2	Does not remain in seat when required (meals, classroom)							
3	Is constantly moving, rarely still							
4	Runs/climbs when inappropriate							
5	Has difficulty playing/performing activities quietly							

KEY:
Y = Yes; O = Often; S = Sometimes; R = Rarely; ? = Unknown; N = No; P = In Past Only

Item	Indicator	Y	O	S	R	?	N	P
6	Speaks excessively, annoys others with talking, often asked to be quiet							
7	Interrupts or blurts/calls out							
8	Struggles to wait turn, impatient							
9	Barges into others' conversations/ activities (Mayo Clinic Staff, 2017, August 16a).							
	Calculate column totals here							

Record when symptoms began:_____

Predominantly Hyperactive/Impulsive ADHD Presentation

To qualify, the child or adolescent will have six or more (five or more for ages 17 and older) symptoms on this checklist. Some symptoms should occur prior to age 12, have persisted for at least six months, are present in two or more settings, and affect their functioning (Centers for Disease Control and Prevention, 2017, August). This condition without inattention problems occurs typically in younger children who are not yet required to demonstrate concentration and attention abilities consistently.

Combined Inattentive and Hyperactive/Impulsive ADHD Presentation

To qualify, they will meet criteria for both inattentive and hyperactive/ impulsive presentations.

CDASS Checklist for **ADHD Indicators**

YES_____   NO_____   Unknown or Unclear_____

The following difficulties are often associated with and can be suggestive of true ADHD. The more items checked, the greater the likelihood that true ADHD may exist, particularly for older children and adolescents. Some younger children may have ratings of higher frequencies (more "Often" and

"Sometimes") that are developmentally appropriate based on their age and comparisons to neurotypical peers. Clinicians should also explore if these indicators are related to or better explained by other conditions besides ADHD.

KEY:
Y = Yes; O = Often; S = Sometimes; R = Rarely; ? = Unknown; N = No; P = In Past Only

Item	Indicator	Y	O	S	R	?	N	P
	Early Childhood Indicators							
1	Had poor health during infancy							
2	Had early childhood delays in motor and language skills (Barkley, 2013)							
3	Early Indicators of Combined ADHD *(Only rate these items if they occurred or occur now between ages 3 to 5)*							
a	Had increased hyperactivity and/or inattention levels persisting for at least one year							
b	Had increased levels of parent-child conflict							
c	Had increased levels of maternal negativity and directiveness with child							
d	Had greater than normal defiant behavior							
e	Had resistance to parental control							
f	Had higher emotional reactivity to events							
g	Experienced preschool behavioral difficulties (excessively out of seat, talking, noisy, disruptive) (Barkley, 2015, March 19a)							
h	Had social problems with peers							

KEY:
Y = Yes; O = Often; S = Sometimes; R = Rarely; ? = Unknown; N = No; P = In Past Only

Item	Indicator	Y	O	S	R	?	N	P
i	Was easily upset/overwhelmed							
j	Was demanding							
k	Had high intensity							
l	Demonstrated negative mood (angers quickly, irritable)							
m	Had low adaptability, struggles with change (Barkley, 2013)							
n	Had significant temper tantrums and temper loss (occur daily or every other day, last longer than 5 minutes, aggression may occur, happen with non-parent adults, can occur without known triggers). The more frequent, severe, and intense, the greater risk of developing behavioral/emotional difficulties and ADHD. 84% of male and female preschoolers have temper tantrums occasionally, and older preschoolers are less likely to tantrum. About 10% of ages 3–5 had concerning daily tantrums (Wakschlag et al., 2012).							
	Executive Functioning Deficits (common with Combined & Inattentive ADHD)							
4	Initiating tasks difficulties (problems starting activities/tasks)							
a	Has problems/delays initiating homework							
b	Has problems/delays initiating reading							

KEY:

Y = Yes; O = Often; S = Sometimes; R = Rarely; ? = Unknown; N = No; P = In Past Only

Item	Indicator	Y	O	S	R	?	N	P
c	Has problems/delays initially acting upon parental requests/instructions							
d	Has problems/delays initiating chores/assigned tasks							
e	Has problems/delays initiating bathroom hygiene tasks (teeth brushing, bathing, hair)							
f	Has problems/delays initiating dressing in mornings/bedtimes							
5	Selective and sustained attention difficulties (once started, trouble with focusing upon and maintaining focus)							
a	Has difficulties focusing upon homework							
b	Has difficulties focusing upon reading							
c	Has difficulties focusing on conversations/discussions							
d	Has difficulties focusing on parental requests/instructions							
e	Has difficulties focusing on chores/assigned tasks							
f	Has difficulties focusing on bathroom hygiene tasks							
g	Has difficulties focusing on meals							
h	Has difficulties focusing upon family activities and events							
i	Has difficulties focusing upon dressing during mornings/bedtimes							

KEY:

Y = Yes; O = Often; S = Sometimes; R = Rarely; ? = Unknown; N = No; P = In Past Only

Item	Indicator	Y	O	S	R	?	N	P
6	Experiences shifting attention difficulties (problems shifting focus fluidly; unable to move focus from one task to another easily)							
7	Struggles with being flexible/ adaptable to changes/new things							
8	Has problems persisting with/completing tasks/activities they do not like or enjoy							
9	Struggles following directions							
10	Has difficulties adhering to rules/ expectations							
11	Has difficulties completing tasks (particularly multi-step tasks)							
12	Has improved attention to new, interesting, or highly stimulating activities/events							
13	Has working or short-term memory deficits (trouble recalling what was read, forgets to submit homework, struggles to recall what parents requested, forgets what others said)							
14	Is easily bored, loses interest quickly							
15	Daydreams							
16	Has trouble planning ahead							
17	Poorly anticipates consequences of actions							
18	Has poor organizational and/or time management skills; difficulties prioritizing activities/tasks; loses track of time; underestimates how long tasks take							

KEY:

Y = Yes; O = Often; S = Sometimes; R = Rarely; ? = Unknown; N = No; P = In Past Only

Item	Indicator	Y	O	S	R	?	N	P
19	Makes poor choices							
20	Is over-reactive, excessively reacts to others/situations (more common with Combined ADHD)							
21	Has self-control difficulties (trouble inhibiting actions, restraining comments/actions) (more common with Combined ADHD)							
22	Has excessive activity levels (Combined ADHD)							
23	Has poor frustration tolerance (easily overwhelmed, irritable, aggressive, escalates, angry when asked to do things or told no)							
24	Has slow processing speed and deficits (moves/react slower, thinks less quickly, memory difficulties, takes longer to initiate/complete tasks; 61% of children with ADHD experience this) (Braaten & Wolloughby, 2014)							
25	Appears selfish, self-centered or insensitive to others' needs/requests (more common with Combined ADHD)							
26	Has lower self-awareness (lacks understanding of how they impact others)							
	Difficulties at Home (*some items may also occur at other settings;* common with Combined & Inattentive ADHD)							
27	Does not complete expected chores or home tasks consistently							
28	Tasks are left unfinished/incomplete							

KEY:

Y = Yes; O = Often; S = Sometimes; R = Rarely; ? = Unknown; N = No; P = In Past Only

Item	Indicator	Y	O	S	R	?	N	P
29	Has inconsistent/fluctuating performance of daily activities/tasks							
30	Procrastinates; rushes to complete things last minute							
31	More productive with close supervision and when instructions are repeated							
32	Has self-esteem deficits							
33	Is oppositional/defiant with parents (more common with Combined ADHD)							
34	Has messy room/closet; leaves trail of belongings around house							
35	Has difficulty leaving home on-time for school/appointments							
36	Is late when coming home or for appointments							
37	Lies							
38	Misplaces items							
39	Resists/dislikes reading							
	Academic and School Difficulties (common with Combined & Inattentive ADHD)							
40	Has significant academic underachievement in current or most recent grade (D or F mid-term/final grades)							
41	Has fluctuations in academic performance (variable test/quiz grades, changes in final grades over academic year)							

KEY:
Y = Yes; O = Often; S = Sometimes; R = Rarely; ? = Unknown; N = No; P = In Past Only

Item	Indicator	Y	O	S	R	?	N	P
42	Teachers comment about under-performance ("not living up to potential," "could be doing better," "not applying self")							
43	Has problems/delays initiating class-room activities							
44	Has difficulties focusing upon class-room activities							
45	Has homework difficulties (trouble organizing, completing, comprehending, and submitting; rushes; makes errors/mistakes)							
46	Has reading problems (poor reading skills, comprehension, recall)							
47	Has difficulties learning/mastering new school materials or topics							
48	Has messy book bag/desk							
49	Is tardy to school/classes							
50	Makes errors/mistakes on tests and schoolwork (may rush through work)							
51	Complains of/struggles with boredom with school and academics							
52	Has school behavioral problems (more common with Combined ADHD)							
	Social Difficulties (unless indicated, below are more common with Combined ADHD)							
53	Relationship problems/interpersonal difficulties with:							
a	Parents							
b	Siblings							

KEY:

Y = Yes; O = Often; S = Sometimes; R = Rarely; ? = Unknown; N = No; P = In Past Only

Item	Indicator	Y	O	S	R	?	N	P
c	Friends outside of school							
d	Peers and friends at school							
e	Others							
54	Dominates/controls social interactions (including speaking excessively, lesser turn-taking in conversations)							
55	Is rejected by others							
56	Is socially reserved/withdrawn (more common with Inattentive ADHD)							
57	Has few or no friends (occurs with Combined & Inattentive ADHD)							
58	Bullies peers							
59	Is bullied by peers (occurs with Combined & Inattentive ADHD)							
60	Prefers to play with younger children (occurs with Combined & Inattentive ADHD)							
61	Makes hurtful/offensive comments							
62	Is aggressive with others							
63	Interacts with some adults as if they are peers							
64	Is tangential in conversations and/or explanations							
65	Misses/misperceives social/non-verbal cues during interactions							
	Adolescent Difficulties (*some items may occur earlier than adolescence;* unless indicated, below are more common with Combined ADHD)							

KEY:

Y = Yes; O = Often; S = Sometimes; R = Rarely; ? = Unknown; N = No; P = In Past Only

Item	Indicator	Y	O	S	R	?	N	P
66	Views inappropriate content and/or spends excessive time on internet (occurs with Combined & Inattentive ADHD)							
67	Sends or receives inappropriate electronic messages (occurs with Combined & Inattentive ADHD)							
68	Has problematic/excessive social media use (occurs with Combined & Inattentive ADHD)							
69	Has problematic/excessive video-gaming (occurs with Combined & Inattentive ADHD)							
70	Has problematic substance use (nicotine, marijuana, alcohol, other drugs; may start earlier than others)							
71	Has had risky/concerning sexual activity (frequency; lack of birth control use; began earlier; sexually transmitted disease/infection)							
72	Exhibits other risky behaviors (shoplifting, vandalism, skipping school, violating curfews)							
73	Has a greater number of automotive moving violations (occurs with Combined & Inattentive ADHD)							
74	Has a greater number of automotive accidents (occurs with Combined & Inattentive ADHD)							
75	Has employment difficulties (trouble maintaining job, late, learning or performance issues, conflicts at work)							
	Calculate column totals here							

CDASS Checklist for **Risk Factors Associated with ADHD**

YES_____   NO_____   Unknown or Unclear_____

This checklist is intended to help identify the risk factors that can contribute to the development of ADHD, and may help to suggest if true ADHD exists. The more checklist items indicated, the greater the risk and likelihood that true ADHD may exist. However, due to the complexity of its development, true ADHD can occur without the clear presence of these items. The references for this checklist are listed in the References section of Chapter 3. Refer to Chapter 3 for more information about these items.

KEY:
Y = Yes; ? = Unknown; N = No

Item	Indicator	Y	?	N
1	Family history of ADHD exists (highly suspected or confirmed)			
a	Father (highest risk of transmission)			
b	Mother (highest risk of transmission)			
c	Sibling/s (higher risk)			
d	Grandparents, uncles, aunts, cousins			
2	Had premature birth			
a	Moderate preterm birth (born between 33 weeks to 36 weeks) (Chu et al., 2012; Lindstrom, Lindblad, & Hjern, 2011; Sucksdorff et al., 2015)			
b	Very preterm birth (born between 26 to 32 weeks; higher risk of developing ADHD than moderate preterm) (Chu et al., 2012; Johnson & Marlow, 2011; Lindstrom, Lindblad, & Hjern, 2011; Sucksdorff et al., 2015)			
c	Extremely preterm birth (born at 25 weeks or earlier; higher risk than moderate preterm) (Lindstrom, Lindblad, & Hjern, 2011; Sucksdorff et al., 2015)			
3	Had post-term birth (born at 42 weeks or later) (Marroun et al., 2012)			
4	Had high birth weight of over 10 lbs. (Sucksdorff et al., 2015)			

KEY:
Y = Yes; ? = Unknown; N = No

Item	Indicator	Y	?	N
5	Had low birth weight			
a	Low birth weight (children born weighing between 3 pounds 5 ounces to 5 to 5 pounds 7 ounces) (Chu et al., 2012; Johnson & Marlow, 2011)			
b	Very low birth weight (children born weighing between 3 pounds 4 ounces to 2 pounds 4 ounces) (Johnson & Marlow, 2011)			
c	Extremely low birth weight (children born weighing 2 pounds 3 ounces and under) (Chu et al., 2012; Johnson & Marlow, 2011)			
6	Had prenatal fetal substance exposure			
a	Alcohol in-utero exposure			
b	Tobacco/nicotine exposure (maternal cigarette use, secondhand smoke exposure, other nicotine exposure)			
c	Illict/prescribed drug in-utero exposure: marijuana, cocaine, opioids (heroin and abused prescription opioids), methamphetamine and amphetamine, other substances			
7	Certain pregnancy and birth complications occurred			
a	Maternal gestational diabetes (maternal diabetes during pregnancy only)			
b	Moderate to significant prenatal maternal anxiety (Adamson, Letourneau, & Lebel, 2018), stress, and stressful life events (divorce, housing move) (Ronald, Pennell, & Whitehouse, 2011)			
c	Repeated infections during pregnancy (Barkley, 2013)			
d	Fetal distress during pregnancy or labor			
e	Unusually short or long labor			
f	Low forceps delivery (head is on pelvic floor; forceps can damage brain) (Singh, Yeh, Verma, & Das, 2015)			
8	Experienced situations before, during, or just after birth that caused oxygen deprivation (ischemic-hypoxic conditions)			

KEY:

Y = Yes; ? = Unknown; N = No

Item	Indicator	Y	?	N
a	Preeclampsia/toxemia in pregnant mother (pregnancy induced high blood pressure with leakage of toxins in the blood and swelling in face, feet, or hands)			
b	Birth asphyxia (breathing problems just before, during, or after birth causing decreased oxygen to brain and possible brain injury; can involve very long/problematic delivery, difficulties with umbilical cord during delivery and cord around neck, severe infection in mother or baby, blocked airway in newborn, other situations)			
c	Neonatal respiratory distress syndrome (breathing disorder in premature newborns due to lack of fully developed lungs) (Getahun et al, 2013).			
9	Moderate to severe jaundice occurred as newborn infant (particularly for male, preterm and low-birth weight infants with jaundice) (Wei et al., 2015)			
10	Experienced head injury (traumatic brain injury). Multiple injuries increase risks.			
11	Experienced near drowning, severe smoke inhalation, or carbon monoxide poisoning (these can cause brain oxygen deprivation)			
12	Early pathogenic care experienced during first 5 years of life, including significant/severe neglect (see checklist in Chapter 11 if necessary). This item should exclude prenatal substance exposure.			
13	Raised by single parent, lesser maternal education, and lower parental socioeconomic status (Barkley, 2013)			
14	Childhood neurotoxic exposure. *Besides recent lead exposure, most of these items may be difficult to determine, and can be long-term rule out factors. Because of these challenges, many families may choose to not explore these items. This category should exclude maternal fetal substance exposure.* See this section in Chapter 3 for more information.			
a	Lead			
b	Mercury			

KEY:
Y = Yes; ? = Unknown; N = No

Item	Indicator	Y	?	N
c	Endocrine disruptors: Bisphenol A (BPA), Polybrominated diphenyl ethers (PBDEs), Polychlorinated biphenyls (PCBs), and others (Lu, 2015)			
d	Certain chemicals used in the home: cleaning products with alcohol, trichloroethylene, xylene, and other neurotoxins (Koger, Schettler, & Weiss, 2005)			
e	Certain pesticides and lawn chemicals including pyrethroids, an insecticide (Lu, 2015)			
f	Cadmium, manganese, and certain industrial hazardous toxins (Koger, Schettler, & Weiss, 2005)			
15	Certain mineral and vitamin deficiencies. *Without specific testing, these items will not be adequately identified. See this section in Chapter 3 for more information.*			
a	Zinc deficiency			
b	Magnesium deficiency			
c	Iron deficiency (see this checklist in Chapter 14 if necessary)			
d	B vitamin deficiency (particularly B6)			
e	D vitamin deficiency			
16	Walsh biochemical imbalances. *Without specific testing, these items will not be adequately identified. See this section in Chapter 3 for more information.*			
a	Overmethylation (over and under conditions cause imbalances in histamine, plasma, zinc, copper, and certain neurotransmitters, causing a range of symptoms)			
b	Undermethylation			
c	Copper overload			
d	Zinc deficiency			
e	Folate deficiency			
f	Folate overload			

KEY:

Y = Yes; ? = Unknown; N = No

Item	Indicator	Y	?	N
g	Pyrrole disorder (a genetic condition that limits sufficient serotonin production)			
h	Glucose dyscontrol			
i	Toxic heavy-metal overload (lead, mercury, cadmium)			
j	Toxic substance exposure (pesticides, chemicals)			
k	Malabsorption (stomach, digestion, intestine problems)			
l	Essential fatty acids imbalances (insufficient omega-3 and excessive omega-6 levels, but sometimes the converse) (Walsh, 2015; Walsh Research Institute, 2005-2016b)			
17	Exposure to artificial food colorings (particularly red, yellow, and blue), preservatives (sodium benzoate, sodium nitrate and nitrite, BHA, BHT, calcium propionate), additives (aspartame, MSG) in foods and beverages. *Because this exposure is so pervasive for most children, without elimination diets focused on these items, it will be hard to determine if these are a factor.*			
	Calculate column totals here			

CDASS Checklist for **Common Coexisting Conditions with ADHD**

While other conditions and disorders frequently coexist with ADHD, the following are some of the most common.

YES_____   NO_____   Unknown or Unclear_____

KEY:

Y = Yes; O = Often; S = Sometimes; R = Rarely; ? = Unknown; N = No; P = In Past Only

Item	Indicator	Y	O	S	R	?	N	P
1	Has insomnia or problems initiating sleep (see this checklist if necessary)							
2	Has inadequate hours of sleep/partial sleep deprivation (see this checklist if necessary)							

KEY:

Y = Yes; O = Often; S = Sometimes; R = Rarely; ? = Unknown; N = No; P = In Past Only

Item	Indicator	Y	O	S	R	?	N	P
3	Has speech and articulation deficits (see this checklist if necessary)							
4	Has expressive and/or receptive language delays and disorders (see checklists if necessary)							
5	Has fine motor skills deficits/delays (difficulties with drawing, buttoning, use of scissors or zippers, tying shoes)							
6	Has dysgraphia (significantly messy and impaired handwriting) (see this checklist if necessary)							
7	Has gross motor skills deficits/delays (difficulties kicking running, sport activities, using a ball, riding a bike)							
8	Has reading learning disorder (see this checklist if necessary)							
9	Has mathematics learning disorder (see this checklist if necessary)							
10	Experiences nocturnal enuresis (nighttime bedwetting)							
11	Has oppositional defiant disorder (see this checklist if necessary)							
12	Has conduct disorder (see this checklist if necessary)							
13	Has gaming disorder (video game addiction; see this checklist if necessary)							
14	Has depression symptoms or disorder (see this checklist if necessary)							
15	Has anxiety symptoms or disorder (see this checklist if necessary)							

KEY:
Y = Yes; O = Often; S = Sometimes; R = Rarely; ? = Unknown; N = No; P = In Past Only

Item	Indicator	Y	O	S	R	?	N	P
16	Has substance abuse or problematic use (for older children and adolescents; see this checklist if necessary)							
17	Has prenatal fetal alcohol spectrum disorder or fetal drug exposure (see these checklists if necessary)							
18	Has sensory processing disorder/s (see these checklists if necessary)							
19	Is obese {ADHD is more prevalence with obesity. Obesity is associated with shorter sleep duration and time in bed, sleep-disordered breathing, other sleep disorders, and impulsive eating (Hvolby, 2015), and may be related to lesser activity levels, increased screen time, and/or poor food choices)							
20	Has been exposed to traumatic experiences or abuse (see this checklist if necessary)							
	Calculate column totals here							

REFERENCES

Barkley, R. (2013). *Taking charge of ADHD* (3rd ed.). New York: Guilford Press.

Barkley, R. (2015, March 19a). *ADHD: Nature, course, outcomes, and comorbidity.* Retrieved from www.continuingedcourses.net/active/courses/course003.php

Braaten, E., & Willoughby, B. (2014). *Bright kids who can't keep up.* New York: Guilford Press.

Centers for Disease Control and Prevention. (2017, August 31). *Attention-deficit/hyperactivity disorder (ADHD)–Symptoms and diagnosis.* Retrieved from https://www.cdc.gov/ncbddd/adhd/diagnosis.html

Hvolby, A. (2015, March). Associations of sleep disturbance with ADHD: Implications for treatment. *Attention Deficit and Hyperactivity Disorders, 7*(1), 1–18. doi: 10.1007/s12402-014-0151-0

Mayo Clinic Staff. (2017, August, 16a). *Attention-deficit/hyperactivity disorder (ADHD) in children—Symptoms & causes.* Retrieved from https://www.mayoclinic.org /diseases-conditions/adhd/symptoms-causes/syc-20350889

Wakschlag, L. S., Choi, S. W., Carter, A. S., Hullsiek, H., Burns, J., McCarthy, K., Leibenluft, E., & Briggs-Gowan, M. J. (2012, November). Defining the developmental parameters of temper loss in early childhood: Implications for developmental psychopathology. *Journal of Child Psychology and Psychiatry, 53*(11), 1099–108.

Chapter 14

THE COMPREHENSIVE DIAGNOSTIC ADHD SCREENINGS SYSTEM (CDASS) CHECKLISTS FOR CONDITIONS

MEDICAL CONDITIONS CHECKLISTS

The references for these checklists are listed in the References section of Chapter 4.

CDASS Checklist for **Vision Difficulties**

YES_____   NO_____   Unknown or Unclear_____

When indicated, ask the child or adolescent if they have these items below. Parents will only know about the items below if the child has been diagnosed or has complained about these items.

KEY:
Y = Yes; O = Often; S = Sometimes; R = Rarely; ? = Unknown; N = No; P = In Past Only

Item	Indicator	Y	O	S	R	?	N	P
1	Has been prescribed glasses							
2	Has been prescribed eye glasses and recommended to wear consistently, but does not wear regularly (*ask child/teen and parent*)							
3	Cannot see board/teacher in class (*ask child/teen*)							

KEY:

Y = Yes; O = Often; S = Sometimes; R = Rarely; ? = Unknown; N = No; P = In Past Only

Item	Indicator	Y	O	S	R	?	N	P
4	Has symptoms or diagnosis of near sightedness (myopia), a common condition where near objects can be seen clearly but distant objects are harder to see							
5	Has symptoms or diagnosis of farsightedness (hyperopia), where distant objects can be seen clearly but near objects are not							
6	Has symptoms or diagnosis of astigmatism (which causes distorted images due to an eye defect), including headaches or eye strain after reading, frequent squinting, objects are blurry, and small print is difficult to read							
7	Has symptoms or diagnosis of color blindness (*ask child/teen if has difficulty seeing colors*)							
8	Has blurry vision (*ask child/teen*)							
9	Child/teen reports they have any other experiences of vision problems not listed above (*Ask child/teen "Do you have any kind of strange or unusual vision problems?"*)							
	Calculate column totals here							

Record when symptoms began:_____

If vision condition has been diagnosed, list condition/s and when diagnosed:

_____

_____

CDASS Checklist for **Hearing Difficulties**

YES_____ NO_____ Unknown or Unclear_____

KEY:

Y = Yes; O = Often; S = Sometimes; R = Rarely; ? = Unknown; N = No; P = In Past Only

Item	Indicator	Y	O	S	R	?	N	P
1	Has suspected hearing deficits							
2	Has speech and language problems							
3	Has learning problems							
4	Has chronic congestion from allergies, colds, sinus, ear infections							
5	Has one or more of following risk factors: hearing concerns from parents, family history of hearing deficits, 5 or more days of neonatal intensive care, in-utero infections, certain syndromes (including Waardenburg), neurodegenerative disorders, certain infectious diseases (especially meningitis), head trauma, damaging sound level exposures, nervous system trauma, toxic drugs, ear abnormalities, and global developmental delays (Harlor & Bower, 2009)							
	Calculate column totals here							

Record when symptoms began:_____

If hearing condition has been diagnosed, list condition/s and when diagnosed:

_____

_____

CDASS Checklist for **Nasal Allergies and Allergy Medication Use**

YES_____   NO_____   Unknown or Unclear_____

KEY:

Y = Yes; O = Often; S = Sometimes; R = Rarely; ? = Unknown; N = No; P = In Past Only

Item	Indicator	Y	O	S	R	?	N	P
1	While experiencing allergies or during allergy season, has ADHD-like or increased ADHD symptoms							
2	After taking allergy medications, appears drowsy or has ADHD-like symptoms							
3	Has red/dark circles under the eyes							
4	Has mood difficulties only with allergy symptoms							
5	Has breathing problems							
6	Has mouth breathing (see this checklist if necessary)							
7	Experiences poor quality of sleep related to allergies							
8	Has sinus difficulties							
9	Wheezes							
10	Frequent rubs of the nose							
11	Has nasal stuffiness							
12	Frequent has runny nose							
13	Has irritated, red, watery or itchy eyes							
14	Congestion causes hearing problems							
15	Sneezes							
16	Family history of allergies							
Calculate column totals here								

Record when symptoms began:_____

If allergy condition has been diagnosed, list condition/s and when diagnosed:

_____

_____

If allergy medications are used, list medication/s: _____

_____

CDASS Checklist for **Chronic Sinus Problems**

YES_____   NO_____   Unknown or Unclear_____

KEY:
Y = Yes; O = Often; S = Sometimes; R = Rarely; ? = Unknown; N = No; P = In Past Only

Item	Indicator	Y	O	S	R	?	N	P
1	ADHD-like symptoms occur during sinus problems							
2	Has enlarged adenoids (see this checklist if necessary)							
3	Sinus problems impact sleeping							
4	Has chronic breathing problems during day							
5	Has mouth breathing (see this checklist if necessary)							
6	Sinus problems appear to cause hearing difficulties							
	Calculate column totals here							

Record when symptoms began:_____

If chronic sinus conditions exist, including recurrent colds, sinus infections, and allergies, list condition and when diagnosed:_____

_____

If sinus medications are used, list medication/s:_____

CDASS Checklist for **Asthma Problems**

YES_____   NO_____   Unknown or Unclear_____

KEY:
Y = Yes; O = Often; S = Sometimes; R = Rarely; ? = Unknown; N = No; P = In Past Only

Item	Indicator	Y	O	S	R	?	N	P
1	ADHD-like symptoms occur during asthma problems							
2	Asthma appears to cause breathing problems during day/night							
3	Asthma appears to impact sleeping							
4	After taking asthma medications has ADHD-like symptoms							
5	Has nasal allergies (see this checklist if necessary)							
6	Family history of asthma							
Calculate column totals here								

Record when symptoms began:_____

If asthma condition has been diagnosed, list when:_____

If asthma medications are used, list medication/s:_____

CDASS Checklist for **Enlarged Tonsils and Adenoids**

YES_____   NO_____   Unknown or Unclear_____

KEY:
Y = Yes; O = Often; S = Sometimes; R = Rarely; ? = Unknown; N = No; P = In Past Only

Item	Indicator	Y	O	S	R	?	N	P
1	Snores							
2	Has mouth breathing (see this check-list if necessary)							
3	Has obstructive sleep apnea (see this checklist if necessary)							
4	Has sinus problems (see this checklist if necessary)							
5	Has nasal allergies (see this checklist if necessary)							
	Calculate column totals here							

If tonsils and adenoids were removed, indicate when:_____

CDASS Checklist for **Diabetes**

YES_____   NO_____   Unknown or Unclear_____

KEY:
Y = Yes; O = Often; S = Sometimes; R = Rarely; ? = Unknown; N = No; P = In Past Only

Item	Indicator	Y	O	S	R	?	N	P
1	Has recent weight loss or gain							
2	Has increased/persistent urination							
3	Has new onset of bed-wetting							
4	Has unusual thirst							
5	Exhibits irritability							
6	Sweats excessively							

KEY:
Y = Yes; O = Often; S = Sometimes; R = Rarely; ? = Unknown; N = No; P = In Past Only

Item	Indicator	Y	O	S	R	?	N	P
7	Displays confusion							
8	Is excessively hunger (Garber, Garber, & Spizman, 1996)							
9	Has moodiness							
10	Has hypoglycemia (see this checklist if necessary)							
11	Family history of diabetes							
	Calculate column totals here							

Record when symptoms began:_____

If diabetes was diagnosed, list type and when:_____

CDASS Checklist for **Hypoglycemia**

YES_____   NO_____   Unknown or Unclear_____

KEY:
Y = Yes; O = Often; S = Sometimes; R = Rarely; ? = Unknown; N = No; P = In Past Only

Item	Indicator	Y	O	S	R	?	N	P
1	Has brief or intermittent periods of loss of attention							
2	Exhibits aggression, hostility, or acting out							
3	Has persistent difficulties with being tired, lethargy							
4	Has skin paleness (Garber, Garber, & Spizman, 1996)							
5	Demonstrates irritability							

KEY:
Y = Yes; O = Often; S = Sometimes; R = Rarely; ? = Unknown; N = No; P = In Past Only

Item	Indicator	Y	O	S	R	?	N	P
6	Has anxiety							
7	Is drowsy after meals							
8	Trembles							
9	Craves for sweets (Walsh Research Institute, 2005–2016b)							
10	Has diabetes or other conditions causing hypoglycemia							
11	Displays confusion							
	Calculate column totals here							

Record when symptoms began:_____

If hypoglycemia condition has been determined, list when:_____

_____

CDASS Checklist for **Anemia and Iron Deficiency**

YES_____   NO_____   Unknown or Unclear_____

KEY:
Y = Yes; O = Often; S = Sometimes; R = Rarely; ? = Unknown; N = No; P = In Past Only

Item	Indicator	Y	O	S	R	?	N	P
1	Exhibits irritability							
2	Has impaired cognitive skills (attention, learning, memory, comprehension)							
3	Has fatigue/physical weakness							
4	Has pale skin							
5	Experiences shortness of breath							
6	Has headaches							

KEY:
Y = Yes; O = Often; S = Sometimes; R = Rarely; ? = Unknown; N = No; P = In Past Only

Item	Indicator	Y	O	S	R	?	N	P
7	Experiences lightheadedness							
8	Complains of cold hands/feet							
9	Has tongue inflammation/soreness							
10	Has poor appetite							
11	Has brittle nails							
12	Has restless legs syndrome (see this checklist if necessary)							
13	Has unusual cravings for non-nutritive substances (such as ice)							
14	Family history of heritable anemia (such as sickle cell)							
	Calculate column totals here							

Record when symptoms began:_____

If anemia was diagnosed, list when:_____

CDASS Checklist for **Thyroid Disorders**

YES_____   NO_____   Unknown or Unclear_____

KEY:
Y = Yes; O = Often; S = Sometimes; R = Rarely; ? = Unknown; N = No; P = In Past Only

Item	Indicator	Y	O	S	R	?	N	P
	Hypothyroidism							
1	Exhibits "brain fog," sluggishness, confusion							
2	Has short-term memory problems							
3	Is constipated							

KEY:
Y = Yes; O = Often; S = Sometimes; R = Rarely; ? = Unknown; N = No; P = In Past Only

Item	Indicator	Y	O	S	R	?	N	P
4	Has depression symptoms							
5	Has recent weight gain or loss							
6	Has dry and itchy skin							
7	Experiences hair loss or thinning							
8	Has voice hoarseness							
9	Complains of cold sensitivity/intolerance, feels cold when others do not							
10	Experiences more frequent/heavier menstrual periods							
	Hyperthyroidism							
11	Has muscle weakness							
12	Has brittleness of hair							
13	Sweats							
14	Complains of heat sensitivity/intolerance, feels hot when others do not							
15	Has vision difficulties or changes							
16	Has increased appetite							
17	Has heart palpitations							
18	Experiences less frequent/lighter menstrual periods							
19	Thyroid gland is enlarged (a goiter, or bulge, fullness or tenderness in neck)							
	Hypo and Hyperthyroidism							
20	Has sleep difficulties							
21	Has anxiety symptoms							
22	Is irritable							
23	Exhibits mood swings							

KEY:

Y = Yes; O = Often; S = Sometimes; R = Rarely; ? = Unknown; N = No; P = In Past Only

Item	Indicator	Y	O	S	R	?	N	P
24	Family history of thyroid disorders							
	Calculate column totals here							

Record when symptoms began:_____

If thyroid condition was diagnosed, list type and when:_____

_____

CDASS Checklist for **Seizures**

YES_____　　　　　NO_____　　　　　Unknown or Unclear_____

KEY:

Y = Yes; O = Often; S = Sometimes; R = Rarely; ? = Unknown; N = No; P = In Past Only

Item	Indicator	Y	O	S	R	?	N	P
1	After taking seizure medications has ADHD-like symptoms							
2	Has brief memory loss episodes (inability to remember what happened)							
3	Excessively blinks							
4	Has staring episodes							
5	Appears to blank/zone out							
6	When name is called does not respond							
7	Has repeated loss of awareness							
8	Makes slight tasting movements of mouth							
9	Makes odd hand movements (rubbing fingers together, hand scratching)							
10	Contracts/relaxes of muscles							

KEY:

Y = Yes; O = Often; S = Sometimes; R = Rarely; ? = Unknown; N = No; P = In Past Only

Item	Indicator	Y	O	S	R	?	N	P
11	Smacks lips							
12	Flutters/raises eyelids							
13	Eyes roll upward							
14	Makes chewing movements							
15	Is suddenly motionless							
16	Has forward/backward leaning behaviors							
17	Makes licking/swallowing movements							
18	Is unaware of surroundings							
19	Has daydreaming episodes							
20	Has twitching episodes (eyelids, mouth corners, arms)							
21	Does not respond to others unless touched/spoken to							
22	Has poor listening skills with staring/daydreaming episodes							
23	Family history of seizures in first degree relatives							
24	History of moderate/severe traumatic brain injury (one or more)							
	Calculate column totals here							

Record when symptoms began:_____

If seizure condition was diagnosed, list type, when diagnozed, and medications:

_____

_____

OTHER MEDICAL CONDITIONS ASSOCIATED WITH HIGHER RISKS OF ADHD OR ADHD-LIKE PRESENTATIONS

The following items do not have checklists. Print YES, NO, or Unknown/ Unclear next to each item if the child/adolescent has or has had:

_____ **Low Blood Count**

_____ **Food Sensitivities and Allergies:** List these and when determined:

_____

_____

_____ **Persistent/Recurrent Ear Infections**

_____ **Conditions Causing Chronic Bodily Pain or Discomfort**

List identified conditions and when diagnosed:_____

_____

_____ **Hunger, Food Insecurity or Malnutrition**

_____ **Other Prescription or Over-the Counter Medication Use:** Do not list medications already addressed. List other medications and when began using these:

_____

_____

_____ **Other Medical Conditions:** List conditions and when diagnosed:

_____

_____

_____ **Phenylketonuria (PKU)**

_____ **Stroke**

_____ **Meningitis, Encephalitis, or other Brain Diseases/Infections/Tumors**

_____ **Lyme Disease**

_____ **Celiac Disease**

_____ **Leukemia, Head and Neck Cancer Treatments**

_____ **Fragile X Syndrome**

SLEEP CONDITIONS CHECKLISTS

The references for these checklists are listed in the References section of Chapter 5.

CDASS Checklist for **Persistent Mouth Breathing**

YES_____   NO_____   Unknown or Unclear_____

Parents may be initially unaware if mouth breathing exists, and can require additional time to explore this topic. These items may need review after parental monitoring of breathing during day and night for 2–4 weeks.

KEY:
Y = Yes; O = Often; S = Sometimes; R = Rarely; ? = Unknown; N = No; P = In Past Only

Item	Indicator	Y	O	S	R	?	N	P
1	* Breathes with open mouth during the day, mouth is open when not talking							
2	* Sleeps with mouth open at night (*ask parents and child*)							
3	* Has chronic allergies							
4	* Has chronic sinus or congestion problems							
5	Has obstructive sleep apnea symptoms (see this checklist if necessary)							
6	Breathing is raspy, shallow							
7	Has dark circles under eyes							
8	Has bad breath							
9	Has overlapping teeth, teeth were removed due crowding							
10	Gums are excessively visible when smiles							
11	Has night sweating							
12	Was failure to thrive baby/child							
13	Has visibly protruding jaw							

KEY:

Y = Yes; O = Often; S = Sometimes; R = Rarely; ? = Unknown; N = No; P = In Past Only

Item	Indicator	Y	O	S	R	?	N	P
14	Has high arched, narrow mouth palate (roof of the mouth)							
15	Has long-term pacifier use or thumb sucking							
16	Exhibits social problems							
17	Has depression symptoms, excessively moody/emotional							
18	Has anxiety symptoms (Sinha & Guilleminault, 2010)							
19	* Has crossbite/malocclusion (upper and lower jaws are misaligned, upper teeth bite inside or behind lower teeth on front/sides of mouth); may have had correcting orthodontia							
20	* Has excessively long/narrow face in older children and teens							
21	Has crooked or overlapping teeth							
22	Has shorter upper lip							
23	Complains of headaches when waking							
24	Has restlessness during sleep							
25	Is smaller in size or height							
26	Has behavioral problems							
27	Snores							
28	Has runny/stuffy nose							
29	Sneezes							
30	Displays tongue posture changes during speaking, resting, chewing, swallowing							
31	Complains of dry mouth; thirsty when waking or during night							
32	Has deviated or swollen nasal septum							

KEY:

Y = Yes; O = Often; S = Sometimes; R = Rarely; ? = Unknown; N = No; P = In Past Only

Item	Indicator	Y	O	S	R	?	N	P
33	Exhibits daytime sleepiness							
34	Is irritable (Thome Pacheco et. al., 2015, May/June)							
35	Drools on pillow							
36	Easily tires							
37	Has anterior open bite in older children/teens (front teeth don't touch or close properly, opening exists between upper and lower front teeth)							
38	Has gingivitis in upper front teeth (gum inflammation disease) (Thome Pacheco et. al., 2015, July/August)							
39	Is obese							
40	Has unrefreshing sleep; wakes up tired after sufficient hours							
41	Experiences insomnia							
42	Is aggressive (Spruyt & Gozal, 2011)							
43	Has small jaw (Fischman, Kuffler, & Bloch, 2015)							
44	Has voice hoarseness							
	Calculate column totals here							

* = Important common item

Record when symptoms began:_____

_____ **Snores** *(This may fluctuate or occur inconsistently. This item does not have a checklist. Print Yes, No, or Unknown/Unclear. Some parents may need to check on child while sleeping over 1–2 weeks if unsure).*

CDASS Checklist for **Obstructive Sleep Apnea**

YES_____   NO_____   Unknown or Unclear_____

KEY:
Y = Yes; O = Often; S = Sometimes; R = Rarely; ? = Unknown; N = No; P = In Past Only

Item	Indicator	Y	O	S	R	?	N	P
1	* While sleeping, stops breathing, gasps/snorts, begins breathing again							
2	* Snores (may fluctuate or occur inconsistent)							
3	* Has mouth breathing while sleeping							
4	Has mouth breathing during day							
5	Exhibits additional mouth breathing symptoms besides open mouth (see this checklist if necessary)							
6	Wets bed							
7	Is excessively sleepy during day							
8	Has behavioral problems							
9	Is obese							
10	Complains of morning headaches (O'Brien, n.d.)							
11	Exhibits oppositional behavior							
12	Has decreased academic performance							
13	Experiences peer social difficulties (Greene, 2014)							
14	Is aggressive (Breus, 2013)							
15	Has unrefreshing sleep; wakes up tired after sufficient hours							
16	Experiences insomnia (Spruyt & Gozal, 2011)							

KEY:
Y = Yes; O = Often; S = Sometimes; R = Rarely; ? = Unknown; N = No; P = In Past Only

Item	Indicator	Y	O	S	R	?	N	P
17	Has bruxism (jaw clenching, teeth grinding during sleep) (Idzikowski, 2013)							
18	Has difficulty waking in morning							
19	* Family history of OSA							
20	Is restless during sleep							
21	Drools							
22	Has smaller jaw (Fischman, Kuffler, & Bloch, 2015)							
23	Arouses in morning with agitation							
24	Has swallowing difficulty							
25	Exhibits atypical sleeping positions (neck extended oddly, sleeps on knees/hands)							
26	Sweats when sleeping (Foldvary-Schaefer, 2006)							
27	Is smaller in height/size							
28	Is easily winded from sports							
29	Has nasal voice							
30	Has chronic allergies							
31	Is irritable							
32	Has mood symptoms or problems							
	Calculate column totals here							

* = Important common item

Record when symptoms began:_____

CDASS Checklist for **Increased Nocturnal Motor Activity**

YES_____   NO_____   Unknown or Unclear_____

KEY:

Y = Yes; O = Often; S = Sometimes; R = Rarely; ? = Unknown; N = No; P = In Past Only

Item	Indicator	Y	O	S	R	?	N	P
1	Moves excessively while sleeping (*if present, screen for periodic limb movement disorder & restless legs syndrome with these checklists*)							
2	Bed sheets/blankets are significantly disrupted in morning							
3	Is heard hitting things near bed, banging wall while sleeping							
4	Talks in sleep							
5	Has daytime sleepiness							
6	Has difficulty waking in morning							
7	Is irritable							
	Calculate column totals here							

Record when symptoms began:_____

CDASS Checklist for **Periodic Limb Movement Disorder**

YES_____   NO_____   Unknown or Unclear_____

KEY:
Y = Yes; O = Often; S = Sometimes; R = Rarely; ? = Unknown; N = No; P = In Past Only

Item	Indicator	Y	O	S	R	?	N	P
1	* While sleeping, makes repetitive jerking/rhythmic and involuntary movements in one/both legs or upward flexing of feet that occurs about every 20 to 40 seconds in clusters of minutes/several hours							
2	* Sleeps during the leg/arm movements							
3	Makes frequent leg movements that disrupt sleep							
4	The frequent leg movements cause multiple/brief awakenings from sleep (arousals may unknown to parents)							
5	Experiences daytime drowsiness or sleepiness							
6	Is irritable (The Cleveland Clinic Foundation, n.d.)							
7	Has high levels of motor activity/restlessness in legs and/or arms while sleeping (however not movements in item #1)							
8	Has inadequate hours of sleep symptoms (see this checklist if necessary)							
9	Tosses/turns while sleeping							
10	Bed sheets/blankets are significantly disrupted in morning							

KEY:
Y = Yes; O = Often; S = Sometimes; R = Rarely; ? = Unknown; N = No; P = In Past Only

Item	Indicator	Y	O	S	R	?	N	P
11	Is heard hitting things near bed/banging the wall while sleeping							
	Calculate column totals here							

* = Important common item

Record when symptoms began:_____

CDASS Checklist for **Restless Legs Syndrome**

YES_____   NO_____   Unknown or Unclear_____

KEY:
Y = Yes; O = Often; S = Sometimes; R = Rarely; ? = Unknown; N = No; P = In Past Only

Item	Indicator	Y	O	S	R	?	N	P
1	* Has overwhelming need to move legs when resting, lying down, sitting							
2	* Has strange sensations/discomfort in legs (children may have difficulty describing this); feels like pins, needles, crawling insects, itchy							
3	* Has repeated urges to move after having leg sensations/discomfort							
4	* Leg sensations/discomfort stop when they move							
5	* Has trouble falling asleep due to leg sensations/discomfort							
6	Urges to move typically occur in evening or worse at night							
7	Has trouble staying in bed due to leg sensations/discomfort							

KEY:

Y = Yes; O = Often; S = Sometimes; R = Rarely; ? = Unknown; N = No; P = In Past Only

Item	Indicator	Y	O	S	R	?	N	P
8	After sleeping, wakes up in middle of night and has difficulties falling back to sleep due to leg sensations/discomfort							
9	Has daytime sleepiness							
10	Experiences trouble waking up/starting day in morning							
11	Is irritable (Martin, 2013)							
12	Resists bedtime (from expecting RLS discomfort)							
13	Has unpleasant sensations in legs when in bed at night (*ask child this question*)							
14	Experiences restlessness that prevents falling asleep at night (*ask child this question*) (Konofal, Lecendreux, & Cortese, 2010)							
15	Family history of RLS							
16	Has iron deficiency (see this checklist if necessary)							
17	Has inadequate hours of sleep symptoms (see this checklist if necessary)							
Calculate column totals here								

* = Important common item

Record when symptoms began:_____

Identify the Types of Insomnia

Print Yes, No, or Unknown/Unclear before insomnia types. Ask child/teen and parent these questions. Frequencies of once or more a week can be significant, but fluctuating or less frequent occurrences may also be impactful.

_____ **Has sleep onset/initial insomnia:** Child/teen struggles to fall asleep while in bed with head on pillow, lights off, and it takes 30 minutes or more to fall asleep.

A. How often does this occur? List number of nights per week or month child/teen struggles to fall asleep when it takes 30 minutes or more to fall asleep:

_____

B. When falling asleep problems occur, what is the range of times it takes to fall asleep?

   • Shortest amount of time that is greater than 30 minutes: _____

   • Longest amount of time to fall asleep: _____

C. When falling asleep problems occur, what is the most common amount of time it takes to fall asleep when it takes 30 or more minutes to fall asleep?

_____

D. List when insomnia began and reasons why they believe this occurs:

_____

_____

_____

_____ **Has sleep maintenance/middle insomnia:** Child/teen has difficulties once a week or more with waking in middle of night and cannot return to sleep after 30 minutes or more. The additional questions above from sleep onset insomnia may also be used.

• How often does this occur? List number of nights per week or month child/teen wakes in middle of night and struggles to return to sleep, and it takes 30 minutes or more to fall back asleep:

_____

_____ **Has early morning awakening/terminal insomnia:** Child/teen wakes in the morning 30 minutes or more before they plan or expect to wake up. The additional questions above from sleep onset insomnia may also be used.

- How often does this occur? List number of early mornings per week or month child/teen wakes before they are expected to wake and struggles to return to sleep, and it takes 30 minutes or more to fall back asleep:

_____

CDASS Checklist for **Insomnia and Sleep Initiation Difficulties**

YES_____   NO_____   Unknown or Unclear_____

KEY:
Y = Yes; O = Often; S = Sometimes; R = Rarely; ? = Unknown; N = No; P = In Past Only

Item	Indicator	Y	O	S	R	?	N	P
1	Does not have restful or refreshing sleep							
2	Has difficulties waking up or getting out of bed in morning							
3	Is sleepy or fatigued during morning or day							
4	Has anxiety symptoms							
5	Is irritable							
6	Has depression symptoms							
7	Has psychological trauma symptoms							
8	Has other psychological condition/s that affect sleep							
9	Worries before going to bed or in bed (including sleeping problems)							
10	Lays in bed with mind racing, unable to stop thinking							
11	Has distractions in bedroom at night (including siblings)							
12	Environmental factors impact sleep (excessive hot, cold, light, noise)							

KEY:
Y = Yes; O = Often; S = Sometimes; R = Rarely; ? = Unknown; N = No; P = In Past Only

Item	Indicator	Y	O	S	R	?	N	P
13	Uses electronic screen devices just before bed, in bed, or left on while sleeping							
14	Has inconsistent bedtimes							
15	Experiences poor sleep quality							
16	Snores							
17	Has mouth-breathing at night or day (see this checklist if necessary)							
18	Has obstructive sleep apnea symptoms (see this checklist if necessary)							
19	Uses medication that impacts sleep (prescribed or over-the-counter)							
20	Has medical conditions that cause discomfort, breathing difficulties, or impact sleep (asthma, allergies, chronic pain)							
21	Exhibits behavioral problems or bedtime refusal/resistance before bed (transitioning to bed, arguing)							
22	Lacks quiet time or routines to "wind down" before bed							
23	Has dysfunctional family factors that impact sleep							
24	Naps during the day							
25	Has inconsistent sleep arrangements (sleeps in various places)							
26	Regularly co-sleeps with parents or siblings, does not remain in their own bed							
27	Has restless legs syndrome (see this checklist if necessary)							

KEY:

Y = Yes; O = Often; S = Sometimes; R = Rarely; ? = Unknown; N = No; P = In Past Only

Item	Indicator	Y	O	S	R	?	N	P
28	Has periodic limb movement disorder (see this checklist if necessary)							
29	Has increased nocturnal motor activity during sleep (see this checklist if necessary)							
30	Does physical activity/exercise close to bedtime							
31	Has night wakings							
32	Has delayed sleep-phase disorder (see this checklist if necessary)							
33	Drinks caffeinated beverages, particularly in afternoons/evenings							
	Calculate column totals here							

Record when symptoms began:_____

Calculate Number of Hours of Sleep Per Night

To calculate the number of typical hours of sleep per night a child or teen obtains, ask when the child/teen typically goes to bed, when they actually fall asleep, and when they awaken. These can be averages or ranges over the prior months. Two sets of sleep hours should be calculated, one for school nights, and the other for non-school nights (weekends, summers, and holidays).

A. What time does child/teen go to bed on school nights typically? (give a range if necessary):

_____

B. What time does child/teen wake on school days typically? (give a range if necessary):

_____

C. What time does child/teen go to bed on weekends or nonschool nights typically? (give a range if necessary):

_____

D. What time does child/teen wake on weekends or non-school days typically? (give a range if necessary):

_____

E. Does the child/teen nap? If so calculate the total amount of time child/teen naps each day (give a range if necessary):

_____

F. Calculate typical number of hours of sleep per night child/teen obtains on school nights from A, B & E (include naps, give a range if necessary, and state when this amount began):

_____

_____

G. Calculate typical number of hours of sleep per night child/teen obtains on nonschool nights from C, D & E (include naps, give a range if necessary, and state when this amount began):

_____

_____

_____ Inadequate Hours of Sleep from Sleep Guidelines

Print *Yes, No, or Unknown/Unclear* on the short line above by comparing the calculated numbers of typical sleep hours (F and G in above section) to the following sleep guidelines:

Children ages 3 to 5 should consistently obtain 10 to 13 hours of sleep per 24 hours (including naps), and most do not require a nap after age 5. Children ages 6 to 12 consistently require 9 to 12 hours of sleep per night. Adolescents ages 13 to 18 consistently require 8 to 10 hours of sleep per night (American Academy of Pediatrics, 2016). The range of hours of sleep are guidelines, but needs may vary. Even if a child is obtaining the lower end of the range, they may still need more than this minimum number due to individual differences.

_____

CDASS Checklist for **Inadequate Hours of Sleep/Chronic Inadequate Sleep Duration**

Note: There can be an overlap of symptoms with insomnia and inadequate sleep duration, so there may be similarly checked items on both checklists.

YES_____   NO_____   Unknown or Unclear_____

KEY:
Y = Yes; O = Often; S = Sometimes; R = Rarely; ? = Unknown; N = No; P = In Past Only

Item	Indicator	Y	O	S	R	?	N	P
1	* Obtains inadequate hours of sleep based on sleep guidelines							
2	Has chronic difficulties waking/getting out of bed in morning							
3	Has difficulties becoming alert after awakening, struggles with morning tasks							
4	Has initial insomnia							
5	Has middle insomnia							
6	Has terminal insomnia							
7	Experiences poor quality of sleep							
8	Has delayed sleep-phase disorder (see this checklist if necessary)							
9	Goes to bed later than normal/ expected							
10	Has restlessness during sleep							
11	Obtains lower or poor school grades							
12	Has depression symptoms							
13	Is irritable							
14	Has low energy, fatigue							
15	Is sleepy/tired during day							
16	Has poor frustration tolerance							

KEY:

Y = Yes; O = Often; S = Sometimes; R = Rarely; ? = Unknown; N = No; P = In Past Only

Item	Indicator	Y	O	S	R	?	N	P
17	Lacks consistent enforced bedtime; bedtime varies							
18	Uses electronic screen devices in bed at night							
19	Snores							
20	Has mouth-breathing at night/day (see this checklist if necessary)							
21	Has obstructive sleep apnea symptoms (see this checklist if necessary)							
22	Takes medication that impacts sleep							
23	Has medical conditions that cause discomfort, breathing difficulties, or impact sleep							
24	Exhibits behavioral problems at night that impacts bedtime (difficulties transitioning, arguing, bedtime resistance)							
25	Has dysfunctional family factors that impact sufficient sleep							
26	Naps during day (for older children and teens)							
27	Has inconsistent sleep arrangements (sleeps in various places)							
28	Has restless legs syndrome (see this checklist if necessary)							
29	Has periodic limb movement disorder (see this checklist if necessary)							
30	Wakes during night							
	Calculate column totals here							

* = Important common item

Record when symptoms began:_____

CDASS Checklist for **Delayed Sleep-Phase Disorder**

YES_____   NO_____   Unknown or Unclear_____

KEY:
Y = Yes; O = Often; S = Sometimes; R = Rarely; ? = Unknown; N = No; P = In Past Only

Item	Indicator	Y	O	S	R	?	N	P
1	* Prefers/enjoys going to bed later than normal							
2	* Prefers to wake later							
3	Complains not tired or cannot sleep at normal bedtime							
4	Argues, resistant to going to bed, or has behavioral problems before bedtime							
5	Has difficulties waking in morning, getting out of bed							
6	Struggles with alertness/sluggish in mornings							
7	Dislikes mornings							
8	Grumpy or irritable in morning							
9	Sleepy during the day							
10	Obtains inadequate hours of sleep (see this checklist if necessary)							
	Calculate column totals here							

* = Important common item

Record when symptoms began:_____

CDASS Checklist for **Parasomnias**

YES_____   NO_____   Unknown or Unclear_____

KEY:
Y = Yes; O = Often; S = Sometimes; R = Rarely; ? = Unknown; N = No; P = In Past Only

Item	Indicator	Y	O	S	R	?	N	P
1	Has nocturnal enuresis (bedwetting)							
2	Has nightmares							
3	Sleep walks							
4	Talks in sleep							
5	Has sleep terrors (while sleeping the child screams, is highly upset, may move about but typically has no recall in morning)							
6	Has confusional arousals (child acts confused or strange as they wake or just after waking)							
7	Has bruxism (nighttime teeth grinding and clenching)							
8	Has sleep paralysis (a brief frightening experience of not being able to move or speak when falling asleep or waking)							
9	Has rhythmic movement disorder (making repeated involuntary body movements during/before sleep, frequently involving the neck and head, with humming/sounds accompanying movements)							
	Calculate column totals here							

Record when symptoms began:_____

NEURODEVELOPMENTAL CONDITIONS CHECKLISTS

The references for these checklists are listed in the References section of Chapter 6.

CDASS Checklist for **Reading Learning Disorder**

YES_____   NO_____   Unknown or Unclear_____

KEY:
Y = Yes; O = Often; S = Sometimes; R = Rarely; ? = Unknown; N = No; P = In Past Only

Item	Indicator	Y	O	S	R	?	N	P
1	* *Single basic screening question for reading LD:* Has concerning reading difficulties, including inadequately sounding out and pronouncing words and does not understand meaning of what is read (significantly below age/grade/educational level)							
2	* Only has inattention during reading tasks, and no focusing problems during non-reading tasks (positive answer could suggest reading LD and no true ADHD) (Barkley, 2015, March 19b)							
3	* Family history of diagnosed/ suspected significant reading problems or LD (poor academic performance not from ADHD)							
4	* Did not develop fluent reading by end of third grade or later that is below their age/educational experiences							
5	* Struggles with word recognition, below what is expected for age/grade/educational experiences							
6	* Has deficit spelling abilities below what is expected for age/grade/educational experiences							

KEY:

Y = Yes; O = Often; S = Sometimes; R = Rarely; ? = Unknown; N = No; P = In Past Only

Item	Indicator	Y	O	S	R	?	N	P
7	* Has deficit decoding ability, below what is expected for age/grade/educational experiences (does not read and pronounce words properly) (Tannock & Brown, 2009)							
8	* Has difficulties with basic reading skills by end of first grade or later							
9	Has hearing impairments							
10	Learned poor/minimal reading skills or received inadequate reading instructions during preschool years (Drummond, 2005–2007)							
11	Has speech articulation difficulties after age 5–6							
12	Has difficulties naming letters in kindergarten ("can you show me the letter E?")							
13	Has problems attaching sounds to letters by early first grade ("G is for go"); difficulties learning the connections between sounds and letters (Kutscher, 2014)							
14	Has word-find/word recall difficulties (trouble finding right word to say)							
15	Has difficulties learning the names of colors							
16	Has difficulties remembering phone numbers/addresses							
17	Has problems mis-sequencing syllables ("donimos" for "dominoes" or "aminals" or "animals")							

KEY:

Y = Yes; O = Often; S = Sometimes; R = Rarely; ? = Unknown; N = No; P = In Past Only

Item	Indicator	Y	O	S	R	?	N	P
18	Has difficulties following directions							
19	Lesser speech production							
20	Has expressive language difficulties (not just speech articulation) (see this checklist if necessary)							
21	Has difficulties with peer relations related to language deficits; interpersonal expression problems, aggression, withdrawal (Parker, 2000)							
22	Was delayed speaking words and using full sentences							
23	* Has poor reading comprehension by end of third grade or later							
24	Transposes sequence of numbers (43 is read 34)							
25	Learns new skills slowly							
26	Has letter/number recognition problems							
27	Reads very slowly							
28	Has lesser vocabulary for age							
29	Resists sounding out unrecognized words							
30	Has problems reading single words without pictures/visual cues							
31	Struggles reading new/pseudo words (Dr. Seuss words)							
32	Dislikes reading aloud (Kemp, Smith, & Segal, 2012)							
33	Is slow to remember facts							
34	Confuses basic words when reading (walk, go, sleep, want)							

KEY:

Y = Yes; O = Often; S = Sometimes; R = Rarely; ? = Unknown; N = No; P = In Past Only

Item	Indicator	Y	O	S	R	?	N	P
35	Relies on memorization for reading skills							
36	Makes letter inversions errors (w/m)							
37	Makes letter reversal errors (d/b)							
38	Makes transpositions of letters within words (left for felt)							
39	Makes letter substitutions within words (broom for doom)							
40	Has difficulties telling time (Coordinated Campaign for Learning Disabilities, 1997)							
41	Struggles with open-ended test questions							
42	Avoids/dislikes reading							
43	Struggles with math word problems							
44	Has difficulties reading longer passages							
45	Obtains poor grades related to reading, teacher reports reading deficits							
	Difficulties associated with reading LD:							
46	Has organizational problems with writing assignments							
47	Dislikes/avoids writing							
48	Has poor/sloppy handwriting or dysgraphia (see this checklist if necessary)							
49	Has fine motor coordination problems							
50	Has difficulties with rhyming/recognizing rhyming words (Kemp, Smith, & Segal, 2012)							

KEY:
Y = Yes; O = Often; S = Sometimes; R = Rarely; ? = Unknown; N = No; P = In Past Only

Item	Indicator	Y	O	S	R	?	N	P
51	Has had injuries, illnesses, or other factors that impacted hearing and auditory processing within the first 3 years (Bellis, 2002)							
52	Has auditory processing disorder (see this checklist if necessary)							
	Conditions which may cause reading deficits without true LD:							
53	Has visual processing disorder deficits (see this checklist if necessary)							
54	Has sleep-disordered breathing difficulties (see these checklists if necessary)							
	Calculate column totals here							

* = Important common item

Record when symptoms began:_____

CDASS Checklist for **Mathematics Learning Disorder**

YES_____   NO_____   Unknown or Unclear_____

KEY:
Y = Yes; O = Often; S = Sometimes; R = Rarely; ? = Unknown; N = No; P = In Past Only

Item	Indicator	Y	O	S	R	?	N	P
1	** Single basic screening question for math LD:* Has concerning math difficulties, including inadequately performing math skills and operations (significantly below age/grade/educational level)							

KEY:
Y = Yes; O = Often; S = Sometimes; R = Rarely; ? = Unknown; N = No; P = In Past Only

Item	Indicator	Y	O	S	R	?	N	P
2	* Only has inattention when performing math tasks, and no focusing problems during non-math or number related tasks (positive answer could suggest math LD and no true ADHD) (Barkley, 2015, March 19b)							
3	Has difficulties with addition skills, beyond what is expected for age/grade/educational level							
4	Has difficulties with subtraction skills							
5	Has difficulties with multiplication skills							
6	Has difficulties with division skills							
7	Is slow to learn math skills; has difficulties learning basic math concepts							
8	Has problems with organization of numbers							
9	Has difficulties memorizing math facts (multiplication tables)							
10	Has difficulties using operation signs (+ or x)							
11	Has difficulties borrowing/carrying numbers in addition/multiplication							
12	Has difficulties with sequencing complex math operations							
13	Has trouble learning counting principles (by 5s or 10s)							
14	Makes excessive math mistakes							
15	Erases frequently with math problems							
16	Has difficulties using/counting money or making change (Kemp, Smith, & Segal, 2012)							

KEY:

Y = Yes; O = Often; S = Sometimes; R = Rarely; ? = Unknown; N = No; P = In Past Only

Item	Indicator	Y	O	S	R	?	N	P
17	Transposes sequence of numbers (43 is read 34)							
18	Confuses/struggles to understand arithmetic signs (-, +, x, =, /)							
19	Has difficulties telling time (Coordinated Campaign for Learning Disabilities, 1997)							
20	Obtains poor math grades, teacher reports math deficits							
21	Family history of diagnosed math LD or significant math difficulties (including poor academic performance not from ADHD)							
	Difficulties associated with math LD can include:							
22	Has reading LD or significant reading deficits							
23	Dislikes/avoids writing							
24	Has poor/sloppy handwriting or dysgraphia (see this checklist if necessary)							
25	Has fine motor coordination problems (Kemp, Smith, & Segal, 2012)							
26	Has had injuries, illnesses, or other factors that impacted hearing and auditory processing within the first 3 years (Bellis, 2002)							
27	Has speech and language delays/conditions							
28	Has expressive language deficits (see this checklist if necessary)							
29	Has hearing deficits/impairments							

KEY:
Y = Yes; O = Often; S = Sometimes; R = Rarely; ? = Unknown; N = No; P = In Past Only

Item	Indicator	Y	O	S	R	?	N	P
30	Has auditory processing disorder (see this checklist if necessary)							
	Conditions which may cause math deficits without true LD:							
31	Has visual processing disorder deficits (see this checklist if necessary)							
32	Has sleep-disordered breathing difficulties (see these checklists if necessary)							
	Calculate column totals here							

* = Important common item

Record when symptoms began:_____

CDASS Checklist for **Written Expression Learning Disorder**

YES_____   NO_____   Unknown or Unclear_____

KEY:
Y = Yes; O = Often; S = Sometimes; R = Rarely; ? = Unknown; N = No; P = In Past Only

Item	Indicator	Y	O	S	R	?	N	P
1	* Has difficulties expressing themselves in handwriting and keypad typing; difficulties expressing thoughts/ideas on paper or screen							
2	Family history of diagnosed or suspected significant written expression difficulties							
3	Avoids/dislikes writing activities/tasks							
4	Makes punctuation errors							
5	Makes grammatical errors							
6	Makes spelling errors							

KEY:
Y = Yes; O = Often; S = Sometimes; R = Rarely; ? = Unknown; N = No; P = In Past Only

Item	Indicator	Y	O	S	R	?	N	P
7	Struggles with writing sentences; poor sentence organization/clarity							
8	Has poor organization or clarity when writing paragraphs							
9	Writes excessively slow							
10	Makes numerous writing mistakes							
11	Leaves words unfinished when writing							
12	Mixes letter sizes when writing							
13	Has handwriting difficulties or dysgraphia (see this checklist if necessary)							
	Conditions which may cause written expression deficits without true LD:							
14	Has expressive language symptoms or disorder (see this checklist if necessary); written expression LD cannot be diagnosed if expressive language disorder exists							
15	Has visual processing disorder (see this checklist if necessary)							
	Calculate column totals here							

* = Important common item

Record when symptoms began:_____

CDASS Checklist for **Concentration Deficit Disorder (CDD)**

YES_____   NO_____   Unknown or Unclear_____

KEY:
Y = Yes; O = Often; S = Sometimes; R = Rarely; ? = Unknown; N = No; P = In Past Only

Item	Indicator	Y	O	S	R	?	N	P
1	Lacks energy							
2	Moves slowly							
3	Daydreams							
4	Is confused easily							
5	Is spacey/mind seems far away							
6	Has trouble staying alert/awake							
7	Stares							
8	Is less active							
9	Does not seem to understand questions/explanations correctly							
10	Has sleepy presentation							
11	Is indifferent, withdrawn							
12	Appears absorbed in thoughts							
13	Is slow to finish tasks							
14	Lacks drive to start, effort decreases during tasks/activities							
15	Has depression symptoms (see this checklist if necessary)							
16	Has anxiety symptoms (see this checklist if necessary)							
17	Has academic problems							
18	Has social problems (Barkley, 2015)							

KEY:

Y = Yes; O = Often; S = Sometimes; R = Rarely; ? = Unknown; N = No; P = In Past Only

Item	Indicator	Y	O	S	R	?	N	P
19	Has slow processing speed deficits (see this checklist if necessary)							
	Calculate column totals here							

Record when symptoms began:_____

CDASS Checklist for **Nonverbal Learning Disorder**

YES_____   NO_____   Unknown or Unclear_____

KEY:

Y = Yes; O = Often; S = Sometimes; R = Rarely; ? = Unknown; N = No; P = In Past Only

Item	Indicator	Y	O	S	R	?	N	P
	Neuropsychological Difficulties							
1	Has difficulties with multi-step instructions							
2	Is accident prone, clumsy							
3	Has poor fine motor coordination (buttoning, zippers, drawing, playing, tying shoes)							
4	Has poor gross motor coordination (running, throwing, kicking, riding a bike; dislikes/avoids playground or sports)							
5	Has difficulties applying learned information to new situations							
6	Gets lost							
7	Is late							
8	Verbally labels events to understand them							

KEY:

Y = Yes; O = Often; S = Sometimes; R = Rarely; ? = Unknown; N = No; P = In Past Only

Item	Indicator	Y	O	S	R	?	N	P
9	Has visual-spatial problems (Non-Verbal Learning Disabilities, 2001-2) (doing dance moves, telling how far objects are, navigating around, playground activities)							
10	Has excellent vocabulary and verbal expression skills							
11	Has poor abstract reasoning							
12	Pays attention to details but misses "big picture"							
13	Exhibits more concrete/literal thinking							
14	Has anxiety symptoms (especially in adolescence)							
15	Has depression symptoms (especially in adolescence)							
16	Has low self-esteem							
17	Lacks common sense							
18	Has trouble adjusting to/dislikes changes (Tanguay, 1998)							
19	Has strong memory abilities							
20	Is fearful of new situations (Boyse, 2012)							
21	Rote linguistic skills are normal (repetition, fluency, naming) but poor social language use							
22	Has sensory processing deficits (see these checklists if necessary)							
23	Has sloppy, poor handwriting or dysgraphia (see this checklist if necessary)							
24	Has poorly modulated affect							

KEY:
Y = Yes; O = Often; S = Sometimes; R = Rarely; ? = Unknown; N = No; P = In Past Only

Item	Indicator	Y	O	S	R	?	N	P
25	Exhibits unusual/strange thinking							
26	Has rituals or routines (may be rigid about these)							
27	Does stereotypic behaviors (purpose-less, repetitive actions like head banging, nail biting, hand waving)							
28	Has perfectionism							
29	Has rigid thinking (Dinklage, n.d.)							
30	Has poor frustration tolerance							
31	Exhibits tantrums							
32	Becomes emotionally overwhelmed							
33	Has dyspraxia symptoms (see this checklist if necessary)							
	Academic Difficulties							
34	Was early reader							
35	Had early reading difficulties							
36	Has reading comprehension difficul-ties (these may begin later, in upper elementary grades) (Tanguay, 1998); may have good reading decoding and spelling skills							
37	Has disorganized/lesser content when writing paragraphs, often despite good grammar/vocabulary							
38	Has academic difficulties							
39	Math is first problematic subject							
40	Math facts are memorized but strug-gles with word math problems (Dinklage, n.d.)							

KEY:

Y = Yes; O = Often; S = Sometimes; R = Rarely; ? = Unknown; N = No; P = In Past Only

Item	Indicator	Y	O	S	R	?	N	P
41	Dislikes or has difficulties with art/art projects							
	Social Difficulties							
42	* Lacks basic social skills							
43	Withdrawals from others (Tanguay, 1998)							
44	Asks excessive questions							
45	Has difficulties with nonverbal communication (reading body language, facial expressions, tone/volume of voice) (Non-Verbal Learning Disabilities, 2001-2)							
46	* Has relational difficulties with peers							
47	Prefers to play with much older/younger children							
48	Stands too close to others							
49	Stares inappropriately							
50	Makes poor eye contact							
51	Is oblivious to others' reactions							
52	Interacts better with adults							
53	Affect does not match their speech							
54	Lacks empathy (Dinklage, n.d.)							
55	Has trouble making/maintaining friendships							
56	Lacks a sense of humor							
57	Seems immature/naive for age							
	Calculate column totals here							

* = Important common item

Record when symptoms began:_____

_____

CDASS Checklist for **Slow Processing Speed and Deficits**

YES_____ NO_____ Unknown or Unclear_____

KEY:

Y = Yes; O = Often; S = Sometimes; R = Rarely; ? = Unknown; N = No; P = In Past Only

Item	Indicator	Y	O	S	R	?	N	P
1	Moves/reacts slower than most others							
2	Thinks less quickly							
3	Has memory difficulties, trouble recalling words/facts							
4	Once started, takes longer to complete tasks (homework, writing assignments, tests, chores, bathroom activities)							
5	Has trouble/delays initiating tasks							
6	Has difficulties completing tasks							
7	Has social problems							
8	Had motor delays as younger child							
9	Had language delays as younger child							
10	Has trouble maintaining conversations							
11	Is slower responding to others or in interpersonal interactions							
12	Reads slowly							
13	Struggles with longer reading tasks							
14	Is slow to wake and get ready in morning							
15	Has difficulties going to bed							
16	Obtains lower grades, academic underachiever							
17	Has difficulties following directions							
18	Seems confused (Braaten & Wolloughby, 2014)							

KEY:

Y = Yes; O = Often; S = Sometimes; R = Rarely; ? = Unknown; N = No; P = In Past Only

Item	Indicator	Y	O	S	R	?	N	P
	Potential sources of processing speed deficits (see these checklists if necessary):							
19	Has concentration deficit disorder							
20	Has combined or inattentive ADHD							
21	Has reading learning disorder							
22	Has math learning disorder							
23	Has expressive language learning disorder							
24	Has non-verbal learning disorder							
25	Has autism spectrum disorder							
26	Has anxiety disorder							
27	Has depressive disorder							
28	Has experienced psychological trauma							
29	Has psychological stressors (Braaten & Wolloughby, 2014)							
30	Has sensory processing or sensory based motor disorder							
31	Had fetal substance exposure							
	Calculate column totals here							

Record when symptoms began:_____

CDASS Checklist for **Dysgraphia**

YES_____   NO_____   Unknown or Unclear_____

KEY:

Y = Yes; O = Often; S = Sometimes; R = Rarely; ? = Unknown; N = No; P = In Past Only

Item	Indicator	Y	O	S	R	?	N	P
1	* *Basic screening question for hand-writing difficulties:* Has concerning handwriting problems; writing is significantly messy, sloppy, hard to read							
2	Avoids/dislikes writing or writing assignments							
3	Does not form letters correctly							
4	Has unstable/unusual pencil grip							
5	Has excessively tight pencil grip							
6	Has trouble writing within spaces or staying on lines							
7	Is inaccurate in copying letters/words							
8	Spells inconsistently							
9	Writes slowly, takes excessive time for writing assignments							
10	Makes frequent mistakes when writing							
11	Mixes letter shapes/sizes							
12	Has poor spelling							
13	Forgets what they wanted to write (Somers, n.d.)							
14	Has poor fine motor coordination problems (buttoning, using zipper, drawing, playing with Legos)							
15	Has poor gross motor skills (jumping, throwing, catching, running, biking)							

KEY:
Y = Yes; O = Often; S = Sometimes; R = Rarely; ? = Unknown; N = No; P = In Past Only

Item	Indicator	Y	O	S	R	?	N	P
16	Teacher reports poor handwriting							
17	Has dyspraxia symptoms (see this checklist if necessary)							
18	Has visual processing deficits (see this checklist if necessary)							
19	Has immature STNR symptoms (see this checklist if necessary)							
	Calculate column totals here							

* = Important common item

Record when symptoms began:_____

CDASS Checklist for **Speech and Articulation Deficits**

YES_____   NO_____   Unknown or Unclear_____

KEY:
Y = Yes; O = Often; S = Sometimes; R = Rarely; ? = Unknown; N = No; P = In Past Only

Item	Indicator	Y	O	S	R	?	N	P
1	* Has lack of clarity in speech							
2	* Speech is difficult to understand							
3	* Has pronunciation or articulation problems							
4	Parents/others ask child to repeat themselves because difficult to understand							
5	Clinician notices speech deficits with child							
6	Mumbles							
7	Has lisp							

KEY:

Y = Yes; O = Often; S = Sometimes; R = Rarely; ? = Unknown; N = No; P = In Past Only

Item	Indicator	Y	O	S	R	?	N	P
8	Stutters							
9	Voice is raspy or hoarse							
10	Pitch of voice changes while speaking							
11	Has hypernasal quality to speech							
12	Has robotic or monotone vocal quality							
13	Speaks too quietly							
14	Speaks too loudly							
15	Speaks too quickly							
16	Speaks too slowly							
17	Is embarrassed about their speech							
18	Avoids speaking							
19	Struggles to use lips, mouth, jaw to produce intelligible speech (may indicate verbal/speech apraxia)							
20	Substitutes one sound for another, such as "w" or "r"							
21	Has consistent pattern of pronunciation errors (such as words with "st" or "sp" are spoken without the "s" so "state" is said as "tate")							
22	Family history of language or speech deficits							
23	Has expressive language deficits (see this checklist if necessary)							
	Calculate column totals here							

* = Important common item

Record when symptoms began:_____

From *Evaluating ADHD in Children and Adolescents: A Comprehensive Diagnostic Screening System* by Gene Carroccia, 2020, from Charles C Thomas, Publisher, Ltd. Permission to photocopy this form is granted to the purchaser of this book for personal use only.

CDASS Checklist for **Expressive Language Disorder**

YES_____   NO_____   Unknown or Unclear_____

KEY:

Y = Yes; O = Often; S = Sometimes; R = Rarely; ? = Unknown; N = No; P = In Past Only

Item	Indicator	Y	O	S	R	?	N	P
1	* Has difficulties clearly expressing what they wish to say							
2	Has limited production of words, speaks less than others							
3	Has limited vocabulary							
4	Has problems learning new words							
5	Has word-find/word retrieval difficulties, struggles to find or say words							
6	Makes inaccurate word substitutions, misnames "chair" for "bed"							
7	Omits essential parts of sentences when speaking							
8	Had slower language development, spoke later than others (PsychCentral, 2010)							
9	Has difficulties with writing abilities and tasks, poor written skills							
10	Dislikes reading out loud							
11	Has difficulties answering questions accurately							
12	Makes grammatical mistakes							
13	Uses standard simple phrases							
14	Speaks in basic, shorter, or immature sentences below their age							
15	Struggles to start/maintain a conversation							

KEY:
Y = Yes; O = Often; S = Sometimes; R = Rarely; ? = Unknown; N = No; P = In Past Only

Item	Indicator	Y	O	S	R	?	N	P
16	Is socially reluctant, reserved, shy							
17	Has few or no friends							
18	Has social problems							
19	Points to things, relies on non-verbal gestures, smiles to avoid talking							
20	Family history of language and/or speech deficits							
21	Had injuries, illnesses, or other factors that impacted hearing and auditory processing within the first three years (Bellis, 2002)							
22	Has deficit spelling skills							
23	Has trouble describing/discussing events, experiences, telling stories							
24	Has delays in responses when spoken to							
25	Verbally responds in odd/inappropriate ways							
26	Has reading deficits							
	Calculate column totals here							

* = Important common item

Record when symptoms began:_____

CDASS Checklist for **Tourette's Disorder and Tic Disorders**

YES_____   NO_____   Unknown or Unclear_____

KEY:
Y = Yes; O = Often; S = Sometimes; R = Rarely; ? = Unknown; N = No; P = In Past Only

Item	Indicator	Y	O	S	R	?	N	P
1	Makes repeated and uncontrollable sudden bodily movements (blinking, squinting, sniffing, shoulder shrugging, arm jerking)							
2	Has repeated and uncontrollable twitches							
3	Makes repeated and uncontrollable vocal sounds (humming, clearing the throat, yelling words or phrases)							
4	Makes repeated and uncontrollable movements involving several different body parts, possibly in a pattern (head bobbing while jerking arm and jumping) (Centers for Disease Control and Prevention, 2014)							
5	Symptoms began suddenly or became worse up to 6 months after a streptococcal infection (strep throat or scarlet fever), often with other symptoms including mood fluctuations, severe anxiety, irritability, ODD, regressive behaviors, academic decline, sensory problems, restrictive eating, sleep or bedwetting difficulties; called Pediatric Autoimmune Neuropsychiatric Disorders Associated with Streptococcal Infections or PANDAS (PANDAS Network, 2017)							
	Calculate column totals here							

Record when symptoms began:_____

CDASS Checklist for **Giftedness**

YES_____   NO_____   Unknown or Unclear_____

KEY:
Y = Yes; O = Often; S = Sometimes; R = Rarely; ? = Unknown; N = No; P = In Past Only

Item	Indicator	Y	O	S	R	?	N	P
1	Has unusual ideas							
2	Has advanced vocabulary for age							
3	Speaks like adult							
4	Asks unusual/complex questions							
5	Is highly observant							
6	Identifies complex patterns/relationships							
7	Has excellent memory							
8	Learned numbers/letters before others							
9	Read before taught in school							
10	Is strong-willed							
11	Is impatient with themselves							
12	Is impatient/frustrated with others, particularly if others don't understand their ideas							
13	Is perfectionistic							
14	Exhibits talent/s in specific area (science, math, art, music, writing, drama) (National Association for Gifted Children and Supporting Emotional Needs of the Gifted, 2007)							
15	Is curious							
16	Becomes physically/mentally involved with projects/discussions							
17	Elaborates/discusses things in detail							

KEY:

Y = Yes; O = Often; S = Sometimes; R = Rarely; ? = Unknown; N = No; P = In Past Only

Item	Indicator	Y	O	S	R	?	N	P
18	Is advanced, beyond the class							
19	Has strong feelings/opinions							
20	Masters concepts quickly							
21	Prefers adults to children their age							
22	Draws inferences quickly							
23	Initiates projects							
24	Is intense with others							
25	Is creative							
26	Is insightful							
27	Enjoys learning							
28	Loves complexity							
29	Is keen observer							
30	Is highly self-critical (Tennessee Association for the Gifted, n.d.)							
31	Complains schoolwork is too easy/boring							
	Calculate column totals here							

Record when symptoms began:_____

_____ **Has Intellectual Disability:** *Print YES, NO, OR Unknown/Unclear on line. There is no checklist for this item.*

CDASS Checklist for **Autism Spectrum Disorder–Level 1** **(formerly Asperger's Syndrome)**

YES_____   NO_____   Unknown or Unclear_____

KEY:
Y = Yes; O = Often; S = Sometimes; R = Rarely; ? = Unknown; N = No; P = In Past Only

Item	Indicator	Y	O	S	R	?	N	P
	Difficulties with Communication and Social Skills {this section also contains social (pragmatic) communication disorder symptoms}							
1	Lacks empathy							
2	Does not understand jokes, sarcasm, metaphors							
3	Only uses literal language (does not use metaphors, humor, sarcasm)							
4	Has difficulties with flow and turn-taking in conversations							
5	Speech has flat tone; lacks tone, pitch or accent							
6	Has formal style of speaking that seems advanced for age							
7	Talks excessively/one-sided conversations about favorite subjects							
8	Internal thoughts are verbalized							
9	Does not make eye contact							
10	Stares at others							
11	Has difficulties interacting with others							
12	Is awkward in social situations							
13	Has difficulties initiating/maintaining conversations							

KEY:
Y = Yes; O = Often; S = Sometimes; R = Rarely; ? = Unknown; N = No; P = In Past Only

Item	Indicator	Y	O	S	R	?	N	P
14	Has difficulties adjusting conversational styles with peers and adults, and at different settings							
15	Has difficulties perceiving or understanding body language, non-verbal cues, facial expressions or gestures							
16	Has difficulties making/maintaining friendships							
17	Does not seek out others to share interests/achievements							
18	Does not seem to enjoy being with others							
	Eccentric or Repetitive Behaviors							
19	Makes odd/repetitive movements (hand flapping or motions, finger twisting)							
20	Has odd/repetitive speech							
21	Has unusual facial expressions/bodily postures							
	Rituals, Routines, and Limited but Intense Interests							
22	Exhibits rituals; may be rigid about these or refuse to alter							
23	Has intense, obsessive, or unusual interests in one/few areas (dinosaurs, weather, maps, specific movies, objects)							
24	Has limited activities/interests							
25	Is exceptionally talented/skilled in particular area (such as music, math)							

KEY:

Y = Yes; O = Often; S = Sometimes; R = Rarely; ? = Unknown; N = No; P = In Past Only

Item	Indicator	Y	O	S	R	?	N	P
	Coordination Difficulties							
26	Had delayed motor development							
27	Has difficulties with fine motor skills (utensils, pencils, zippers)							
28	Has difficulties with gross motor skills (sports, bike riding, use of balls)							
29	Has poor handwriting							
30	Makes awkward/clumsy movements							
31	Walk appears stilted, bouncy, unusual							
32	Has dyspraxia symptoms (see this checklist if necessary)							
	Sensory Processing Deficits							
33	Has sensory processing deficits (see these checklists if necessary)							
	Calculate column totals here							

Record when symptoms began:_____

SENSORY PROCESSING AND MOTOR DISORDERS CHECKLISTS

The references for these checklists are listed in the References section of Chapter 7.

CDASS Checklist for **Auditory Processing Disorder**

YES_____   NO_____   Unknown or Unclear_____

KEY:
Y = Yes; O = Often; S = Sometimes; R = Rarely; ? = Unknown; N = No; P = In Past Only

Item	Indicator	Y	O	S	R	?	N	P
	Common Auditory Processing Symptoms							
1	* Has hearing difficulties despite normal hearing tests							
2	Refuses/reluctant to participate in classroom							
3	Makes off-topic/unrelated comments							
4	Has poor singing or musical skills							
5	Has social difficulties (poor communication, struggles with friends, withdraws)							
6	Is easily frustrated							
7	Has poor problem-solving abilities (Bellis, 2002)							
8	* Inconsistently responds when spoken to							
9	* Struggles to follow verbal directions/instructions							
10	Is slow to respond when spoken to							
11	Asks others to repeat themselves; says "huh?," "what?"							
12	* Struggles with conversations							
13	Is easily distracted by sounds							
14	* Has trouble recalling verbally presented information or instructions, auditory memory deficits							

KEY:

Y = Yes; O = Often; S = Sometimes; R = Rarely; ? = Unknown; N = No; P = In Past Only

Item	Indicator	Y	O	S	R	?	N	P
15	Has reading and spelling problems							
16	Has written expression difficulties							
17	Needs visual cues during conversations, watches faces excessively							
18	Struggles locating source of sounds							
19	Has history of chronic middle ear infections (more than 5 or 6)							
20	Has history of chronic colds and/or sinus problems							
21	Has lower self-esteem (Johnson, Benson, & Seaton, 1997)							
22	Has significant trouble hearing with background noise							
23	Is sensitive to noises							
24	Has poor listening skills							
25	* Misunderstands others							
26	Has improved focusing in quiet environments							
27	"Runs" words together							
28	Drops end of words (Scherer, 2004)							
29	Has problems discriminating between similar sounding words ("cat" & "cap," "bag" & "bad")							
	Difficulty Modulating Auditory Sensations/Auditory Over-Responders (Auditory Defensiveness)							
30	Asks others to be quiet							

KEY:

Y = Yes; O = Often; S = Sometimes; R = Rarely; ? = Unknown; N = No; P = In Past Only

Item	Indicator	Y	O	S	R	?	N	P
31	Is upset by environmental sounds (outdoor equipment, machines) ("Sensory Processing Disorder Checklist: Signs and Symptoms of Dysfunction," n.d.)							
32	Dislikes louder noises, covers ears (alarms, music, TV)							
33	Dislikes noisy environments (restaurants, crowds, stores)							
34	Reacts to sounds others don't hear							
35	Has excessive reactions to specific sounds (appliances, vacuums, phones, certain voices) (Biel & Peske, 2009)							
	Auditory Under-Responders and Auditory Sensory Seeking (When Hearing is Adequate)							
36	Desires music/sounds excessively loud							
37	Gets too close to speakers/sounds							
38	Does not respond when called (Kranowitz, 2016)							
39	Asks others to speak louder							
40	Makes loud noises							
41	Dislikes softer, quiet sounds (Biel & Peske, 2009)							
	Auditory Discrimination Deficits							
42	Has difficulties recognizing certain sounds							
43	Has difficulties tracking sounds (Kranowitz, 2005)							

KEY:
Y = Yes; O = Often; S = Sometimes; R = Rarely; ? = Unknown; N = No; P = In Past Only

Item	Indicator	Y	O	S	R	?	N	P
	Other Possible Coexisting Items							
44	Has expressive language deficits (see this checklist if necessary)							
45	Has speech and articulation deficits (see this checklist if necessary)							
	Calculate column totals here							

* = Important common item

Record when symptoms began:_____

CDASS Checklist for **Visual Processing Disorder**

YES_____   NO_____   Unknown or Unclear_____

KEY:
Y = Yes; O = Often; S = Sometimes; R = Rarely; ? = Unknown; N = No; P = In Past Only

Item	Indicator	Y	O	S	R	?	N	P
	For items 1 to 8, ask child/teen and parent/s *"During or after reading or electronic screen use, do you experience:"*							
1	Dizziness							
2	Blurry/fuzzy words							
3	Double vision							
4	Headaches							
5	Words that seem too close together on page/screen							
6	Words that move/vibrate							
7	Eye strain or discomfort							
8	Rubbing your eyes (Kranowitz, 2005)							

KEY:
Y = Yes; O = Often; S = Sometimes; R = Rarely; ? = Unknown; N = No; P = In Past Only

Item	Indicator	Y	O	S	R	?	N	P
	Common Visual Processing Symptoms							
9	Is fatigued during reading, academics, sports							
10	Has difficulties with size/spacing of letters/words							
11	Uses fingers during reading							
12	Has poor visual memory							
13	Has short attention span when reading/copying							
14	Moves head instead of eyes when reading							
15	Has dysgraphia (see this checklist if necessary)							
16	Is excessively slow reading/completing assignments (Kranowitz, 2005)							
17	Has visual analysis problems (struggles with mazes, puzzles, seek-find pictures)							
18	Has difficulties finding/locating objects (items in closets/drawers) (Biel & Peske, 2009)							
19	Is easily distracted by visual information							
20	Confuses or misunderstands letters/number/symbols							
21	Has difficulties with depth perception, judging distances (places objects too close to edge, bumps into things)							
22	Has difficulties with fluid movements (knocks over things, clumsy)							

KEY:
Y = Yes; O = Often; S = Sometimes; R = Rarely; ? = Unknown; N = No; P = In Past Only

Item	Indicator	Y	O	S	R	?	N	P
23	Struggles to write on lines/within margins							
24	Reads inaccurately, reading/homework difficulties							
25	Has difficulties recalling directions to locations							
26	Has trouble finding things on page (numbers, phrases)							
27	Struggles with identifying information from maps, charts, pictures (National Center for Learning Disabilities, 2003b)							
28	For teens: has driving difficulties, car accidents (Kranowitz, 2016)							
	Visual Over-Responder							
30	Squints (Kranowitz, 2005)							
31	Dislikes/avoids bright lights, sunshine; prefers dim lights and darkness							
32	Is sensitive to florescent lights							
33	Dislikes visually busy settings (stores) (Biel & Peske, 2009)							
34	Dislikes electronic screen activities							
	Visual Under-Responder or Sensory-Seeking							
35	Enjoys watching visual activities (doors opening, cars)							
36	Reacts slowly to gestures or things thrown at them (Kranowitz, 2016)							
37	Seeks moving, shiny, or spinning objects							

KEY:
Y = Yes; O = Often; S = Sometimes; R = Rarely; ? = Unknown; N = No; P = In Past Only

Item	Indicator	Y	O	S	R	?	N	P
38	Craves intense visual experiences (active movies, videogames)							
39	Prefers bright lights, dislikes dim lights (Biel & Peske, 2009)							
	Poor Visual Motor Skills							
40	Has poor fine/gross motor abilities							
41	Has poor eye-hand/eye-foot coordination							
42	Has difficulties with sports/rhythmic movements (Kranowitz, 2005)							
	Seven Main Components of Visual Processing							
43	*Visual Discrimination Deficits:*							
a	Has difficulties searching for things (in refrigerators, drawers, closets) (Kranowitz, 2016)							
b	Has difficulties recognizing similarities/differences between shapes, letters, objects, colors, patterns (National Center forLearning Disabilities, 2003a)							
44	*Visual Figure-Ground Discrimination Deficits:*							
a	Has difficulties finding specific information on printed pages							
b	Has trouble seeing image within a background (National Center for Learning Disabilities, 2003a)							
45	*Visual Sequencing Deficits:*							
a	Has difficulties seeing/distinguishing the order of words, symbols, images							

KEY:

Y = Yes; O = Often; S = Sometimes; R = Rarely; ? = Unknown; N = No; P = In Past Only

Item	Indicator	Y	O	S	R	?	N	P
b	Has difficulties staying in correct place while reading							
c	Skips words, lines, paragraphs while reading							
d	Re-reads lines							
e	Misreads similar letters, words, numbers (like hat and mat)							
f	Reverses letters, words, numbers for children older than age 7 (m for w; 41 read as 14) (National Center for Learning Disabilities, 2003a)							
46	*Visual Motor Processing Deficits:*							
a	Has difficulties using eyes to coordinate movements with other body parts (writing within the lines, copying from a book, sports)							
b	Bumps into things, clumsy							
c	Struggles with sports, physical activities (National Center for Learning Disabilities, 2003a)							
47	*Visual Short-Term and Long-Term Memory Deficits:*							
a	Has difficulties with reading comprehension							
b	Struggles to recall things learned visually							
c	Has trouble using a keyboard/calculator with accuracy/speed							
d	Has difficulties recalling familiar words with irregular spellings (National Center for Learning Disabilities, 2003a)							

KEY:
Y = Yes; O = Often; S = Sometimes; R = Rarely; ? = Unknown; N = No; P = In Past Only

Item	Indicator	Y	O	S	R	?	N	P
48	*Visual Closure Deficits:*							
a	Has difficulties knowing what an object is when only some parts are visible							
b	Is unable to identify a word when letter is missing (National Center for Learning Disabilities, 2003a)							
49	*Spatial Relationships Deficits:*							
a	Has difficulties getting from/to places							
b	Has trouble spacing words/letters on paper							
c	Has problems telling time with non-digital clocks							
d	Has difficulties reading maps, charts, graphs (National Center for Learning Disabilities, 2003a)							
	Calculate column totals here							

Record when symptoms began:_____

CDASS Checklist for **Tactile and Gustatory Processing Disorders**

YES_____   NO_____   Unknown or Unclear_____

KEY:
Y = Yes; O = Often; S = Sometimes; R = Rarely; ? = Unknown; N = No; P = In Past Only

Item	Indicator	Y	O	S	R	?	N	P
	Tactile and Gustatory Over-Responders (Tactile Defensiveness)							
1	Prefers long sleeves/pants to avoid air on skin							

KEY:
Y = Yes; O = Often; S = Sometimes; R = Rarely; ? = Unknown; N = No; P = In Past Only

Item	Indicator	Y	O	S	R	?	N	P
2	Is a fussy eater, prefers mushy/soft foods							
3	Dislikes hair brushing/hats							
4	Is uncomfortable with kisses/physical affection (Kranowitz, 2016)							
5	Is overly sensitive to touch							
6	Is irritated with clothing/fabrics on skin (National Center for Learning Disabilities Editorial Team, n.d.b)							
7	Avoids being close to others/groups due to fear of touch							
8	Becomes nervous/angry when touched							
9	Dislikes stiff/new clothes, rough/certain textures or clothes							
10	Becomes upset by certain clothes on skin							
11	Wants to wear t-shirts/shorts all year							
12	Dislikes fingernails cut/hair cuts							
13	Fears/dislikes dental visits							
14	Resistant to eating new foods ("Sensory Processing Disorder Checklist: Signs and Symptoms of Dysfunction," n.d.)							
15	Dislikes washing/showers							
16	Dislikes teeth brushing							
17	Is particular about clothing/shoes							
18	Is uncomfortable walking barefoot							
19	Avoids becoming messy							
20	Experiences pain more than others							

KEY:
Y = Yes; O = Often; S = Sometimes; R = Rarely; ? = Unknown; N = No; P = In Past Only

Item	Indicator	Y	O	S	R	?	N	P
21	Is sensitive to temperatures (Biel & Peske, 2009)							
	Tactile and Gustatory Under-Responders							
22	Is unaware if clothes fall down/twist							
23	Is not affected by bruises, cuts, pain, injuries							
24	Is unaffected by cold/hot temperatures							
25	Is unaffected by cold/hot weather (Kranowitz, 2016)							
26	Craves crispy/crunchy foods							
27	Enjoys intense vibrations							
28	Requires intensive touch to register sensations (Biel & Peske, 2009)							
29	Desires intense flavored foods							
30	Chews/licks objects ("Sensory Processing Disorder Checklist: Signs and Symptoms of Dysfunction," n.d.)							
	Tactile and Gustatory Sensory Seeker							
31	Excessively touches people/objects (Kranowitz, 2016)							
32	Seeks very hot/cold temperatures/showers (Kranowitz, 2005)							
33	Seeks physical touches/affection							
34	Craves strong/intense food/beverage flavors, spices, or temperatures							
35	Prefers walking barefoot (Biel & Peske, 2009)							

KEY:
Y = Yes; O = Often; S = Sometimes; R = Rarely; ? = Unknown; N = No; P = In Past Only

Item	Indicator	Y	O	S	R	?	N	P
	Tactile and Gustatory Sensory Discrimination Problems							
36	Has messy hair/face							
37	Is messy dresser, wears clothing incorrectly							
38	Does not notice taste/texture differences in food (sweet, hot, crunchy)							
39	Drops things							
40	Has trouble identifying size, shape, temperatures when holding things (Kranowitz, 2016)							
41	Has poor fine motor abilities							
42	Fears dark ("Sensory Processing Disorder Checklist: Signs and Symptoms of Dysfunction," n.d.)							
	Calculate column totals here							

Record when symptoms began:_____

CDASS Checklist for **Olfactory Processing Disorder**

YES_____   NO_____   Unknown or Unclear_____

KEY:
Y = Yes; O = Often; S = Sometimes; R = Rarely; ? = Unknown; N = No; P = In Past Only

Item	Indicator	Y	O	S	R	?	N	P
	Olfactory Over-Responders (Olfactory Defensiveness)							
1	Is a fussy eater							

KEY:

Y = Yes; O = Often; S = Sometimes; R = Rarely; ? = Unknown; N = No; P = In Past Only

Item	Indicator	Y	O	S	R	?	N	P
2	Is excessively sensitive to specific odors (body odors, perfume, cleaning products) (Kranowitz, 2016)							
3	Complains of food smells							
4	Becomes upset by smells others don't notice ("Sensory Processing Disorder Checklist: Signs and Symptoms of Dysfunction," n.d.)							
5	Is overly sensitive to specific foods, kitchen, garbage smells							
6	Eats small range of foods							
7	Becomes nauseous/gags easily							
8	Holds nose closed (Biel & Peske, 2009)							
	Olfactory Under-Responders							
9	Is unaware of unpleasant odors							
10	Is unable to smell food/odors (Kranowitz, 2005)							
	Olfactory Sensory-Seekers							
11	Excessively smells objects, food, people (Kranowitz, 2016)							
12	Craves strong/intense smells (Beil & Peske, 2009)							
	Olfactory Sensory Discrimination Problems							
13	Cannot distinguish specific scents (soap, oranges, vinegar) (Kranowitz, 2005)							
	Calculate column totals here							

Record when symptoms began:_____

CDASS Checklist for **Vestibular Processing Disorder**

YES_____   NO_____   Unknown or Unclear_____

KEY:
Y = Yes; O = Often; S = Sometimes; R = Rarely; ? = Unknown; N = No; P = In Past Only

Item	Indicator	Y	O	S	R	?	N	P
1	Has poor coordination (Kranowitz, 2016)							
2	Has history of repeated ear infections							
	Vestibular Over-Responder/ Intolerance for Movement (Vestibular Defensive)							
3	Is uncomfortable with elevators, rocking chairs, boats, airplanes (Kranowitz, 2016)							
4	Moves too carefully/slowly							
5	Fears/avoids heights							
6	Dislikes using stairs							
7	Loses balance quickly (trouble riding bikes)							
8	Does not like/avoids playground activities (slides, ladders, swings) ("Sensory Processing Disorder Checklist: Signs and Symptoms of Dysfunction," n.d.)							
9	Dislikes spinning/fast movements							
10	Becomes nauseous/dizzy in cars, rides (Biel & Peske, 2009)							
11	Is fearful of falling during normal activities/play							
12	Prefers activities with lesser movement							
13	Has social problems							

KEY:
Y = Yes; O = Often; S = Sometimes; R = Rarely; ? = Unknown; N = No; P = In Past Only

Item	Indicator	Y	O	S	R	?	N	P
14	Has difficulties with group activities							
15	Is aggressive/explosive/hostile during movement/playground activities							
16	When overstimulated becomes anxious, clingy, withdrawn, rigid (Hanft, Miller, & Lane, 2000)							
	Gravitational Insecurity							
17	Dislikes bending over for shoes, car travel, turning body around (Kranowitz, 2016)							
18	Prefers to sit/lay near ground							
19	Avoids physical activities							
20	Becomes upset when moved							
21	Dislikes feet leaving the ground							
22	Avoids/dislikes playground activities							
23	Is afraid of stairs, heights, falling (Biel & Peske, 2009)							
	Vestibular Sensory Disregarder with Under-Responsiveness							
24	Does not notice/extend hand when falling (Kranowitz, 2016)							
25	Does not notice when moved							
26	Lacks desire to move							
27	Has unusually low activity levels (Kranowitz, 2005)							
	Vestibular Sensory-Seeking Child with Increased Tolerance/ Hyposensitivity to Movement							

KEY:

Y = Yes; O = Often; S = Sometimes; R = Rarely; ? = Unknown; N = No; P = In Past Only

Item	Indicator	Y	O	S	R	?	N	P
28	Craves intense, high action activities (skateboarding, bikes, swings, spinning, rides)							
29	Prefers to be in motion/difficulties being still (Kranowitz, 2016)							
30	Loves movements/activities when feet leave the ground							
31	Is fearless of falling, heights, movements (Biel & Peske, 2009)							
32	Jumps on things							
33	Enjoys upside down positions							
34	Prefers to hop, jump run instead of walk							
	Calculate column totals here							

Record when symptoms began:_____

CDASS Checklist for **Proprioceptive Sensory Processing Disorder**

YES_____   NO_____   Unknown or Unclear_____

KEY:

Y = Yes; O = Often; S = Sometimes; R = Rarely; ? = Unknown; N = No; P = In Past Only

Item	Indicator	Y	O	S	R	?	N	P
	Proprioceptive Over-Responders							
1	Is inactive (Kranowitz, 2005)							
2	Avoids/dislikes sports, playgrounds, intense movements (Biel & Peske, 2009)							

KEY:
Y = Yes; O = Often; S = Sometimes; R = Rarely; ? = Unknown; N = No; P = In Past Only

Item	Indicator	Y	O	S	R	?	N	P
	Proprioceptive Under-Responders							
3	Sits in "W" position on floor with knees close, feet out							
4	When walking, slaps feet on ground (Kranowitz, 2016)							
5	Lacks motivation to play/move							
6	Is clumsy							
7	Sits in uncomfortable positions							
8	Has low muscle/body tone							
9	Holds elbow to ribs when writing							
10	Knees are close together when standing (Kranowitz, 2005)							
	Proprioceptive Sensory Seeking							
11	Chews on objects, pens, fingernails, hair							
12	Enjoys intense hugs							
13	Crashes/bumping into people, things (Kranowitz, 2016)							
14	Stomps feet while walking							
15	Kicks chairs/floor when seated							
16	Desires very tight clothing (shirts, pants, shoelaces, belts)							
17	Is excessively rough/aggressive with peers							
18	Bites/sucks objects							
19	Jumps excessively							

KEY:
Y = Yes; O = Often; S = Sometimes; R = Rarely; ? = Unknown; N = No; P = In Past Only

Item	Indicator	Y	O	S	R	?	N	P
20	Enjoys being wrapped tightly ("Sensory Processing Disorder Checklist: Signs and Symptoms of Dysfunction," n.d.)							
21	Bangs head							
22	Rub hands on tables							
23	Has unusually high activity levels							
24	Has social problems (Kranowitz, 2005)							
25	Enjoys risky play (climbing, jumping from heights) (Biel & Peske, 2009)							
26	Stands too close to others, poor boundaries							
	Other Signs of Proprioceptive Dysfunction							
28	Has difficulties dressing due to coordination deficits (Kranowitz, 2016)							
29	Uses too little effort/force/pressure for activities/tasks (writes too lightly, trouble with buttons)							
30	Uses too much effort/force/pressure for activities/tasks (writes too hard, breaks things)							
31	Is physically weaker than peers							
32	Looks at feet when moving							
33	Has poor fine motor skills (drawing, buttoning, writing)							
34	Slumps over when reading/doing academic work							
35	Moves stiffly/awkwardly (Beil & Peske, 2009)							

KEY:
Y = Yes; O = Often; S = Sometimes; R = Rarely; ? = Unknown; N = No; P = In Past Only

Item	Indicator	Y	O	S	R	?	N	P
36	Has poor gross motor skills (running, kicking, throwing balls)							
37	Posture seems odd/incorrect							
38	Has vestibular sensory deficits (see this checklist if necessary)							
39	Has tactile sensory deficits (see this checklist if necessary)							
	Calculate column totals here							

Record when symptoms began:_____

CDASS Checklist for **Sensory-Based Motor Disorder–Dyspraxia**

YES_____   NO_____   Unknown or Unclear_____

KEY:
Y = Yes; O = Often; S = Sometimes; R = Rarely; ? = Unknown; N = No; P = In Past Only

Item	Indicator	Y	O	S	R	?	N	P
1	Had extremely low birth weight							
2	Was born prematurely (Gibbs, Appleton, Appleton, 2007)							
3	As young child had difficulties with milestones (sitting, crawling, standing, walking, toilet training)							
4	Has speech or articulation deficits							
5	Has trouble dressing/putting on coats							
6	Has gross motor skills difficulties (walking, jumping, swimming)							
7	Has difficulties using stairs							

KEY:
Y = Yes; O = Often; S = Sometimes; R = Rarely; ? = Unknown; N = No; P = In Past Only

Item	Indicator	Y	O	S	R	?	N	P
8	Takes longer/struggles to learn new skills							
9	Has social problems							
10	Is excessively slow, hesitates							
11	Dislikes playground/sports or physical activities							
12	Takes excessive time to complete writing assignments							
13	Has organizational difficulties							
14	Struggles to recall instructions							
15	Struggles with smooth/coordinated movements, makes awkward motions (Nordqvist, 2007)							
16	Has fine motor skills deficits (buttoning, drawing, using toothbrush)							
17	Has weak/unusual pencil grip							
18	Has difficulties forming letters/ numbers							
19	Has slow/messy handwriting (see dysgraphia checklist)							
20	Has gross motor problems (playing sports, riding a bike)							
21	Struggles with/dislikes grooming activities (teeth/hair brushing)							
22	Is overly sensitive to touch, irritation with clothing on skin							
23	Has difficulties establishing left- and right-hand preference							
24	Demonstrates obsessive/phobic behaviors							

KEY:

Y = Yes; O = Often; S = Sometimes; R = Rarely; ? = Unknown; N = No; P = In Past Only

Item	Indicator	Y	O	S	R	?	N	P
25	Has poor frustration tolerance							
26	Has behavioral problems (National Center for Learning Disabilities Editorial Team, 2012, n.d.b)							
27	Is clumsy, bumps into/drops things, trips							
28	Breaks things, accident prone							
29	Has poor self-esteem							
30	Has anxiety symptoms							
31	Has depression symptoms (National Center for Learning Disabilities Editorial Team, n.d.a)							
32	Is a fussy eater							
33	Has chewing/swallowing difficulties (Kranowitz, 2005)							
34	Has specific preferences about food textures							
35	Avoids/dislikes new foods (Biel & Peske, 2009)							
36	Is a sloppy eater							
37	Has messy appearance							
38	Has sensory seeking symptoms (see these checklists)							
39	Has postural disorder symptoms (Miller, 2007) (see this checklist if necessary)							
40	Has trouble with balance							
41	Has difficulties with tasks requiring multiple steps (chores, grooming, dressing)							

KEY:
Y = Yes; O = Often; S = Sometimes; R = Rarely; ? = Unknown; N = No; P = In Past Only

Item	Indicator	Y	O	S	R	?	N	P
42	Has immature symmetric tonic neck reflex (STNR) symptoms (see this checklist if necessary)							
	Calculate column totals here							

Record when symptoms began:_____

CDASS Checklist for **Sensory-Based Motor Disorder–Postural Disorder**

YES_____   NO_____   Unknown or Unclear_____

KEY:
Y = Yes; O = Often; S = Sometimes; R = Rarely; ? = Unknown; N = No; P = In Past Only

Item	Indicator	Y	O	S	R	?	N	P
1	Is clumsy							
2	Has poor coordination							
3	Has poor gross motor skills (kicking, using balls, swimming)							
4	Desires to be inactive, low activity levels							
5	Has difficulties sitting/remaining upright (Kranowitz, 2016)							
6	Moves awkwardly							
7	Sits on edge of chair/one foot on floor for stability							
8	Fidgets							
9	Has poor/unusual posture							
10	Has poor fine motor skills							

KEY:
Y = Yes; O = Often; S = Sometimes; R = Rarely; ? = Unknown; N = No; P = In Past Only

Item	Indicator	Y	O	S	R	?	N	P
11	Has difficulties turning doorknobs/handles							
12	Has loose grasp on pencils/cutlery							
13	Has overly tight grasp on objects							
14	Has difficulties jumping							
15	Did not crawl/crawling difficulties as baby (Kranowitz, 2005)							
16	Becomes easily tired, struggles with endurance							
17	Has balance problems							
18	Has difficulties climbing							
19	Falls easily							
20	Has lesser muscle/body tone							
21	Has limp/weak appearance							
22	Slumps/leans when sitting/writing at table/desk							
23	Is slow with/dislikes physical tasks/activities							
24	Has dyspraxia symptoms (see this checklist if necessary)							
25	Has visual-motor difficulties (hitting balls, copying information from board) (Miller, 2007) (see this checklist if necessary)							
26	Struggles with gym classes, play-ground activities							
	Calculate column totals here							

Record when symptoms began:_____

CDASS Checklist for **Immature Symmetric Tonic Neck Reflex**

YES_____   NO_____   Unknown or Unclear_____

KEY:
Y = Yes; O = Often; S = Sometimes; R = Rarely; ? = Unknown; N = No; P = In Past Only

Item	Indicator	Y	O	S	R	?	N	P
1	* Did not crawl at all as baby							
2	Crawled for less than 6 months							
3	* Did not crawl properly as baby							
4	* Was in playpens/walkers/braces for lengthy time when young							
5	Walked before age one							
6	* Has difficulties sitting properly at desk with elbows/hips bent at same time							
7	Prefers slouching, slouches when sitting							
8	Prefers sitting on feet							
9	Has difficulties sitting long periods							
10	Has difficulties sitting properly							
11	Wraps feet around chair legs							
12	Changes position frequently							
13	Lies down when reading/writing/watching screens							
14	Reaches outward when sitting, attempts to write with arms extended							
15	Writes/reads with head resting on arms							
16	Stands with one knee/leg on chair							
17	Has difficulties writing							
18	Writes sloppily/illegibly							

KEY:
Y = Yes; O = Often; S = Sometimes; R = Rarely; ? = Unknown; N = No; P = In Past Only

Item	Indicator	Y	O	S	R	?	N	P
19	Writes very large/small							
20	Tries to write standing up							
21	Avoids/dislikes writing							
22	Has difficulties with directions							
23	Confuses left, right							
24	Reverses letters/numbers							
25	Lacks coordination							
26	Is clumsy							
27	Has trouble running							
28	Has difficulties with sports							
29	Struggles with/rushes through home work (O'Dell & Cook, 1997)							
30	Struggles to relax/feel comfortable							
31	Squirms							
32	Difficulties completing academic work (Pederson, 2016)							
	Calculate column totals here							

* = Important common item

Record when symptoms began:_____

PRENATAL SUBSTANCE EXPOSURE CHECKLISTS

The references for these checklists are listed in the References section of Chapter 8.

CDASS Checklist for **Fetal Alcohol Spectrum Disorders**

YES_____   NO_____   Unknown or Unclear_____

KEY:
Y = Yes; O = Often; S = Sometimes; R = Rarely; ? = Unknown; N = No; P = In Past Only

Item	Indicator	Y	O	S	R	?	N	P
	Items about Mothers							
1	* Any maternal report of alcohol use during pregnancy (*add details below*)							
2	* Maternal report of alcohol use during pregnancy and child had significant behavior problems and/or marked developmental delays in the first three years (this suggests FASD)							
3	Mother currently has/had known excessive alcohol use							
4	Mother has other children with FASD							
5	Mother had treatment/s for excessive alcohol use							
6	Mother has history of medical/social/legal problems related to alcohol use (Eme & Millard, 2012)							
	Items About Children and Adolescents							
	Items about Infants							
7	Infant was difficult-to-settle/slow-to-warm temperaments, followed by early-onset ADHD-like symptoms							
8	Infant had self-soothing, irritability, mood difficulties							
9	Infant had state regulation difficulties							
10	Infant had hyperactivity							

KEY:

Y = Yes; O = Often; S = Sometimes; R = Rarely; ? = Unknown; N = No; P = In Past Only

Item	Indicator	Y	O	S	R	?	N	P
11	Infant had hypersensitivity to sensory stimuli (O'Malley & Nanson, 2002)							
12	Infant had sleep/sucking difficulties							
	Partial or Full Fetal Alcohol Syndrome Physical Signs							
13	Has abnormal facial features including absence of the vertical ridge between the nose and upper lip							
14	Has very small/thin upper lips							
15	Has short horizontal openings between the eye lids/lack of normal openings for eyes							
16	Has smaller head size							
17	Has lower body weight							
18	Has below average height							
19	Has vision problems							
20	Has hearing problems							
21	Has heart, kidney, bones difficulties							
	Additional FASD Indicators							
22	Has poor coordination							
23	Has academic difficulties (particularly math)							
24	Has speech problems							
25	Has learning difficulties (particularly learning new material)							
26	Has mathematics learning disorder							
27	Has lower/below average IQ score							
28	Has poor reasoning abilities							

KEY:
Y = Yes; O = Often; S = Sometimes; R = Rarely; ? = Unknown; N = No; P = In Past Only

Item	Indicator	Y	O	S	R	?	N	P
29	Demonstrates poor judgement skills (Centers for Disease Control and Prevention, 2015, April 16)							
30	Has non-verbal learning disorder symptoms (see this checklist if necessary)							
31	Possesses lesser emotional regulation abilities (Eme & Millard, 2012)							
32	Has language difficulties, particularly both expressive and receptive (see expressive language disorder checklist if necessary)							
33	Has lesser daily living skills							
34	Has poor planning, organization abilities							
35	Uses alcohol/substances							
36	Has depression symptoms							
37	Has anxiety symptoms							
38	Is sexually promiscuous							
39	Has sexual behavior problems							
40	Has poor problem-solving skills							
41	Experiences difficulties with change							
42	Is gullible, easily influenced or manipulated							
43	Has difficulties understanding/conforming to social norms (Tao et al., 2013)							
44	Lacks guilt for misbehavior/inappropriate actions							
45	Acts younger/immature							

KEY:

Y = Yes; O = Often; S = Sometimes; R = Rarely; ? = Unknown; N = No; P = In Past Only

Item	*Indicator*	Y	O	S	R	?	N	P
46	Exhibits delinquent behaviors							
47	Shows cruelty to others/animals							
48	Lies							
49	Steals in/outside home (Nash et al., 2006)							
50	Has difficulty interpreting/understanding other's facial reactions, emotions							
51	Has persistent social/relational problems (Alcoholism: Clinical & Experimental Research, 2009)							
52	Had earlier onset of ADHD-like symptoms							
53	Has difficulties with shifting attention							
54	Has working memory deficits							
55	Has atypical stimulant medication response							
56	Has medical conditions							
57	Has developmental conditions							
58	Has diagnostically complex presentation (O'Malley & Nanson, 2002)							
59	Has oppositional defiant symptoms (see checklist if necessary)							
60	Has conduct disorder symptoms (see checklist if necessary)							
61	Is aggressive							
62	Has sleeping problems (see these checklists if necessary)							
63	Has eating problems							

KEY:
Y = Yes; O = Often; S = Sometimes; R = Rarely; ? = Unknown; N = No; P = In Past Only

Item	Indicator	Y	O	S	R	?	N	P
64	Has sensory processing deficits (see these checklists if necessary)							
65	Has fine/gross motor difficulties							
66	Has poor frustration tolerance							
	Calculate column totals here							

* = Important common item

Record when symptoms began:_____

Details about Maternal Alcohol Use:
If there was maternal report of alcohol use during pregnancy, indicate details of use, including amount drank, frequency, and for how long during pregnancy:

_____

_____

_____

CDASS **Prenatal Nicotine Exposure**

YES_____   NO_____   Unknown or Unclear_____

If so, indicate details of use, including amount, frequency, and for how long during pregnancy:

_____

_____

_____

CDASS Checklist for **Prenatal Maternal Use of Illicit Drugs and Abuse of Opioid Prescriptions**

YES_____   NO_____   Unknown or Unclear_____

KEY:

Y = Yes; O = Often; S = Sometimes; R = Rarely; ? = Unknown; N = No; P = In Past Only

Item	Indicator	Y	O	S	R	?	N	P
1	Any maternal report of illicit drug use during pregnancy							
2	Child was found positive for drugs after birth from testing by hospital							
3	Mother currently has or in the past had known illict drug use							
4	Mother has one or more other children that were found to be drug exposed at birth							
5	Mother has history of treatment for drug use							
6	Mother has history of medical/social/legal problems related to drug use (Eme & Millard, 2012)							
7	Had lower birthweight							
	Indicate which drugs were believed to be used prenatally by the mother:							
8	Marijuana							
9	Cocaine							
10	Opioids (heroin and abused opioid medications)							
11	Methamphetamine and Amphetamine							
12	Other Substances							
	Calculate column totals here							

If illicit or prescription drugs were used, indicate details of use, including what drugs were used, amount, frequency, and for how long during pregnancy:

_____

_____

_____

PSYCHOLOGICAL CONDITIONS CHECKLISTS

The references for these checklists are listed in the References section of Chapter 9.

CDASS Checklist for **Anxiety Disorders**

YES_____   NO_____   Unknown or Unclear_____

KEY:
Y = Yes; O = Often; S = Sometimes; R = Rarely; ? = Unknown; N = No; P = In Past Only

Item	Indicator	Y	O	S	R	?	N	P
1	* Exhibits nervous/anxious mood							
2	* Excessively worries							
3	Has more than normal fears for age							
4	Has restlessness							
5	Has tantrums							
6	Has excessively high expectations for self							
7	Has school refusal							
8	Is resistant going to bed							
9	Avoids activities, withdraws							
10	Complains of stomach aches, headaches, bodily discomfort without medical causes (Matheis, 2016)							

KEY:

Y = Yes; O = Often; S = Sometimes; R = Rarely; ? = Unknown; N = No; P = In Past Only

Item	Indicator	Y	O	S	R	?	N	P
11	Has concentration difficulties related to worry/anxiety							
12	Is irritable, cranky, easily upset							
13	Is tired							
14	Has trouble falling to sleep (30 minutes or longer), insomnia							
15	Has difficulties remaining asleep							
16	Experiences poor sleep quality							
17	Has nightmares							
18	Has perfectionism							
19	Lacks confidence, self-doubting, needs reassurance often							
20	Has excessive separation anxiety							
21	Experiences panic attacks/severe anxiety attacks							
22	Family history of significant anxiety							
	Calculate column totals here							

* = Important common item

Record when symptoms began:_____

CDASS Checklist for **Social Anxiety Disorder**

YES_____   NO_____   Unknown or Unclear_____

KEY:
Y = Yes; O = Often; S = Sometimes; R = Rarely; ? = Unknown; N = No; P = In Past Only

Item	Indicator	Y	O	S	R	?	N	P
1	* Has intense fear of situations when they don't know others							
2	* Fears situations where they believe they will be judged							
3	* Worries about being embarrassed/humiliated							
4	Fears others will notice their anxiety							
5	Fears/dreads upcoming events							
6	Has panic attacks triggered by social interactions/situations							
7	Has trembling hands							
8	Blushes							
9	Profusely sweats							
10	Has muscle tension							
11	Has racing heart							
12	Understands fear is out of proportion to situation but cannot control it							
13	Has anxiety when interacting with strangers							
14	Has anxiety during conversations							
15	Has anxiety after making eye contact with others (Cuncic, 2014)							

KEY:
Y = Yes; O = Often; S = Sometimes; R = Rarely; ? = Unknown; N = No; P = In Past Only

Item	Indicator	Y	O	S	R	?	N	P
16	Has excessive, persistent, and concerning social media use (social media anxiety disorder)							
	Calculate column totals here							

* = Important common item

Record when symptoms began:_____

CDASS Checklist for **Obsessive Compulsive Disorder**

YES_____   NO_____   Unknown or Unclear_____

KEY:
Y = Yes; O = Often; S = Sometimes; R = Rarely; ? = Unknown; N = No; P = In Past Only

Item	Indicator	Y	O	S	R	?	N	P
1	Has checking obsessions (repeatedly checks homework, book bags, door locks, injuries)							
2	Has counting obsessions (counts objects/footsteps)							
3	Has symmetry obsessions (repeatedly straightens/orders things for symmetry, repeatedly adjusts clothing, must walk in certain patterns, counts symmetrical things)							
4	Has perfection obsessions (very upset over mistakes, repeatedly writes/erases words)							
5	Has contamination obsessions (avoids contact with people/objects, washes hands/cleaning frequently, frequent bathroom trips, avoids messy things)							

KEY:
Y = Yes; O = Often; S = Sometimes; R = Rarely; ? = Unknown; N = No; P = In Past Only

Item	Indicator	Y	O	S	R	?	N	P
6	Exhibits reassurance seeking obsessions (repeatedly asks obsession-related questions from parents but doubts answers)							
7	Has hoarding/collecting obsessions (cannot throw things away, reluctance to clean room/book bag, saves/collects things, repeatedly talks and thinks about collections)							
8	Has repeating rituals (repeatedly reads things, checks/counts letters and numbers that look a certain way, skips words containing certain letters)							
9	Has scrupulosity/religious obsessions (overfocused on right and wrong/fairness issues, over-focused on religious topics, overconcerned about being good/evil, persistent worries/feels guilty about actions/thoughts, confesses to behaviors not done, excessive focus on injustices)							
10	Has aggression/sexual obsessions (fears will be aggressive or sexual without doing these actions, avoids sharp objects, over-focus on disturbing words/images) ("Checklist of OCD Symptoms," 2005)							
11	Has excessive paper towels/soap usage							
12	Has chapped/raw hands from repeated washing							
13	Excessive erases causing holes/rips in school work							
14	Increase in utility bills due to excessive water use/laundry							

KEY:

Y = Yes; O = Often; S = Sometimes; R = Rarely; ? = Unknown; N = No; P = In Past Only

Item	Indicator	Y	O	S	R	?	N	P
15	Has irrational/frequent fears							
16	Requests parents to participate in OCD rituals/activities; upset if they don't participate							
17	Takes excessive time doing tasks/activities, homework, tests							
18	Repeated asks about family members' health							
19	Performs rituals before leaving house/going to bed ("Obsessive-Compulsive Disorder," 2012)							
20	Family history of OCD							
21	OCD symptoms began suddenly/became worse up to 6 months after streptococcal infection (strep throat or scarlet fever), often with other symptoms including mood fluctuations, severe anxiety, irritability, oppositionality, defiance, regressive behaviors, academic decline, sensory problems, restrictive eating, sleep or bedwetting difficulties; called Pediatric Autoimmune Neuropsychiatric Disorders Associated with Streptococcal Infections or PANDAS (PANDAS Network, 2017)							
22	Has tic disorder							
23	Experienced abuse/trauma prior to symptom onset							
	Calculate column totals here							

Record when symptoms began:_____

CDASS Checklist for **Children Ages Three to Six with School and/or Nap Transition Difficulties**

YES_____   NO_____   Unknown or Unclear_____

KEY:
Y = Yes; O = Often; S = Sometimes; R = Rarely; ? = Unknown; N = No; P = In Past Only

Item	Indicator	Y	O	S	R	?	N	P
1	Has difficulties transitioning into or from half to full days of preschool, kindergarten, first grade, or daycare							
2	Has difficulties transitioning to shorter to no naps							
3	Has persisting separation anxiety at school or day care							
	Calculate column totals here							

Record when symptoms began:_____

CDASS Checklist for **Depressive Disorders**

YES_____   NO_____   Unknown or Unclear_____

KEY:
Y = Yes; O = Often; S = Sometimes; R = Rarely; ? = Unknown; N = No; P = In Past Only

Item	Indicator	Y	O	S	R	?	N	P
1	* Has depressed/sad mood							
2	Has irritability							
3	Exhibits outbursts of anger							
4	Has loss of interest/enjoyment in activities							
5	Concentration difficulties are related to sadness/depressed mood							
6	Is indecisive							

KEY:

Y = Yes; O = Often; S = Sometimes; R = Rarely; ? = Unknown; N = No; P = In Past Only

Item	Indicator	Y	O	S	R	?	N	P
7	Has insomnia, trouble falling asleep (30 minutes or longer)							
8	Moves about excessively/restlessly							
9	Has energy loss/tiredness							
10	Has poor appetite/eating less, weight loss, underweight							
11	Has increased appetite/excessive eating, weight gain							
12	Has worthlessness feelings							
13	Has guilt feelings							
14	Has suicidal thoughts, behaviors							
15	Walks/moves in slower ways							
16	Has bodily complaints with no medical causes (stomach discomfort, headaches, back pains)							
17	Experiences self-harm behaviors							
18	Has school refusal							
19	Has social withdrawal							
20	Feels hopeless							
21	Family history of depression (Mayo Clinic Staff, 2017)							
22	Has crying episodes							
23	Has lower self-esteem							
	Calculate column totals here							

* = Important common item

Record when symptoms began:_____

CDASS Checklist for **Bipolar Disorder**

YES_____   NO_____   Unknown or Unclear_____

KEY:
Y = Yes; O = Often; S = Sometimes; R = Rarely; ? = Unknown; N = No; P = In Past Only

Item	Indicator	Y	O	S	R	?	N	P
	The Five "Handle Symptoms" Below with Asterisks Are Specific to Bipolar But Not ADHD, So They Can Help With Differentiation							
1	* Has persistent phases of highly elevated/elated mood (excessive/extreme happiness, giddiness, excitement, goofiness, euphoria) that is inappropriate in intensity, duration, or context, and may last for many hours or days							
2	* Has grandiosity (unrealistic belief they are special, better than others, can do things others cannot)							
3	* Exhibits pressured or rapid speech							
4	* Has hypersexuality, excessive sexual interests at earlier age; may exhibit sexual behavior problems							
5	* Has racing thoughts; may struggle to express themselves clearly because thoughts are too fast (Youngstrom et al., 2005)							
	Additional Pediatric Bipolar Symptoms							
6	Has rapid cycling of mood; frequent mood swings; rapid mood changes during one hour or more hours to day/s							
7	Is irritable							

KEY:

Y = Yes; O = Often; S = Sometimes; R = Rarely; ? = Unknown; N = No; P = In Past Only

Item	Indicator	Y	O	S	R	?	N	P
8	Displays explosive temper tantrums or severe rages for 30 minutes or more; occurs when frustrated; during episodes may regress, have irrational thinking, and forget episode later							
9	Has angry moods							
10	Demonstrates verbal/physical aggression							
11	Has separation anxiety							
12	Has difficulty falling asleep							
13	Talks excessively; does not remain on topics							
14	Exhibits oppositional/defiant behaviors							
15	Exhibits deliberate risk-taking behaviors							
16	Is overly enthusiastic/active in games/activities							
17	Hallucinates, has delusions							
18	Has significant distortions/misinterpretations of events/reality							
19	Experiences paranoia							
20	Has poor self-esteem							
21	Is fatigued							
22	Is withdrawn							
23	Has decreased need for sleep, shorter sleep durations							
24	Hoards objects/food							

KEY:

Y = Yes; O = Often; S = Sometimes; R = Rarely; ? = Unknown; N = No; P = In Past Only

Item	Indicator	Y	O	S	R	?	N	P
25	Is easily embarrassed/humiliated; sensitive about others teasing/ laughing at him/her							
26	Exhibits intentional destructive behaviors during angry moods							
27	Has depressed/dysphoric moods							
28	Experiences severe nightmares, night terrors							
29	Has obsessive/compulsive behaviors							
30	Displays bullying, provocative, antagonizing behaviors with peers							
31	Is gifted with talent/abilities, artistic							
32	Has advanced verbal abilities							
33	Has non-lethal self-harming/cutting behaviors							
34	Has suicidal thoughts or behaviors							
35	Has poor organizational skills							
36	Has working memory deficits							
37	Has learning disorders/deficits (Papolos & Papolos, 2006)							
38	Lacks guilt/remorse after rages, aggression, or breaking things							
39	Has social problems with peers							
40	Has relational problems with family members							
41	Has higher activity levels while sleeping (see Increased Nocturnal Motor Activity checklist if necessary)							
42	Uses alcohol/substances							

KEY:
Y = Yes; O = Often; S = Sometimes; R = Rarely; ? = Unknown; N = No; P = In Past Only

Item	Indicator	Y	O	S	R	?	N	P
43	Family history of bipolar disorder							
	Calculate column totals here							

Record when symptoms began:_____

CDASS Checklist for **Intermittent Explosive Disorder**

YES_____   NO_____   Unknown or Unclear_____

KEY:
Y = Yes; O = Often; S = Sometimes; R = Rarely; ? = Unknown; N = No; P = In Past Only

Item	Indicator	Y	O	S	R	?	N	P
1	Exhibits verbal aggression							
2	Is physically aggressive to people/animals but not causing injury							
3	Is physically aggressive to people/animals that causes injury							
4	Causes destruction or damage to others' property or possessions							
5	Has legal involvements/consequences as a result of aggressive behaviors							
	Calculate column totals here							

Record when symptoms began:_____

CDASS Checklist for **Oppositional Defiant Disorder**

YES_____   NO_____   Unknown or Unclear_____

KEY:
Y = Yes; O = Often; S = Sometimes; R = Rarely; ? = Unknown; N = No; P = In Past Only

Item	Indicator	Y	O	S	R	?	N	P
1	Displays temper problems							
2	Is easily annoyed/touchy							
3	Has angry mood or resents others							
4	Is argumentative with adults							
5	Is defiant or does not respect adults' rules/requests							
6	Is intentionally annoying							
7	Blames other people for their mis-behaviors/errors							
8	Is revengeful/cruel (Mayo Clinic Staff, 2015)							
	Calculate column totals here							

Record when symptoms began:_____

CDASS Checklist for **Conduct Disorder**

YES_____   NO_____   Unknown or Unclear_____

KEY:
Y = Yes; O = Often; S = Sometimes; R = Rarely; ? = Unknown; N = No; P = In Past Only

Item	Indicator	Y	O	S	R	?	N	P
1	Breaks rules without specific reasons							
2	Destroys property							
3	Commits vandalism/delinquent/criminal acts							

KEY:
Y = Yes; O = Often; S = Sometimes; R = Rarely; ? = Unknown; N = No; P = In Past Only

Item	Indicator	Y	O	S	R	?	N	P
4	Sets fires intentionally							
5	Steals							
6	Aggressive/cruel to people/animals (fighting, bullying, weapons use, forced sexual activity)							
7	Runs away							
8	Lies to obtain/avoid things							
9	Uses alcohol/substances							
10	Has school truancy							
11	Has social problems							
12	Is oppositional/defiant with adults							
13	Is insincere							
14	Lacks empathy							
15	Lacks guilt/remorse for actions (Rogge & A.D.A.M. Editorial Team, 2015)							
16	Is manipulative							
17	Has significant learning problems/ learning disorder							
	Calculate column totals here							

Record when symptoms began:_____

CDASS Checklist for **Substance Abuse**

YES_____   NO_____   Unknown or Unclear_____

KEY:
Y = Yes; O = Often; S = Sometimes; R = Rarely; ? = Unknown; N = No; P = In Past Only

Item	Indicator	Y	O	S	R	?	N	P
1	Admits to substance use							
2	Exhibits suspected intoxications (inebriated appearance, dilated pupils, bloodshot eyes, smells from substance use)							
3	Has positive drug tests							
4	Alcohol or drug use paraphernalia was found							
5	Has conduct disorder symptoms (see this checklist if necessary)							
6	Has thrill-seeking tendencies							
7	Displays interests in substance use related topics, music, or imagery (posters, clothing)							
8	Visits drug or alcohol-related websites							
9	Friends are known/suspected to use substances							
10	Displays increased secrecy related to their activities/friends							
11	Has had a change in friends							
12	Has had a decreased quality of relationships/interactions with family and prior friends							
13	Has stolen/missing money at home							
14	Comes home later than usual							

KEY:

Y = Yes; O = Often; S = Sometimes; R = Rarely; ? = Unknown; N = No; P = In Past Only

Item	Indicator	Y	O	S	R	?	N	P
15	Avoids parents (particularly when coming home at night), excessively withdrawn							
16	Desires to sleep over friends' houses more often							
17	Makes drug references/jokes							
18	Has had academic performance decline							
19	Misses school classes/days							
20	Displays mood changes, irritability							
21	Exhibits behavioral changes (aggression, running away)							
22	Desires money without specific reasons							
23	Has lack of interest in previously enjoyed activities							
	Calculate column totals here							

Record when symptoms began:_____

CDASS Checklist for **Gaming Disorder**

YES_____   NO_____   Unknown or Unclear_____

KEY:

Y = Yes; O = Often; S = Sometimes; R = Rarely; ? = Unknown; N = No; P = In Past Only

Item	Indicator	Y	O	S	R	?	N	P
1	Plays video games 24 hours a week or more (just over 3 or more hours a day on average)							

KEY:

Y = Yes; O = Often; S = Sometimes; R = Rarely; ? = Unknown; N = No; P = In Past Only

Item	Indicator	Y	O	S	R	?	N	P
2	Is unable to decrease amount of game playing; unsuccessful attempts to stop or reduce							
3	Has decreased sleep due to game playing							
4	Feels compelled to play							
5	Has arguments related to game playing							
6	Misses meals or lateness due to game play							
7	Gaming significantly impacts/interferes with social or family relationships							
8	Gaming interferes with homework/academics							
9	Spends money excessively on games (Warner, 2007)							
10	Has excessive preoccupation with gaming							
11	Exhibits negative mood when attempting to reduce gaming							
12	Neglects activities and/or other interests due to gaming							
13	Displays withdrawal effects when not playing or gaming is removed, including agitation, sadness, anxiety, irritability							
14	Continues excessive gaming despite knowing it causes problems							
15	Deceives others regarding gaming use (Gentile et al., 2017)							

KEY:
Y = Yes; O = Often; S = Sometimes; R = Rarely; ? = Unknown; N = No; P = In Past Only

Item	Indicator	Y	O	S	R	?	N	P
16	Displays irritability, poor frustration tolerance, and lesser focusing and short-term memory abilities immediately after video game use							
17	Has difficulties stopping gaming when requested by parents							
18	Exhibits aggressive episodes after parents stop their game use (Weiss et al., 2011)							
	Calculate column totals here							

Record when symptoms began:_____

PSYCHOLOGICAL TRAUMA AND DISSOCIATION CHECKLISTS

The references for these checklists are listed in the References section of Chapter 10.

Identify The Types of Potential Psychological Trauma

The items below are experiences that may have caused possible traumatic reactions. For each entry line, print "YES" for trauma types that are known, QUESTION MARK (?) for unknown, possible or suspected items, and "NO" for traumas that did not occur.

_____ **Physical Abuse:** This includes exposure to a range of physical aggression, harm, and violence that may include leaving marks or bruises, pushing, shoving, or other types of assault.

_____ **Sexual Abuse:** This includes exposure to a range of unwanted and inappropriate sexualized behavior, including sexual contact or acts, sexual assault, coercion or bribery for sexual contact, exposure to pornography, or inappropriate sexualized comments or behaviors.

_____ **Emotional or Psychological Maltreatment/Abuse:** This includes name calling, being subjected to yelling or cursing, teasing, severe and persistent criticism, threats, or humiliation.

_____ **Neglect:** While sometimes difficult to define, this involves a lack of or inadequate nutrition, housing, clothing, supervision, education, and care (medical, dental, or psychological). Those with neglect often have other traumas, may have poor hygiene and may be inappropriately left alone. Neglect can be intentional, unintentional, or may involve disruptions in care by those who are emotionally or physically unavailable (see the neglect checklist if necessary).

_____ **Bullying Experiences:** These consist of unwanted, deliberate, and repeated emotional, physical, and/or sexual harm, harassment, or threats. It often occurs among similar age children and may be hidden from adults.

_____ **Medical Trauma:** This involves responses to extensive, chronic, frightening, or highly intensive pain conditions, serious illnesses, and medical procedures and/or treatments, as well as other physical injuries, accidents, disfigurements, or serious bodily harm and damage.

_____ **Traumatic Parental Separation or Divorce Experiences:** These can create toxic environments that can impact the child or teen negatively.

_____ **Unstable or Highly Dysfunctional Family Environments:**

    _____ Witness or exposure to domestic violence among parents or other family members (including physical violence or aggressive episodes, sexual violence, verbal abuse, cursing, yelling, screaming)

    _____ Parental substance abuse that negatively impacts child

    _____ Parental mental illness that negatively impacts child

    _____ Excessively permissive parents

    _____ Exposure to adult family members' sexual behaviors

    _____ Other highly dysfunctional family environment factors

_____ **Recent or Current Significant Family Traumas, Stressors, and Experiences:** These include family moves, various parental problems, family financial problems, housing inadequacy or homelessness, food insecurity or hunger, or others traumatic stressors.

_____ **Traumatic Grief:** This is significant, profound, and extended grief from the painful loss or death of important others from a child or adolescent's life.

_____ **Other Types of Trauma:** Additional types include community violence, violence at school, natural disasters, refugee trauma, war zone trauma, and terrorism (The National Child Traumatic Stress Network, 2018).

CDASS Checklist for **Psychological Trauma**

YES_____   NO_____   Unknown or Unclear_____

These items can manifest after trauma exposures, but may also occur for other reasons. Unless trauma is confirmed, a "Yes" above for the "Psychological Trauma" checklist would not necessarily indicate that trauma occurred, but a concern exists. Changes from prior functioning and new items may be significant and potentially suggestive of trauma. For children and teens who experienced significant traumas, particularly more severe and/or chronic trauma, complete the "Dissociation" checklist.

KEY:

Y = Yes; O = Often; S = Sometimes; R = Rarely; ? = Unknown; N = No; P = In Past Only

Item	Indicator	Y	O	S	R	?	N	P
1	Startles easily							
2	Has learning or academic difficulties							
3	Has poor skill development							
4	Exhibits temper problems, easily frustrated							
5	Is irritable							
6	Exhibits behavioral problems/changes							
7	Demands attention through both positive/negative behaviors							
8	Demonstrates regressive behaviors							
9	Is verbally/physically aggressive							
10	Fears separating from caregiver, excessive clinginess							
11	Is unable to trust others							
12	Has difficulties making friends							

KEY:
Y = Yes; O = Often; S = Sometimes; R = Rarely; ? = Unknown; N = No; P = In Past Only

Item	Indicator	Y	O	S	R	?	N	P
13	Blames self for trauma							
14	Fears adults who remind them of trauma							
15	Has disclosed expsoure to trauma/s							
16	Is fearful							
17	Is avoidant, withdrawn							
18	Excessively cries							
19	Bed wets							
20	Urinates/defecates inappropriately after being toilet trained (excludes enuresis)							
21	Demonstrates inappropriate/unusual sexualized behaviors/interests (Symptoms and Behaviors Associated with Exposure to Trauma, 2015)							
22	Complains of stomachaches, headaches, bodily discomfort/pains, somatic concerns with no medical causes							
23	Eats more/less than usual, eating difficulties; eating disorder							
24	Has depression symptoms (see this checklist if necessary)							
25	Has anxiety symptoms (see this checklist if necessary)							
26	Has panic attacks/ intense anxiety attacks							
27	Has obsessive thoughts, compulsive behaviors (see OCD checklist if necessary)							

KEY:

Y = Yes; O = Often; S = Sometimes; R = Rarely; ? = Unknown; N = No; P = In Past Only

Item	Indicator	Y	O	S	R	?	N	P
28	Is angry, resentful							
29	Has had changes in typical routines, activities, interests							
30	Exhibits partial loss/lack of memory (particularly about trauma)							
31	Has increased distractibility							
32	Experiences trauma flashbacks							
33	Experiences nightmares, disturbing dreams							
34	Avoids things associated with trauma							
35	Avoids/disinterested in people/activities previously enjoyed							
36	Has hypervigilance							
37	Experiences intrusive trauma thoughts							
38	Uses alcohol/substances (Emotional and Psychological Trauma: Causes and Effects, Symptoms, and Treatment, 2005)							
39	Re-enacts trauma in play/drawings, trauma-themed play/drawings							
40	Fears trauma may occur again							
41	Demonstrates changes in mood							
42	Has had changes in personality							
43	Experiences difficulties calming down/managing emotions							
44	Has had changes in relationships with others							

KEY:
Y = Yes; O = Often; S = Sometimes; R = Rarely; ? = Unknown; N = No; P = In Past Only

Item	Indicator	Y	O	S	R	?	N	P
45	Has had loss of self-esteem or confidence							
46	Shows lack of eye contact							
47	Exhibits fears related to trauma							
48	Runs away from home							
49	Repeatedly retells/discusses traumatic experience/s							
50	Exhibits increased tension, inability to relax							
51	Has had changes in speech/speech delays							
52	Has difficulties falling/staying asleep, sleeping problems							
53	Exhibits reduced capacity to feel emotions, seems numb							
54	Has adult-like sexual knowledge (Department of Health and Human Services, State of Victoria, 2012a)							
55	Exhibits sexually promiscuous behaviors							
56	Is cruel to/hurts animals							
57	Has pessimistic world-view							
58	Exhibits non-lethal self-harming/cutting behaviors							
59	Has school truancy							
60	Is triggered by trauma reminders							
61	Has suicidal thoughts/behaviors (Department of Health and Human Services, State of Victoria, 2012b)							

KEY:
Y = Yes; O = Often; S = Sometimes; R = Rarely; ? = Unknown; N = No; P = In Past Only

Item	Indicator	Y	O	S	R	?	N	P
62	Exhibits sexual behavior problems, inappropriate touching of other children, excessive masturbation, inappropriate sexualized interactions, exposing themselves, threats/coercing others into sexual acts							
63	Views pornography							
64	Commits vandalism/delinquent acts							
65	Starts fires							
66	Has poor hygiene							
67	Has increased defiance/arguments with adults							
	Calculate column totals here							

Record when symptoms began:_____

CDASS Checklist for **Dissociation**

YES_____   NO_____   Unknown or Unclear_____

KEY:
Y = Yes; O = Often; S = Sometimes; R = Rarely; ? = Unknown; N = No; P = In Past Only

Item	Indicator	Y	O	S	R	?	N	P
	Core Symptoms							
1	* Has blackout experiences							
2	* Has loss of time experiences (for this and blackouts, the more frequent and greater amount of lost time, the more significant; both are key indicators)							
3	Has fugue episodes (no recall of traveling distances alone)							

KEY:
Y = Yes; O = Often; S = Sometimes; R = Rarely; ? = Unknown; N = No; P = In Past Only

Item	Indicator	Y	O	S	R	?	N	P
4	Has passive influence/interference episodes (inability to control behavior after sincere attempts, struggles with compulsive masturbation or self-injurious behaviors despite efforts to stop)							
5	Is unable to recall important personal information or relevant personal history							
6	Lacks memories for a period of years or before age 6							
7	Demonstrates vacant starring spells							
8	Has excessive daydreaming							
9	Exhibits strange freezing episodes							
10	Is forgetfulness for basic information (things in their room, names of friends or pets)							
11	Has inconsistent and fluctuating skills/abilities (athletic, artistic, academic, social)							
12	Has inconsistent and dramatically alternating preferences/habits (different favorite foods, clothes, activities)							
13	Experiences flashbacks							
14	Has intrusive memories							
15	Experiences auditory hallucinations (distinct voices with gender, age, and individual traits, often internalized and heard within their head)							
16	Exhibits rapid behavioral regressions to resemble younger child or baby-like (Putnam, 1997)							

KEY:

Y = Yes; O = Often; S = Sometimes; R = Rarely; ? = Unknown; N = No; P = In Past Only

Item	Indicator	Y	O	S	R	?	N	P
17	Has nonresponsive periods (does not respond when name called or spoken to)							
18	Exhibits trace-like states							
19	Sleeps excessively							
20	Faints							
21	Has amnesia and transient forgetting; while true amnesia for recent behavior is rare, amnesia for past traumatic events is more common; children may say "I forget" as a distraction, due to discomfort, or out of guilt/shame; to discriminate between true amnesia and unwillingness ask child to recall positive experiences (good grades, favorite activities, holidays) or do they only forget certain or angry episodes/misbehavior							
22	Has persistent and vivid imaginary playmates (*if this occurs, clinicians should differentiate between normal and pathological imaginary playmates/fantasy;* pathological fantasy interferes with normal activities, child believes they cannot control fantasy behavior/ playmates, child believes playmates are real, and playmates are in conflict with each other)							
23	Distinct alternate personality states or pathological elaborated identities exist (*clinicians should not be too suggestive with this questioning to encourage child to create these responses*)							

KEY:

Y = Yes; O = Often; S = Sometimes; R = Rarely; ? = Unknown; N = No; P = In Past Only

Item	Indicator	Y	O	S	R	?	N	P
24	Depersonalization occurs (feelings/sense of being detached from one's body; feels not connected to body or like a robot; person feels they are an outside observer to their own thinking, emotions, body; lack of emotional responses; they lack control of their speech or actions)							
25	Derealization occurs (altered experience or perception that external world seems unreal/strange; feels like in movie, dream, another reality; others appear mechanical/unfamiliar)							
26	Has sexual behavior problems (International Society for the Study of Dissociation, 2004)							
	Associated Posttraumatic Symptoms							
27	Has social withdrawal							
28	Has limited range of emotions							
29	Exhibits regressive behaviors							
30	Has loss of developmental milestones/skills							
31	Exhibits new fears							
32	Is aggressive (Putnam, 1997)							
33	Has nightmares							
34	Experiences night terrors (while sleeping child screams, highly upset, moves around but does not recall anything in morning)							

KEY:

Y = Yes; O = Often; S = Sometimes; R = Rarely; ? = Unknown; N = No; P = In Past Only

Item	Indicator	Y	O	S	R	?	N	P
35	Reenacts trauma, trauma-themed play							
36	Seems emotionally numb							
37	Is avoidant (International Society for the Study of Dissociation, 2004)							
	Additional Associated Symptoms							
38	Has depression symptoms							
39	Has anxiety symptoms							
40	Has low self-esteem							
41	Exhibits emotional lability, rapidly fluctuating mood states							
42	Has somatization (fluctuating bodily complaints without causes, stomach aches, headaches, unusual pains)							
43	Has non-suicidal self-injurious/cutting behaviors							
44	Has suicidal thoughts/behaviors							
45	Uses alcohol/substances							
46	Exhibits conduct/behavioral problems							
47	Has had multiple psychological conditions diagnosed							
48	Has academic problems (Putnam, 1997)							
49	Exhibits unpredictable, out of context tantrums (Silberg & Dallam, 2009)							
	Calculate column totals here							

* = Important common item

Record when symptoms began:_____

NEGLECT, ATTACHMENT DISORDERS, AND EARLY PATHOGENIC CARE CHECKLISTS

The references for these checklists are listed in the References section of Chapter 11.

CDASS Checklist for **Neglect**

YES_____   NO_____   Unknown or Unclear_____

KEY:
Y = Yes; O = Often; S = Sometimes; R = Rarely; ? = Unknown; N = No; P = In Past Only

Item	Indicator	Y	O	S	R	?	N	P
1	Has had unmet basic clothing needs							
2	Has had poor hygiene resulting from inadequate care							
3	Experienced malnutrition/insufficient food intake							
4	Has had inadequate medical care							
5	Has had inadequate dental care							
6	Has had emotional neglect, lack of meeting basic psychological needs/affection, caregiver was chronically emotional distant/disengaged							
7	Has experienced inadequate supervision, child was left alone recurrently/inappropriately, or with unsafe/unreliable others							
8	Has had educational neglect, frequent truancy, lack of caregiver's efforts to maintain school attendance, lack of school enrollment							
9	Has had neglect reports to state child protection agency							
10	Has had family involvement in state child protection/foster care system							

KEY:

Y = Yes; O = Often; S = Sometimes; R = Rarely; ? = Unknown; N = No; P = In Past Only

Item	Indicator	Y	O	S	R	?	N	P
11	Has had prenatal substance exposure							
12	Experienced grossly inadequate pre-natal care							
13	Parents had substance abuse condition/s that contributed to neglect							
14	Parents had serious psychological disorders contributing to neglect							
15	Caregivers were highly unstable/unreliable with parenting style or presence							
16	Had significant separations from parent, multiple primary caregivers from parental absence/inconsistency/ problems							
17	Was raised in orphanage/institution where they lacked nurturing attachment figure							
18	Had chronic medical/pain condition and was unable to be soothed by caregiver							
19	Experienced lengthy/multiple hospitalizations causing separations							
20	Caregiver did not protect child from ongoing known abuse/traumas, including domestic violence							
21	Had inadequate protection from harmful siblings/other family members							
22	Highly permissive parents knowingly allowed unsafe behaviors to occur							
	Calculate column totals here							

Record when symptoms began:_____

Attachment Disorders Checklist Using the Parent Relationship Problems Questionnaire (Parent RPQ)
(Minnis, Rabe-Hesketh, & Wolkind, 2002; Minnis et al., 2007; Vervoort et al., 2013) (reproduced with permission)

Significant Score from Parent RPQ

YES_____   NO_____   Unknown or Unclear_____

If responder believes the item is "exactly like" the child, give score of 3 to that item; if it is "like" the child, give score of 2; if it is "a bit like" the child, give score of 1. A score of 7 or higher is a positive screening for an attachment disorder. Because most children do not have these symptoms, even a few positives should be concerning. This checklist incorporates RAD and DSED items.

KEY:
EL = Exactly Like (3); L = Like (2); ABL = A Bit Like (1);
NAAL = Not At All Like (0); ? = Unknown

Item	Indicator	EL	L	ABL	NAAL	?
1	Gets too close physically to strangers					
2	Is too "cuddly" and affectionate with people s/he does not know well					
3	Often asks very personal questions of strangers even though s/he does not mean to be rude					
4	Can be aggressive towards him/herself e.g. using bad language about him/herself, headbanging, cutting					
5	Has problem with conscience					
6	Is too friendly with strangers					
7	Sometimes looks frozen with fear, without an obvious reason					
8	If you approach him/her, s/he often runs away or refuses to be approached					
9	Has a false quality to the affection s/he gives					

KEY:
EL = Exactly Like (3); L = Like (2); ABL = A Bit Like (1);
NAAL = Not At All Like (0); ? = Unknown

Item	Indicator	EL	L	ABL	NAAL	?
10	If you approach him/her, you never know whether s/he will be friendly or unfriendly					
11	Does not tend to go to parents for comfort or soothing					
	Calculate column totals here					

Record when symptoms began:_____

INDEX

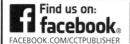